Arthritis

Arthritis

Reverse Underlying Causes of Arthritis with Clinically Proven Alternative Therapies

SECOND EDITION

Ellen Kamhi, Ph.D., R.N.
Eugene R. Zampieron, N.D., M.H. (A.H.G.)

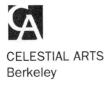

CELESTIAL ARTS
Berkeley

Copyright © 1999, 2006 by InnoVision Health Media Inc.

All rights reserved. Published in the United States by
Celestial Arts, an imprint of the Crown Publishing Group,
a division of Random House, Inc., New York.
www.crownpublishing.com
www.tenspeed.com

Celestial Arts and the Celestial Arts colophon are registered trademarks
of Random House, Inc.

Originally published in the United States in different form as *Arthritis: An Alternative Medicine Definitive Guide* by Future Medicine Pub. [Tiburon, California], in 1999.

Library of Congress Cataloging-in-Publication Data Kamhi, Ellen.
  Alternative medicine definitive guide to arthritis : reverse underlying causes of arthritis with clinically proven alternative therapies / Ellen Kamhi and Eugene R. Zampieron. — 2nd ed.
      p.   cm.
First published under title: Arthritis: an alternative medicine definitive guide / by Eugene R. Zampieron and Ellen Kamhi. Tiburon, Calif. : Future Medicine Pub., 1999.
  Includes bibliographical references and index.
  1. Arthritis — Alternative treatment — Popular works. I. Zampieron., Eugene R.   II. Zampieron., Eugene R. Arthritis.   III. Title.
RC933.Z35 2006
616.7'2206 — dc22   2005032562

ISBN-13: 978-1-58761-258-9

Printed in the U.S.A.

Cover design by Chloe Rawlins

12 11 10 9 8 7 6

Second Edition

Contents

About the Authors

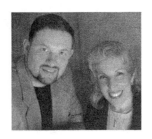

Ellen Kamhi, Ph.D., R.N., H.N.C.
The Natural Nurse

Ellen Kamhi is a clinical instructor at Stony Brook Medical School. In 2004, she received the J.G. Gallimore award for research in science and was nominated for the March of Dimes Woman of Distinction award. A respected authority on natural healing, Dr. Kamhi is a professional member of the American Herbalist Guild (A.H.G.), is nationally board certified as a holistic nurse (H.N.C.), and works to bring together a body of modern and ancient practices and philosophies that use less invasive, less toxic, natural techniques to enhance wellness. She is the author of *Cycles of Life, Herbs for Women, The Natural Guide to Great Sex,* and co-author of *The Natural Medicine Chest.* She hosts health shows on radio and television. Along with Dr. Eugene Zampieron, Ellen is cofounder of Natural Alternatives Health, Education and Multi-Media, Inc., which sponsors international workshops on natural medicine.

Eugene R. Zampieron, N.D., M.H. (A.H.G.)

Dr. Eugene R. Zampieron is a licensed naturopathic physician and an alumnus of Bastyr University of natural health sciences. Dr. Zampieron, aka "Dr. Z," is a medical botanist, herbalist, and professional member of the American Herbalist Guild. He is an expert in the history, folk-lore, phytochemistry, and pharmacology of plant medicines from many areas of the globe. Along with Dr. Ellen Kamhi, Dr. Z has coauthored hundreds of articles and radio programs, as well as several books, including *The Natural Medicine Chest.* He practices in Woodbury, Connecti-cut, with an emphasis on environmental medicine, detoxification, acute and chronic pain management, autoimmune diseases, arthritis, fibro-myalgia, and other inflammatory disorders.

Acknowledgments

In the accomplishment of a project such as this one, we have been shaped, inspired, influenced, motivated, supported, and schooled by many great people, who we now acknowledge and thank.

Ellen Kamhi, Ph.D., R.N., H.N.C.

To my parents, Julius and Sondra, and my children, Brenda, Titus and Ali—thank you, for all your love and support. To my friends, Dr. Michael and Lois Posner, who were occasionally successful at pulling me away from my work marathons, and for providing clinical insight and photography used in this book. To all my wonderful teachers, especially Serafina Corsello, M.D., whose intensity, fortitude, depth of knowledge, and wonderful healthy cooking is always a joy! To Nature's Answer, for providing me with the ongoing opportunity to be involved with the production of wholesome, herbal products; to my business partner and soul brother, Eugene Zampieron, for his ongoing, intense investigations into the highest level of knowledge about natural medicine, and his wife, Kathleen, for always encouraging Eugene and I in our journeys. To G-D, the ultimate source of healing.

Eugene R. Zampieron, N.D., M.H. (A.H.G.)

I wish to thank the creator, for all healing ultimately comes from the infinite. To my wife and soulmate, Kathleen, and our children, Caitlin and Kevin. To Ellen Kamhi, for her unending perseverance, patience, and organization amidst many obstacles to bring our vision of this book to reality. May natural alternatives heal the world! My teachers, friends, and colleagues of natural health who have schooled me in treating the many dimensions of pain and arthritis, including: Ken Bakken, D.O., Joe Pizzorno, N.D., Bill Mitchell, N.D., Douglas Lewis, N.D., Rod Borrie, Ph.D., Kim Vanderlinden, N.D., D.T.C.M., Peter Zilahy, D.C., Ameni Harris, Tom Hudak, L.M.T., Norm Suhu, C.A., Jamba, and Ann Seipt, N.D. To the many hundreds of patients with arthritis and pain whom I coached to wellness and who provided personal and clinical data for this book, thank you for being my patients and teachers, and for your courage and commitment to wellness.

Foreword

Arthritis is among the most common health complaints in America. While various types of arthritis differ, there are some common features. For example, scientific information is accumulating that indicates diet plays a major role in the development, as well as the treatment and prevention, in a wide range of diseases including virtually all types of arthritis. In addition, there is mounting evidence that pharmaceutical drugs may be doing more harm than good. Research indicates drugs such as NSAIDs, which includes aspirin, ibuprofen, and the newer Cox-2 inhibitor drugs such as Vioxx and Celebrex may produce short-term benefits, but actually accelerate the progression of joint destruction, and can cause serious long-term side effects, including death. Conventional physicians prescribe drugs because they are not armed with the knowledge needed to access and administer natural therapies. Drug companies also control, to a very large extent, what is taught at medical schools and continuing education programs. The influence of the drug industry on medical practice was addressed in an editorial that appeared in a major medical journal:

"The overall influence of the industry is to emphasize drug treatment at the expense of other modalities: psychotherapy, social approaches, nutritional, herbal, and natural remedies, rehabilitation, general hygienic measures, nonpatentable drugs, or other alternative approaches. It focuses attention on disorders that are treatable by drugs, and may promote overdiagnosis. It reinforces the practice of dealing with disease by treatment of symptoms, and diverts interest from prevention."

Many doctors are beginning to recognize that drug treatments are not providing the long-term benefit they had hoped to observe. In the treatment of arthritis, they see their patients continuing to suffer with their disease despite stronger and stronger medications. Does medical intervention in some way promote disease progression? Can nutrition and various natural therapies enhance the body's own response toward health? The answer to both of these questions, made evident by the information presented in this book, is clearly yes.

One question that may come up after reading the last statement is: If the natural approach is so effective, why aren't more doctors using this approach? There are some simple answers to this question. Progress is being made and more and more doctors are now recommending natural therapies (e.g., fish oils and glucosamine sulfate), but in most cases, doctors are still uncomfortable with recommending dietary therapy or natural products primarily because they know only what they have been taught. Since the typical medical doctor has less than four hours of training in nutrition, they know very little about how diet might influence arthritis. In fact, the majority of medical schools in the United States do not even offer a required course in nutrition.

Fortunately, nature offers some very effective alternatives. In most cases, the natural approach will provide far greater relief because it addresses the underlying disease process, while rebuilding overall health and vitality, without causing a host of adverse effects. This excellent book provides readers clear direction and recommendations to experience relief from their arthritis without the use of drugs or surgery. If you suffer from arthritis, please take this guidance to heart. My hope is that you will become arthritis-free and that you will share your experience with others, including their physicians, so that even more people can benefit.

—*Michael T. Murray, N.D.*
November 2005

one

Arthritis Can Be Reversed

Although the term *arthritis* is often used as if it encompassed one entity, over 100 types of arthritis have been identified. It is not one disease but an aggregate of illnesses whose common features include joint pain, stiffness, and inflammation. For millions of Americans, arthritis limits everyday movements such as walking, standing, or even holding a pencil. Arthritic conditions can progress to cause joint deformities, brittle bones, loss of mobility, and complete destruction of the protective covering around joints.

Over 66 million Americans (nearly one in three adults) are afflicted with some type of arthritis.[1] Osteoarthritis (OA) is by far the most prevalent form. Under the age of 45, more men than women are diagnosed with OA, often due to accidents and injuries. The disease becomes three times more prevalent in women than in men after the age of 45. Since aging is a factor in this disease, as many more baby boomers turn 50 the number of people afflicted with OA is expected to increase dramatically.

The second most prevalent form of

IN THIS CHAPTER

- Success Story: Out of His Wheelchair with Alternative Medicine

- The Failure of Conventional Arthritis Treatment

- What Alternative Medicine Can Do for Arthritis

- Success Story: A Holistic Approach Alleviates Arthritis

- Undoing Arthritis in Stages: The Scope of This Book

arthritis is rheumatoid arthritis (RA), an inflammatory disease in which the body's immune system attacks its own healthy tissues. RA effects 3% to 4% of the population of the United States, striking people of all ages, including nearly 300,000 children.[2] Women are three times more likely to develop RA than are men. People with a particular genetic marker (HLA-DR4) tend to have a higher incidence of the illness. Other forms of arthritis include gout, which occurs in three out of 1,000 adults, or about two million Americans (the majority of whom are men)[3] and less common forms, such as ankylosing spondylitis, psoriatic arthritis, and infectious arthritis.

The common conventional medical approach to arthritis relies on anti-inflammatory and painkilling drugs. While these drugs provide temporary symptom relief, they also have serious side effects. Alternative medicine, on the other hand, offers a wide range of treatment options for eliminating the often hidden causes of arthritis. As with any disorder, especially chronic ones such as arthritis, more than a single cause is usually involved, as the following patient case history graphically demonstrates.

Success Story: Out of His Wheelchair with Alternative Medicine

Gerald, 45, was so severely affected by ankylosing spondylitis when he first came to see us that he was virtually wheelchair bound. He walked, with great difficulty, with the assistance of two crutches. He also had severe fibromyalgia (SEE QUICK DEFINITION), chronic fatigue, and insomnia. He had spent many years trying to find help with his ailments but had found no relief.

Gerald's health problems started when he was a child. His diet was poor—lots of starches, meat, and sweets, and very few fruits and vegetables—and he was constantly fatigued, had little energy, and complained of muscle pain. He received myriad doses of antibiotics for various ailments throughout his childhood. In his twenties, he began to notice stiffness in his lower back in addition to body-wide pain and inflammation. His diet was still poor at that time, consisting of large quantities of cola and chocolate (to artificially boost his energy levels), hamburgers, fast foods, and very few vegetables.

When Gerald was 28, one morning shortly after battling a severe bout of the flu, he found he couldn't get out of bed because the stiffness and pain in his joints and muscles were so severe. As he continued to try to

Although the term *arthritis* is used as if it encompassed one entity, more than 100 types of arthritis have been identified. It is an aggregate of illnesses whose common features include joint pain, stiffness, and inflammation. For millions of people, arthritis limits everyday movements such as walking, standing, or even holding a pencil.

function, Gerald had to get up earlier every morning, spending several hours stretching and limbering up his body enough to be able to go to work.

Gerald consulted his family physician and specialists in rheumatology, but they were unable to provide a definitive diagnosis of his problem. He was given nonsteroidal anti-inflammatory drugs (NSAIDs) to suppress the pain. He was also referred to a psychiatrist for his condition.

Over the next several years, his health continued to decline. The stiffness and pain, which were made worse by inactivity and rest, prevented him from sleeping more than two to three hours at a time. His hands and feet would stiffen up if he didn't continuously flex them, and his back, shoulder, and other muscles were so tight that he said he felt as if he wore a cement suit. Simple tasks like shaving, bathing, and getting dressed became extremely difficult.

At age 39, Gerald was put on permanent disability leave from his job. He sought help from a string of rheumatologists and pain clinics. His condition was finally diagnosed as ankylosing spondylitis and fibromyalgia, but the therapies offered to him—NSAIDs, psychotherapy, and exhausting physical therapy—provided no relief. It was in this state that Gerald came to the clinic.

The first thing we addressed was

 Fibromyalgia is a multiple-symptom syndrome primarily involving widespread muscle pain (myalgia) that can be debilitating in its severity. The pain seems to be caused by the tightening and thickening of the myofascia, the thin film or tissue that holds the muscle together. Typical tender sites include the neck, upper back, rib cage, hips, and knees. Other symptoms include general fatigue and stiffness, insomnia and sleeping disorders, depression, mood swings, allergies, headaches, a sense of hurting all over, tender skin, numbness, irritable bowel symptoms, and exercise intolerance. Post-traumatic fibromyalgia is believed to develop after a fall, whiplash, or back strain, whereas primary fibromyalgia has an uncertain origin.

 For more **dietary recommendations for arthritis**, see chapter 12, The Arthritis Diet, pages 225–256. For **diagnostic tests for arthritis**, see chapter 3, Diagnosing Arthritis, pages 39–65.

Gerald's diet. We put him on the arthritis diet, a vegetarian, whole foods diet emphasizing fruits and vegetables, raw seeds and nuts, and whole grains. To help him with this transition, Gerald took vegetarian cooking classes and learned about juicing. Almost immediately, he noticed a difference—less fatigue, more joint flexibility, and better sleep patterns.

We ran a stool analysis, blood tests, and a food allergy test on Gerald to get a better picture of his condition. He was in an extreme state of dysbiosis (SEE QUICK DEFINITION), with tests indicating the absence of the friendly bacteria lactobacillus and bifidobacterium in his intestinal tract. Tests found two varieties of pathogenic bacteria, klebsiella and streptococcus, and a severe overgrowth of the yeast candida. Klebsiella is a factor in some ankylosing spondylitis cases because it can escape detection in the body due to a unique genetic marker. Gerald also had allergies to a large number of foods, including bananas, beans, chicken and turkey, clams, cheese and dairy products, eggs, oats, rye, salmon, wheat, and yeast (brewer's and baker's).

To treat the bacterial and yeast infections, we started Gerald on a series of 10 colonic irrigation treatments, which were infused with an herbal antimicrobial formula. He also received additional colonics containing beneficial bacteria, or probiotics, to help repopulate his intestines with friendly bacteria. This therapy had a dramatic impact on Gerald: He had more energy, and his inflammation virtually disappeared after each treatment. He even lost weight. We also gave him a homeopathic preparation, Streptococcinum nosode (SEE QUICK DEFINITION), to decrease his abnormally high numbers of antibodies against streptococcus bacteria.

To address his multiple underlying imbalances, Gerald began taking a number of remedies.

Intestinal dysbiosis refers to an imbalance of intestinal flora. Specifically, these flora are friendly, beneficial bacteria (probiotics), such as *Lactobacillus acidophilus* and *Bifidobacterium bifidum*, and unfriendly bacteria, such as *Citrobacter* spp. and *Clostridium perfringens*. Dysbiosis is considered a primary cause or major cofactor in the development of many health problems, such as yeast overgrowth, chronic fatigue, depression, digestive disorders, food allergies, rheumatoid arthritis, and cancer.

A **nosode** is a superdiluted remedy made as an energy imprint from a disease-causing microorganism, such as bacterial, virus, or protozoa. The nosode, which contains no physical trace of the disease, stimulates the body to remove all "taints" or residues it holds of a particular disease, whether it was inherited or contracted. Only qualified homeopaths may administer a nosode.

For more on **colonic irrigation treatments**, see chapter 5, Detoxifying Specific Organs, pages 88–114.

- To combat the klebsiella bacteria and the yeast infection, we recommended Oregon grape root, which contains berberine, and grapefruit seed extract—both powerful antimicrobials.

- To improve his digestion, we recommended a digestive enzyme supplement. When taken with food, the enzyme supplement helps to improve the body's ability to break down food into easily absorbable components. Enzymes taken between meals also help dissolve circulating immune complexes (CICs); (SEE QUICK DEFINITION), which can be a factor in inflammation in muscles and joints.

> **Circulating immune complexes** (CICs) form in the body when poor digestion results in undigested proteins leaking through the intestinal wall and into the bloodstream. The immune system treats these foreign substances, or antigens, as invaders, causing antibodies to form and couple with them. This antigen and antibody combination is known as a CIC. In a healthy person CICs are neutralized, but in someone with a compromised immune system they tend to accumulate in the blood, where they burden the detoxification pathways or initiate an allergic reaction. If too many CICs accumulate, the kidneys and liver can't excrete enough of them via the urine or stool. The CICs are then deposited in soft tissues, causing inflammation and bringing stress to the immune system. The overload can lead to a variety of chronic health conditions.

- For his chronic pain and inflammation, we gave Gerald the enzyme bromelain (extracted from organic pineapples), along with curcumin, the active constituent in the herb turmeric. Both of these substances have excellent anti-inflammatory properties. We recommended licorice root solid extract (1/4 teaspoon, four times daily on an empty stomach) as a tonic for his stressed adrenal glands, along with valerian root and white willow bark (4 capsules, 1 hour prior to bedtime). We also gave him Rhus tox. 60C (three times daily), a homeopathic remedy specifically for muscular and rheumatic pain and stiffness that is made worse by inactivity.

- As antioxidant support, we recommended vitamin E (200 IU of natural mixed tocopherols with tocotrienols, two times daily with meals) and a combination antioxidant containing selenium, green tea extract (90% polyphenois), tomato extract (5% lycopene), pine bark extract (90% proanthocyanidins), and lutein to decrease the damage from free radicals. Gerald also took a fish oil supplement (3 capsules with each meal), containing the EPA and DHA, two omega-3 essential fatty acids (SEE QUICK DEFINITION, page 6).

- To support his liver as it processed the toxins out of his body, Gerald also took the herb milk thistle in combination with picrorhiza.

Omega-3 and omega-6 fatty acids are the two principle types of essential fatty acids, which are unsaturated fats required in the diet. A balance of these fatty acids in the diet is required for good health. The primary omega-3 fatty acid, alpha-linolenic acid (ALA), is found in flaxseed, canola seeds, pumpkin seeds, walnuts, and soybeans. Fish oils, such as salmon, cod, and mackerel, contain the other important omega-3 fatty acids, DHA (docosahexaenoic acid) and EPA (eicosapentaenoic acid). Omega-3 fatty acids help reduce the risk of heart disease. Linoleic acid, the main omega-6 fatty acid, is found in most plants and vegetable oils, including safflower, corn, peanut, and sesame. The most therapeutic form of omega-6, is gamma-linolenic acid (GLA), is found in evening primrose, black currant, and borage oils. Once in the body, omega-3 and omega-6 fatty acids are converted to prostaglandins, hormonelike substances that regulate many metabolic functions, particularly inflammatory processes.

For more information about **"green" foods**, see chapter 4, General Detoxification, pages 66–87. For more on massage and other physical therapies for arthritis, see chapter 14, Exercises and Physical Therapies, pages 295–320.

After just two months of this regimen, along with the dietary changes and colonics, Gerald made significant progress. He reported that he had gone from feeling 15% functional to 50% functional. Although he had a long way to go, Gerald was excited about experiencing a lessening of symptoms and a tremendous increase in overall energy. In addition, he was optimistic about the potential for a better quality of life, something he hadn't felt before starting the natural therapies. A subsequent stool analysis showed that the klebsiella had been eradicated and that friendly bacterial microflora had reestablished themselves. Gerald received regular massage therapy and chiropractic treatments to help with his pain and stiffness. He then fasted on vegetable juice for seven days, which put an end to his pain. After the fast, he started incorporating "green" foods, such as spirulina and blue-green algae, into his diet. Green foods, which are important for detoxification, helped improve Gerald's energy levels and sleep. Gerald also sought counseling to help with the emotional components of his arthritis.

After embracing this holistic approach 12 years ago, Gerald now shows no signs of ankylosing spondylitis through subjective and objective measurements, though his genetic propensity remains. He is completely functional and engages in physical activities without having to endure days of pain and inflammation. Gerald finds that he must stay on a fairly strict diet and regimen of stress reduction, reporting that if he eats junk food or overexerts himself, he will "wake up with stiff joints and feel lousy." Gerald believes that natural medicine has given him a new lease on life and is well worth the effort.

The Failure of Conventional Arthritis Treatments

As Gerald discovered, conventional medicine prescribes a whole laundry list of pharmaceutical drugs for arthritis. Many of these drugs block the symptoms of pain, often very quickly and with little effort on the part of the patient or doctors. While pain relief is important, these drugs merely hide the symptoms and ignore the underlying causes of the disease.

In addition, conventional drugs have side effects that cause daily discomfort and further remove the patient from an independent, symptom-free life. The first round of pharmaceutical drugs prescribed for most forms of arthritis include NSAIDs, such as aspirin, ibuprofen (Motrin), indomethacin (Indocin), and naproxen (Aleve, Naprosyn). NSAIDs may cause the following side effects: abdominal cramping or pain, gas, constipation, diarrhea, dizziness, fatigue, fluid retention and swelling, headaches, heartburn, loss of appetite, nausea, nervousness, rash, ringing in the ears, skin eruptions, stomach pain, or vomiting.[4] In addition, the National Institutes of Health halted a study on the use of Aleve after patients taking two tablets a day for three years developed a 50% higher risk of heart attack and stroke. The FDA now recommends that naproxen not be taken for more than 10 days in a row.

NSAIDs also contribute to the continuation of degenerative changes by inhibiting the repair of cartilage (the structural support of joints).[5] Studies have clearly illustrated that NSAIDs not only hinder the synthesis of cartilage's base materials but actually accelerate the destruction of cartilage.[6] Furthermore, these drugs destroy the gastrointestinal lining, leading to intestinal permeability and the formation of ulcers, both significant contributing factors to the onset of arthritis.

COX-2 inhibitors are a newer class of NSAIDs that inhibit pro-inflammatory compounds without interfering with the body's natural production of the anti-inflammatory or "good" prostaglandins. These compounds include rofecoxib (Vioxx), celecoxib (Celebrex), and valdecoxib (Bextra). Pharmaceutical companies led consumers to believe that COX-2 inhibitors have fewer side effects than the older NSAIDs. Common adverse effects include diarrhea, nausea, edema, and kidney disorders.[7] More dramatic negative effects surfaced when Vioxx was found to substantially increase the risk of heart attacks and sudden cardiac death.[8] Additional studies showed that Bextra use can be linked to Stevens-Johnson syndrome, a life-threatening skin reaction, and that patients taking Bextra had more than double the risk of suffering a heart attack or

> Conventional medicine prescribes a whole laundry list of pharmaceutical drugs for arthritis. Many of these drugs block the symptoms of pain, often very quickly and with little effort on the part of the patient or doctors. While pain relief is important, conventional drugs merely hide the symptoms and ignore the underlying causes of the disease.

stroke than those patients given placebos. Studies also show that COX-2 inhibitors may be just as detrimental as older NSAIDs in causing an increased risk of gastrointestinal hemorrhage.[9] Due to the severity of the negative cardiovascular effects of these drugs, the American Heart Association advises that all NSAIDs and COX-2 inhibitors be used in the lowest dose possible for short durations, usually no more then 10 days.[10]

Other drug treatments such as injections of corticosteroids control inflammation at a high price. Their side effects can alter a person's personality, causing psychotic behavior, severe depression, or mood swings. High doses cause fluid retention, particularly in the face; this is often referred to as "moon face." Prolonged use causes eye infections, weight gain, fragile skin, muscle weakness, brittle bones, or purplish stripe marks on the skin.

Newer drug therapies for rheumatoid arthritis include infliximab (Remicade), leflunomide (Arava), and etanercept (Enbrel), which function by blocking the action of various inflammatory compounds, such as TNF (tumor necrosis factor) and IL-1 (interleuken-1). Etanercept is injectable, whereas infliximab is given intravenously every two months. Enbrel has been useful for RA patients and shows promise as a drug therapy that can be used effectively along with natural interventions. Adverse reactions to Enbrel include serious infection and sepsis (sometimes fatal), demyelinating disorders of the central nervous system (such as multiple sclerosis), and new onset or exacerbation of seizure disorders.[11]

After experiencing both the benefits and drawbacks of conventional medications, many arthritis sufferers choose to investigate natural therapies. Although these methods don't tout the quick fix promised by conventional drugs, they do offer substantial benefits over time. They require patients to take responsibility for their own health and involve a high level of education, dedication, and lifestyle change.

What Alternative Medicine Can Do for Arthritis

Natural medicine offers arthritis sufferers lasting relief from pain and inflammation. According to the holistic approach, arthritis is a disease that results from multiple causes, many of them with a less-than-obvious connection to the disease or not easily detectable. As you will discover in this book, a number of underlying imbalances, along with accompanying physical, mental, and environmental factors, contribute to all forms of arthritis.

Specifically, arthritis develops as a result of a combination of some of these factors: an accumulation of toxins in the body (from the environment, food, drugs, and other sources); bacterial and yeast infections (often due to excessive use of antibiotics); parasites; leaky gut syndrome; allergies (both food and environmental); nutrient deficiencies leading to slow repair of cartilage; biomechanical stress and imbalances; poor stress-coping abilities and other emotional factors; and immune dysfunction, often resulting in an autoimmune reaction in which the immune system attacks healthy tissues in the body, further worsening arthritic symptoms.

It is essential to understand the factors that went into creating arthritis in each person, because arthritis is never caused by one thing alone and no two people have exactly the same causal factors. Alternative medicine employs a battery of diagnostic tools—physical examination; dietary assessment; tests for immune, digestive, and detoxification function; and emotional evaluation—to build an individualized picture of the patient's condition. Skilled practitioners of alternative medicine take the time needed to find the root causes of arthritis, and the patient becomes actively involved in their own treatment. Alternative medicine not only respects differences between individuals, it also concentrates its diagnosis and treatment plan based on this customized approach.

Alternative medicine draws upon a wide range of therapies to help treat—and even prevent—arthritis. The primary keys are proper diet and nutrition, detoxification, and stress reduction. Diet and nutrition can have a significant impact on pain and inflammation, and special care should be taken to avoid substances that might cause allergic reactions in the body. Vitamins, minerals, herbs, and other natural supplements can provide effective relief, and usually with a far lower rate of adverse effects than conventional drugs.

Removing toxins from the body can be remarkably therapeutic for

> Skilled practitioners of alternative medicine take the time needed to find the root causes of arthritis, and the patient becomes actively involved in their own treatment. Alternative medicine not only respects differences between individuals, it also concentrates its diagnosis and treatment plan based on this customized approach.

arthritis patients, and alternative medicine offers a number of safe and effective detoxification strategies. Mind-body techniques such as meditation, biofeedback, and hypnotherapy can help reduce stress (a key factor in arthritis overlooked by conventional medicine). Skeletal and postural problems can be addressed through a variety of modalities, including bodywork, manipulation, exercises, stretching, and yoga. Alternative medicine restores health to the whole patient rather than simply providing superficial symptom relief. The goal is to help each person achieve balance among physical healing and the emotional, mental, and even spiritual aspects of their life.

In the case history below, we explain the testing procedures, diagnosis of underlying causes, and therapies that enabled Vanessa to reduce her joint pain and discontinue her use of conventional arthritis drugs that caused stomach upset and other gastrointestinal problems.

Success Story: A Holistic Approach Alleviates Arthritis

Vanessa, age 63, had symptoms of both RA and OA, as well as the early stages of osteoporosis (bone loss). Her health survey revealed a number of other problems: diarrhea (which first occurred following a trip abroad), urinary incontinence, other gastrointestinal difficulties, neurological disturbances, and migraine headaches. She was taking medications for her migraines and anti-inflammatory drugs for her arthritis, but she was concerned about possible side effects from prolonged use. Because her conventional medical specialists had been unable to offer lasting relief for her health problems, Vanessa came to us for a holistic evaluation.

A food profile showed that Vanessa's diet was diverse, consisting of tuna, chicken, eggs, oatmeal, yogurt, herbal teas, soups, and generous quantities of vegetables. Sometimes she snacked on chocolate or nuts and other salty snacks. But Vanessa also said that she had multiple food cravings, which alerted us to a possibility of food allergies. (People often crave foods that trigger allergic reactions for them, which may include arthritis pain.) We ordered a test for potential food allergies, and the results revealed sensitivities to wheat, white and brown rice, corn, broccoli, cucumbers, squash, cashews, black pepper, chocolate, coffee, and licorice.

A hair analysis for mineral deficiencies and heavy metal toxicity revealed high levels of calcium, magnesium, aluminum, sodium, and potassium. We interpreted the high calcium and magnesium levels to mean that these minerals were not being absorbed into her cells; deficiencies of calcium and magnesium are common in arthritis patients. The excess levels of aluminum, sodium, and potassium could have been contributing to Vanessa's neurological imbalances because they interfere with nerve signal transmissions. A blood test revealed elevated liver enzymes, indicating a clogged and toxic liver, something we often find in arthritis patients. Her level of the hormone DHEA (dehydro-epiandrosterone), a precursor of the sex hormones, was low normal at 91 (the normal range is 80 to 160); this relatively low level may have been a natural result of aging or caused by chronic stress.

We also performed a darkfield microscopic blood analysis (SEE QUICK DEFINITION) of Vanessa's blood. We could see in the projected image of her blood many long, unidentified tubules, which we have found to correlate with the presence of parasites. The fact that her diarrhea had begun following foreign travel also made us suspect parasites. Her red blood cells were shaped like stop signs, a condition known as echinocytosis, which indicates the possibility of heavy metals in her system. This assumption was supported by the results of the hair analysis, which indicated high levels of aluminum. Vanessa also had a high level of red and yellow crystals in her blood, which we associate with joint pain and

 Darkfield microscopic blood analysis (darkfield microscopy) is a way of studying living whole blood cells under a specially adapted microscope that projects the dynamic image, magnified 1,400 times, onto a video screen. The skilled physician can detect early signs of illness in the form of microorganisms in the blood known to produce disease. Relevant technical features in the blood include color, variously shaped components (spicules, long tubules, and rouleaus), and the size and activity of certain immune cells. The amount of time the blood cells stay viable indicates the overall health of the individual. Darkfield microscopy reveals distortions of red blood cells (which indicate nutritional status), possible undesirable bacterial or fungal life-forms, and blood ecology patterns indicative of health or illness.

swelling. Finally, her neutrophils, a specific type of white blood cells, were static, a sign of suppressed immune function.

Clearly, our treatment of Vanessa needed to employ multiple therapies (as is the case with all our arthritis patients) because of these underlying problems with parasites, nutritional deficiencies, and toxicity that contributed to her arthritis. In consultation with our nutritionist, Vanessa modified her diet to eliminate those foods that she was allergic to, and we supported her with vitamins B_6 and B_{12} as well as folic acid, which help with food allergies. We also wanted her to increase the amount of foods in her diet containing omega-3 essential fatty acids. A deficiency in omega-3s often leads to inflammation (and even arthritis) in the body.

We also recommended a probiotic supplement containing the friendly intestinal bacteria (SEE QUICK DEFINITION) *Lactobacillus acidophilus* and *Bifidobacterium bifidum*. In addition, we gave her a supplement containing fructo-oligosaccharides (FOSs), which act like an intestinal fertilizer, selectively feeding the friendly microflora in the large intestine so that their numbers can increase.

 Friendly intestinal bacteria, or probiotics, refers to beneficial microbes inhabiting the human gastrointestinal tract, where they are essential for proper nutrient assimilation. The human body contains an estimated several trillion beneficial bacteria comprising over 400 species, all necessary for health. Among the more well-known of these are *Lactobacillus acidophilus* and *Bifidobacterium bifidum*. Overly acidic bodily conditions, chronic constipation or diarrhea, dietary imbalances, consumption of highly processed foods, and the excessive use of antibiotics and hormonal drugs can interfere with probiotic function and even reduce the number of these microbes, setting up conditions for illness.

 For more information on **herbs and nutrients for arthritis**, see chapter 13, Supplements for Arthritis, pages 257–294. For more on **fasting**, see chapter 4, General Detoxification, pages 66–87.

Vanessa was given a nutritional supplement that combined B vitamins, magnesium, selenium, potassium, taurine, and antioxidants, along with other nutrients for liver support, including choline, silymarin, shiitake mushroom, burdock, and licorice. She also took buffered vitamin C with bioflavonoids and a special detoxifying tea that was created by holistic nurse Rene Caisse in the 1920s to treat cancer patients; this tea is also good for blood cleansing and general detoxification.

For her digestive disturbances, Vanessa started on the herb cat's claw and a glutamine supplement useful for soothing the intestines. To address her essential fatty acid deficiencies, we recommended black currant seed oil, which provides omega-3s and omega-6s. Since we considered parasites to be a contributing factor to her digestive problems, we put her on an herbal antiparasitic formula that combines barberry root, citrus seed, Chinese goldenseal rhizome (*Coptis*), garlic bulb, black walnut green outer hull, Rangoon creeper fruit (*Quisqualis indica*), quassia wood, cascara sagrada, Chinese wormwood flowering tops (*Artemisia annua*), and volatile oils of thyme, oregano leaf, tea tree, and clove.

Vanessa also started on a fast to cleanse her gastrointestinal tract. For the first three days, we had her eat nothing but a watery soup made of cabbage and other vegetables rich in nutrients important for joint and bone structure. She also took an intestine-cleansing protein powder drink, along with ground flaxseeds as support during the fast. This moderate fast was a good way for Vanessa to give her toxic bowel a rest, begin to cleanse her liver, and experience some days free of joint pain. We normally recommend that patients continue this fast one day per week on an ongoing basis, but Vanessa had such good results that she decided to fast two days per week.

Additional therapeutic support included a weekly intravenous infusion of potassium chloride, magnesium sulfate, manganese, zinc, vitamin B complex,

Ellen Kamhi, PhD., R.N., gives a reflexogy treatment. Reflexology is based on the idea that there are reflex areas in the hands and feet that correspond to every part of the body, including the organs and glands. By applying gentle but precise pressure to these reflex points, reflexologists release blockages that inhibit energy flow and cause pain and disease. Practitioners focus on breaking up lactic acid and calcium crystals accumulated around any of the 7,200 nerve endings in each foot. Eunice Ingham, a physiotherapist, pioneered the discipline in the late 1930s. She mapped out which points on the feet correspond to which areas of the body and developed techniques for inducing healing in those areas.

vitamins B_6 and B_5, calcium, taurine, and glutathione. We also gave her two nutrients specifically to support her arthritic joints: cetyl myristoleate (a fatty acid) and MSM (methylsulfonylmethane, a sulfur compound), both useful for treating inflammation. To reduce Vanessa's heavy metals, we recommended a homeopathic detoxosode program.

Vanessa started receiving monthly massage treatments from a massage therapist. We also encourage arthritis patients to have regular chiropractic adjustments, although Vanessa opted not to do this. She also came with a friend to one of our reflexology classes so that they could perform this specialized massage therapy for each other at no cost.

After three months on this program, Vanessa said she felt much better, and she continued on the program. Now, after five years, her rheumatologist discontinued Vanessa's use of conventional pain medications, which in turn improved her gastrointestinal problems greatly. A subsequent bone density scan showed that she was no longer at high risk for developing osteoporosis. And her migraines have lessened in both frequency and intensity.

Most importantly, Vanessa feels that she is in control of her symptoms and that her quality of life has increased tremendously. Vanessa is now equipped with the tools to restore and maintain her health. She knows which foods invoke arthritis pains and avoids these. Her diet is now tailored to support optimal joint function and prevent further degenerative effects of aging. She plans to continue with the holistic approach to arthritis and stay away from conventional drug therapy and its adverse side effects.

Undoing Arthritis in Stages: The Scope of This Book

Vanessa's case demonstrates many common aspects of treating arthritis with alternative medicine therapies. She, like over 50% of arthritis patients, has a mixed disease process consisting of both osteoarthritis and rheumatoid arthritis. Clearly, no magic pill will correct what many may erroneously think is a natural part of aging. Instead, several therapies are needed to reverse the underlying factors—nutritional deficiencies, infestation by parasites, and liver and digestive dysfunction, among others—that ultimately manifest themselves as arthritis.

When arthritis is viewed through the perspective of alternative medicine, it becomes a correctable disease that requires adjustments to specific organ systems, diet, and lifestyle. This book will describe the tests that alternative medicine practitioners use to determine inadequacies or dysfunction, provide practical solutions for resolving underlying problems, and suggest positive changes (diet, nutritional supplements, stress-relief strategies, and exercises) that you can make to reverse arthritis or prevent its onset.

Types and causes. In chapter 2, What Is Arthritis?, we provide explanations of the various types of arthritis, their predominant symptoms, and their primary causes.

Testing. In order to start an effective treatment plan, you need to know all the components that are contributing to your arthritis. For Vanessa, we tested for nutritional deficiencies, food allergies, heavy metal toxicity, liver function, digestive capacity, and the infestation of parasites, viruses, or bacteria. Chapter 3, Diagnosing Arthritis, covers these and other tests useful for pinpointing underlying factors. Most of the testing involves simple blood, urine, and stool analyses that conventional doctors may not have experience with.

Detoxifying the body. Toxins from environmental and chemical pollutants, stress, poor diet, and food allergies can overwhelm and eventually exhaust the body's ability to process and eliminate harmful substances. These toxins can then accumulate in joint tissues and cause inflammation, free radical damage, and arthritic degeneration. As seen in Vanessa's case, therapies such as fasting cleanse the body of accumulated toxins and relieve the liver of its toxic burden. Chapter 4, General Detoxification, provides step-by-step instructions for all phases of fasting. Chapter 5, Detoxifying Specific Organs, provides therapies to support and tone the organs involved in the detoxification process. Herbal therapies (such as the ones used to treat Vanessa), dietary adjustments, and other therapeutic methods lessen the body's toxic load, reduce joint pain, stop bone and joint deterioration, and boost the efficiency of vital organs.

Viruses, infections, candidiasis, and parasites. Research and clinical evidence have shown that viruses, bacterial infections, candidiasis (infection with the yeastlike fungus *Candida albicans*), and parasites are often present in those afflicted with arthritis, particularly rheumatoid and infectious arthritis. As you will see in chapter 6, Eradicating Bacteria and Yeast, and chapter 7, Eliminating Parasites, these factors both mimic arthritis symptoms and contribute to the toxic load in the body by eroding the lining of the intestines and escaping into the bloodstream.

Intestinal permeability. About 90% of our arthritis patients have intestinal permeability, also known as leaky gut syndrome. Viruses, disease-causing bacteria, candida, parasites, and NSAIDs are the prime culprits of leaky gut. When inappropriate substances cross the intestinal barrier into the circulatory system, the immune system views them as invaders and sends antibodies to attach to the invaders, forming circulating immune complexes. These immune complexes can trigger collagen breakdown in the joints and autoimmune reactions, both factors in arthritis and joint disease. Chapter 8, Alleviating Leaky Gut Syndrome, further explains the effects of intestinal permeability and how to correct it.

Underlying allergies. Hidden allergies to foods may provoke arthritic symptoms of joint tenderness, inflammation, and swelling. Among the most common allergenic foods are wheat, dairy products, and the nightshade family of vegetables. Vanessa's story demonstrates the role of food allergies in arthritis. Once she eliminated problematic foods from her diet, Vanessa experienced a decrease in joint pain. Chapter 9, Allergies and Arthritis, describes other common allergens, testing procedures, and simple therapies for reducing allergic reactions.

The autoimmune response. The autoimmune arthritic diseases (rheumatoid arthritis, ankylosing spondylitis, juvenile rheumatoid arthritis, and lupus) involve destruction of healthy cells by the body's own defensive mechanism, the immune system. Normal cartilage cells that line the joints and ensure smooth motion become the target of repeated attacks by the immune system. In effect, the body has become allergic to its own tissues, causing joint deformities and disabilities. In chapter 10, Desensitizing the Autoimmune Reaction, we discuss safe and effective methods to quell the immune system's aggressive behavior without suppressing its normal activities.

Healing the psychological side of arthritis. A constant state of stress can lead to a number of adverse physiological consequences that can directly affect the severity of your arthritis. Psychological evaluations of our arthritis patients have also defined a specific "arthritis personality," a kind of mental predisposition for arthritis. In chapter 11, Mind-Body Approaches to Arthritis, you will learn how stress, suppressed emotions, and lifestyle choices can contribute to arthritis, how to undo damaging thoughts, and how to develop habits for relaxing and increasing confidence.

Eating away arthritis. It's an old concept, but food as medicine is a powerful tool accessible to everyone. The dietary recommendations in chapter 12, The Arthritis Diet, show you the foods needed in a daily diet to prevent inflammation and improve overall health, the foods that will exacerbate arthritis symptoms, and recipes for making delicious healthy meals.

Nutrients and natural supplements for arthritis. Like most arthritis sufferers, Vanessa had multiple nutritional deficiencies resulting from age (as we grow older, our nutritional reserves decline) and from an infestation of parasites. Eliminating the parasites and improving her digestion made it possible to focus on boosting levels of nutrients needed to synthesize cartilage and connective tissue (to rebuild her joints) and to fight the damaging effects of free radicals. Chapter 13, Supplements for Arthritis, details the nutrients commonly deficient in arthritis sufferers as well as those nutrients useful in promoting joint health. In addition, chapter 13 offers a compendium of Chinese and Western herbs used to decrease inflammation and relieve pain.

Exercises and physical therapies. While daily exercise and physical activity are both important components of a healthy lifestyle, they are an absolute necessity for people who suffer from arthritis. Regular exercise improves energy levels, provides nourishment for muscles and connective tissues, and maintains a healthy weight. By keeping muscles toned and fit so that they can adequately support joints, exercise helps reduce pain and stiffness and halts the progression of the disease. Daily exercise can be further augmented by massage, acupressure, or other physical therapies to promote relaxation and improve the circulation of blood and lymphatic fluid. Therapeutic baths, showers, and other water treatments can improve circulation, clear the body of toxins, and initiate healing of internal organs. In chapter 14, Exercises and Physical Therapies, we discuss some of the most widely available physical therapies so that you and your health-care professional can determine which will be most beneficial for you.

 For **detailed treatment protocols for each type of arthritis**, see Appendix, pages 321–343.

two

What Is Arthritis?

Among the most common types of arthritis are osteoarthritis (degenerative joint disease), rheumatoid arthritis (an autoimmune disease), and gout (usually affecting small joints in the hands and feet). Other types of arthritis include psoriatic arthritis (associated with the skin condition psoriasis), ankylosing spondylitis, and infectious arthritis (caused by bacterial or viral infections). All of these forms of arthritis are a manifestation of similar underlying imbalances that overload the body and impair the normal process of cartilage repair. Specifically, these causes include intestinal imbalances (dysbiosis or parasites), food allergies, heavy metal toxicity, nutritional deficiencies, intake of unhealthy dietary fats, and emotional, psychological, and biomechanical stressors.

IN THIS CHAPTER

- Osteoarthritis
- Rheumatoid Arthritis
- Gout
- Less Prevalent Joint Diseases (Ankylosing Spondylitis, Psoriatic Arthritis, and Infectious Arthritis)

Osteoarthritis

Osteoarthritis (OA) causes the breakdown of cartilage, the smooth, gelatinous tissue that protects the ends of bones from rubbing against each other. Healthy cartilage shields bones against being worn down by friction,

but in those who have OA, the cartilage is worn away, allowing bone ends
to make direct contact. As the disease
progresses, direct contact creates
bone spurs and abnormal bone hardening and leads to inflammation and
severe pain as bones continue to rub
together without proper cushioning.
As a result, bones may become more
brittle and subject to fracture. Over
300,000 knee and hip replacements
are performed in the United States
annually, usually due to OA.

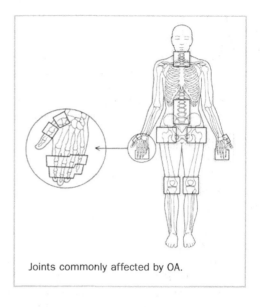

Joints commonly affected by OA.

There are two types of OA: primary and secondary. Primary OA is
considered "wear and tear" arthritis,
due to an unhealthy aging process. It
most commonly develops after age 45 and affects the weight-bearing
joints in the hips, lower back, knees, and feet, as well as the neck and
fingers. It occurs when joints are placed under excessive long-term stress
from supporting too much weight (as seen in obese people with arthritic
knees) or from normal weight demands placed on weak, unhealthy joints.
Genetics can also play a role in several forms of arthritis, a genetic
propensity for the disease runs in families.[1]

Secondary OA is the less common of the two types but has a more
apparent, direct cause: trauma, injury, previous inflammation (even
from rheumatoid arthritis [RA]), congenital joint misalignment, infection, surgery, or prolonged use of medications.[2] It often appears before
the age of 40 and is most commonly caused by sudden or recurring
(chronic) trauma. A fall from a ladder is an example of sudden trauma.
Chronic trauma results from repetitive impact on a particular joint; for
example, the shoulder joint of a baseball pitcher that eventually wears
down due to years of stress from repeated motions. Joe Namath, the
retired New York Jets quarterback, now suffers from arthritis in his knees,
which were repeatedly assaulted by defensive players during football
games. Other examples of secondary OA include an arthritic wrist joint
of a construction worker or worn joints in the feet of a tap dancer. Over
time, repeated motion can lead to a breakdown of cartilage, and that
degeneration often leads to bone deformity.

Anatomy of a Joint

A joint is the area where two bones meet or articulate (that is, move together). The function of the joint is to facilitate mobility and flexibility. Joints are classified into three types, of which arthritis usually affects two—the cartilaginous and synovial joints.

Cartilaginous joints allow only slight movement. The space between adjacent vertebrae in the spine is an example of a cartilaginous joint. Another example of this type of joint allows the pelvis of a pregnant woman to expand. As the name suggests, cartilaginous joints cushion the intersection of two bones with cartilage, a spongelike buffer.

Synovial joints are the freely movable joints in the fingers, arms, legs, hips, and wrists. Their names describe their structure, such as the ball-and-socket joint (which connects the upper leg with the pelvis) or the hinge joint in the elbow and the knee. The wrist joint is called an ellipsoidal joint because it moves in the shape of an ellipse, or oval. And the thumb, or cellar, joint is flexible and gives humans and some primates the ability to manipulate tools. Synovial joints experience more wear and tear than other types of joints.

Synovial joints are made up of numerous components, the most important of which are the synovial membrane, synovial fluid, cartilage, and various types of soft tissue (tendons, ligaments, and muscles). Synovial membrane lines the joint capsule, enclosing all the components of the joint. Dense with nerves, it is the source of much of the pain that people with arthritis experience. The synovial membrane also produces one of the most important substances of the joint, synovial fluid. Synovial fluid, or synovia, coats the joints much like a lubricant coats the parts of a car's engine. It also carries nutrients to the cartilage and removes waste products. The synovial fluid is usually clear, colorless, or pale yellow, resembling blood plasma or serum.

At each joint, cartilage covers the ends of the bones, serving to buffer the bones from rubbing together. Cartilage, one of the smoothest surfaces known to humankind, is rubbery, gel-like, tough, flexible, and slippery. There are two types of cartilage: articular (or moving cartilage) and meniscus (or cushioning cartilage). Both types are very pliable and also act as shock absorbers due to their high water content—cartilage is 65% to 80% water.

Cartilage doesn't contain blood, lymphatic vessels, or nerves. It is nourished entirely through a process that involves contraction and expansion. When pressure is applied to joints, the cartilaginous structures are compressed; as movement stops or the body relaxes, the cartilage reexpands. This compression and relaxation allows the nutrient-bearing synovial fluid to circulate freely in and out of the joint. Moving actually feeds our joints. And conversely, when we stop moving, we begin to starve our joints by shutting down the flow of nutrients. Without synovial fluid, the articular cartilage in joints would begin to wear away like parts of a car engine that isn't adequately lubricated.

Joints are surrounded by soft tissue:

Osteoarthritis Symptoms

The onset of primary OA is gradual, as the disease usually progresses over the course of many years. It most frequently starts with mild pain and stiffness, which can lead to a narrowing of the joint, limited joint mobility, and sometimes a grating sensation and grinding sound called crepitus. This

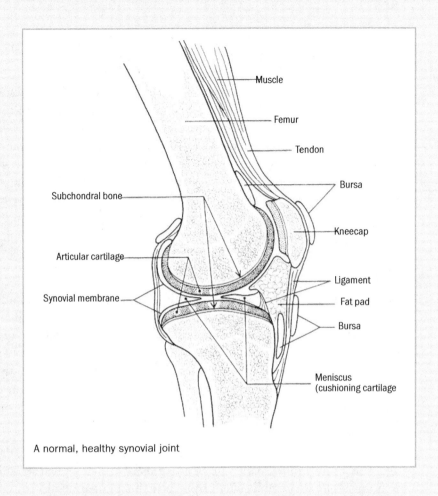

A normal, healthy synovial joint

tendons, which attach muscles to the bone; ligaments, which connect bone to bone with an extremely tough, fibrous tissue known as elastin; and muscles, which make the different parts move as one. To reduce friction during motion, tendons are covered by tendon sheaths, which use a lubricating substance called hyaluronan. To absorb shock during motion, bursa (small sacs filled with synovial fluid), are strategically placed throughout the joints. You may be familiar with the condition called bursitis or tennis elbow, which involves inflammation of the bursa.

additional stress can lead to the development of bone spurs (osteophytes), which in turn cause more friction, further joint breakdown, and pain.

Causes of Osteoarthritis

Although a lifetime of wear and tear on the joints is commonly considered the cause of OA, studies have shown that constant use of the joints by itself doesn't cause bone and cartilage to erode.[3] Many elderly men and women who have been physically active over their entire lifetime experience no debilitating arthritic symptoms. Research now confirms that the degenerative form of arthritis involves ongoing biochemical processes that negatively alter the structure and regeneration of cartilage and joint tissue. These biochemical processes include free radical damage, nutritional deficiencies, imbalances of important hormones, poor dietary and lifestyle choices, food or environmental allergies, genetic predisposition, and even drug treatments prescribed for pain relief. In various combinations, these factors often cause (or contribute to) changes in the biomechanics of the joints and muscles. Changes in the way the joints and muscles interact disturbs the distribution of fluids and nutrients in tissues and cartilage. Consequently, cartilage becomes injured and is unable to repair itself.

Obesity. Obesity is a very strong contributing factor to the development of OA, increasing wear and tear on the joints and negatively influences many biochemical and biomechanical processes. Excess body weight is particularly stressful to the knees and hips, which carry the brunt of the additional weight. For each additional pound of body weight, three pounds of pressure is added to the knees and 6 pounds of pressure is added to the hips. This extra pressure gradually increases the stress on these joints, raising the risk of OA later in life.

Free Radicals. Free radicals are one of the major molecular causes of damage to healthy connective tissue in all kinds of arthritis.[4] A free radical is an unstable, toxic molecule of oxygen with an unpaired electron that steals an electron from another molecule and produces harmful effects. Free radicals are formed when molecules within cells react with oxygen (oxidize) as part of normal metabolic processes. Free radicals are generated by any type of stress, including chemical, physical, biochemical, emotional, and mental. Other sources of free radicals include exposure to environmental toxins in food, air, and water, and also through smoking cigarettes. By the time arthritis sets in, free radicals have been oxidizing cartilage for an extended time.

Imbalanced Hormones. Researchers have investigated the role of hormones, the regulators of bodily functions, in the development of OA. Specifically, imbalances of adrenal, thyroid, and parathyroid hormones have been found to cause or exacerbate OA.[5] The adrenal glands are responsible for the release of many hormones that regulate our reactions to stress and our energy metabolism. These hormones include DHEA (the precursor of estrogen and testosterone), pregnenolone, cortisol, and adrenaline. When the body is under chronic stress, the adrenals produce high levels of steroid hormones (adrenaline and cortisol) instead of DHEA. The result of prolonged exposure to steroid hormones is an increase in bone degeneration, muscle breakdown, accumulation of fat, and an imbalance of important mineral ratios, all of which can lead to the development of arthritis.[6]

Because women experience OA at a rate three times greater than men, estrogen and progesterone imbalances have been investigated as one of the many potential causative factors. Excess levels of estrogen (and decreased levels of progesterone) can cause deficiencies in zinc, magnesium, and the B vitamins, which are involved in hormone maintenance and bone and tissue health. OA sufferers may benefit from using natural substances that help balance estrogen and progesterone levels.

Nutrient Deficiencies. As people age, their levels of many nutrients involved in the synthesis of cartilage become deficient. Although these deficiencies may not directly cause OA, studies have shown that supplementation can often bring pain relief. Vitamin E helps to increase the production of the building blocks of cartilage, as well as to decrease cartilage breakdown and joint pain.[7] Vitamin C levels are often low in OA patients, and this vitamin is vital for repairing joints and building collagen.[8] Vitamin B_3 (niacinamide) has demonstrated good results when used to treat joint pain and stiffness associated with OA.[9] International studies have noted that high levels of OA are found in areas where the mineral boron is deficient in the soil and food supply. Boron supplementation is regularly used for OA patients in Germany, and significant improvement in OA after boron supplementation has been documented.[10]

Diet and Food Allergies. When comparisons are made of particular cultural groups, evidence points to the standard American diet (which is high in fat, sugar, and processed and refined foods) as a major contributing factor to the development of OA.[11] OA is a very rare disease in Japan, where the diet is high in fish and sea vegetables. But an interesting phenomenon occurs when Japanese individuals begin to adopt a standard American diet: There is a marked increase in the development of OA, as well as many other degenerative diseases, after the new diet has been consumed for a number of years. Dietary intake of fats affects the composition of cell membranes and the degree of inflammation and pain that a person experiences. Decreasing hydrogenated oils and fried foods and increasing omega-3 essential fatty acids decreases inflammation.[12]

Food allergies, often a result of poor dietary choices, are also implicated as a causative factor in many cases of arthritis.[13] An allergy to plants in the nightshade family, including tomatoes, peppers, eggplant, potatoes, and tobacco, is common. About one-third of the arthritis sufferers who remove all nightshades from their diet experience some relief of symptoms. Other common food allergens include dairy products, wheat, soy, corn, and eggs.

Biomechanical Changes. OA is more likely to develop if joints lose their full range of motion. Compromised mobility decreases the flow of oxygen and nutrients to the surrounding cartilage and leads to cartilage breakdown. Cartilage can obtain nourishment, repair itself, and get rid of wastes through balanced motion. When a joint is compressed (for example, each time you step forward you compress your knee joint), synovial fluid in the cartilage between the knee bones is pumped out of the area; this is called on-loading. As the joint comes to rest it expands, and fluid rushes back in carrying a fresh supply of oxygen and essential nutrients; this is called off-loading. This exchange of nutrients and waste products is dependent upon balanced (full range), frequent motion. Stress, injury, or lack of activity causes a series of imbalances that alter the interactions of ligaments, tendons, bones, and muscles. As a result, balanced motion is hindered, and the surrounding cartilage starves as the on-loading and off-loading exchange of substances is compromised.

The body also responds to joint and muscle biomechanical imbalances by sending calcium to weak or impaired areas to stabilize the weak joint. This response results in hard, inflexible deposits of calcium where once there were smooth, elastic ligaments, tendons, and even muscle. The joint stiffness that arthritis patients frequently experience is caused by these calcium deposits. Eventually these calcium deposits form spurs that protrude from the joints much like stalactites found inside caves, and the joint ultimately can fuse. The density of calcium spurs is immense, as the following example illustrates: While treating a woman with OA in her neck and shoulder, we inserted an acupuncture needle into a muscle on the front of her neck and hit one of these calcium deposits. The deposit was so impenetrable that it actually bent the needle.

Fibrosis (an excess accumulation of fibrous tissue) can also set in as waste products build up in the muscle and joint area, and further restrict motion. These impediments deprive joints of key nutrients needed to build new cartilage as old cells die. As a result, cartilage physically wears away, exposing bone and leading to the onset of arthritis. Arthritis can actually be transferred to neighboring joints when surrounding muscles and cartilage attempt to compensate for the weakened joint's immobility.

Traumatic injury to cartilage caused by sports, accidents, chronic obesity, or any other means can initiate the development of OA. The injury site may remain slightly sensitive and then develop OA many years later. Trauma has been associated with the onset of OA in young individuals, especially those who participate in contact sports. Rapid compression and excessive torque can tear or damage cartilage or bone, leaving a weakened area that may later develop into arthritis. Damage to ligaments, tendons, and muscles can cause either hypermobility or hypomobility of the joints. Repetitive impact loading is a specific type of trauma we often see in major league baseball pitchers. We also see it in people in other occupations involving repetitive motion, like carpenters or jackhammer operators. Repetitive motion causes an accumulation of microtraumas and subsequent calcifications that, over a long span of time, can contribute to OA.

Insulin Resistance/Deficiency. Patients with OA often display insulin resistance or deficiency. Insulin resistance, often considered a precursor to adult-onset diabetes, is a blood sugar disorder that occurs when the body fails to recognize the effects of insulin in the blood. This makes it more difficult for the body to use sugar (glucose) for energy. The body then begins to break down protein as an alternative energy source, which negatively affects the connective tissue and leads to further destruction within the joints. A diet high in carbohydrates, especially sugars and wheat products, tend to increase insulin resistance, leading to a further imbalance in both intracellular and blood sugar levels.

Rheumatoid Arthritis

Rheumatoid arthritis (RA) is an inflammatory disease in which the body's immune system attacks its own healthy tissues. This is called an autoimmune response. The disorder affects many organs throughout the body, but it's most noted for significantly disabling, deforming, and inflaming the joints and other structures comprised of connective tissue, which supports and binds together other tissues and forms ligaments and tendons. RA can be crippling.

Arthritis: The Breaking Down of Cartilage

The kinds, symptoms, and causes of arthritis are numerous and almost too varied to be grouped under one term. But there is a common factor among the various arthritic diseases—the erosion of cartilage. Under healthy conditions, old or damaged cartilage is replaced by new cartilage constructed by chondrocytes, a specialized type of cell.

Chondrocytes make the constituent parts of cartilage, collagen, and proteoglycans. The quality or type of cartilage created is a function of the raw materials—vitamins, minerals, proteins, amino acids, and GAGs (glycosaminoglycans)—available to the chondrocytes and the stresses being placed on the joints. This stress can be physical, toxic, immunological, emotional, or any other type that produces biochemical inflammatory agents and free radicals that attack joints.

Collagen, the structural protein of cartilage that forms the "scaffolding" of the body, is a major part of bone, skin, ligaments, tendons, and all tissues and organs, giving us shape and form. Strong and resilient, it has qualities like an elastic band. When the molecular components of collagen are changed—due to the aging process, increased free radical production, or poor nutrition—the collagen protein becomes less structured and begins to sag. The structure of the collagen molecules, normally a triple-helix shape, begins to unwind. As the degeneration of collagen progresses, the molecular bonds that create strong connective tissue begin to weaken and dissolve, a process that can lead to arthritis.

Proteoglycans are attached to and cover the framework of collagen fibers. Proteoglycans have the consistency of gelatin and tend to swell up and absorb water like a sponge. They fill in the gaps between collagen molecules. Under a microscope, they look like a long-handled brush used to clean bottles; their long protein core resembles the handle of the bottle brush and the chains of sugar that radiate from the core resemble the bristles of the brush.

Symptoms of Rheumatoid Arthritis

The onset of RA symptoms can be slow, with mild discomfort in the joints, morning stiffness, low-grade fevers systemically or in the affected joints, and a gradual increase of symptoms. People can also develop RA seemingly overnight. The onset of symptoms can be extremely rapid and debilitating; one day a patient of ours went bike riding, and the next day she couldn't get out of bed because the inflammation and pain in her joints were so severe. We've found that RA sets in more quickly if there are multiple causative factors, such as infections, nutritional deficiencies, and heavy metal toxicity.

 For **detailed treatment protocols for each type of arthritis**, see Appendix, pages 321–343.

In the early stages of the RA, the synovial membrane (which secretes synovial fluid, the lubricant in joints) swells and begins to grow rapidly

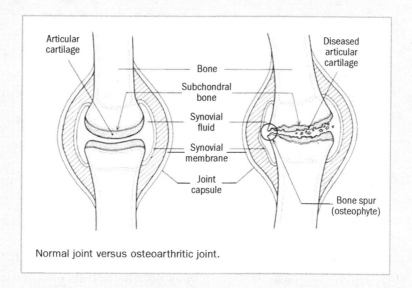

Normal joint versus osteoarthritic joint.

Proteoglycans maintain the content and direct the flow of fluids circulating throughout the cartilage as well as in the joints. The sulfur found in proteoglycans has a negative charge, so that, like a magnet, sulfur attracts water molecules to the cartilage, giving the cartilage a cushion to protect the ends of the bones from premature wear. But the bonds between water and cartilage tend to be weak and easily broken by stress or shock. When these bonds are broken, the water (and cushioning) flows out of the cartilage.

(it can increase over a hundredfold in weight).[14] As a result, the entire joint swells and is inflamed. RA may sometimes affect only one side of the body, but typically it is found on both sides. It is common for RA to strike the same joints on both sides of the body simultaneously—the elbows, for instance. Other symptoms include chronic aches, stiffness, loss of appetite and weight loss, muscle weakness, fatigue, fever, and depression.

Later in the development of the disease, the affected joints become thicker and deformed. The deformity usually comes from contraction of the muscles and tendons that causes them to deviate from their normal shape and pattern. Joint linings become inflamed, and in that chronic state, they thicken and eventually infiltrate cartilage and other local connective tissue (ligaments and tendons). For reasons yet unknown, the synovial cells in patients with RA become altered in such

 For more information about **diagnosing and eradicating bacterial infections**, see chapter 6, Eradicating Bacteria and Yeast, pages 115–133.

> Rheumatoid arthritis is an inflammatory disease in which the body's immune system attacks its own healthy tissues. This is called an autoimmune response. The disorder affects many organs throughout the body, but it's most noted for significantly disabling, deforming, and inflaming the joints.

a way that they begin to produce large amounts of destructive enzymes, which contribute to the breakdown of healthy tissues, leading to joint fusion.

Underlying Causes of Inflammation in Rheumatoid Arthritis

In various combinations and to various degrees, food allergies, nutritional deficiencies, toxicity, intestinal permeability, and microorganisms cause inflammation (the immune system's attack on foreign substances). For someone who has RA, inflammation amplifies, becoming the more destructive autoimmune response, in which the immune system begins to attack healthy tissues.

Viruses and Bacteria. Many symptoms of viral diseases are almost identical to RA. Mumps, viral hepatitis, rubella, and viruslike organisms such as mycoplasmas are capable of creating an arthritis-like syndrome. In addition, there are cases of direct viral infection of the joints.[15] Mounting evidence points more convincingly to the role of bacterial infections in RA's autoimmune response. Bacteria, such as streptococcus, gonococcus, pneumococcus, propionibacterium, salmonella, staphylococcus, and *Borrelia burgdorferi* (the spirochete implicated in Lyme disease), can cause illnesses similar to RA.

Intestinal Permeability. Many scientific studies have documented that a significant number of patients with autoimmune disease and arthritis have increased permeability in their intestinal walls.[16] The intestinal lining becomes inflamed because of use of alcohol, drugs, NSAIDs, allergens, lectins (SEE QUICK DEFINITION, page 29), and imbalance of intestinal microorganisms. During inflammation, chemicals are released that actually dissolve the barrier-like membrane of the intestines, allowing undigested proteins and intestinal microorganisms to enter the general blood circulation, where they trigger more inflammation throughout the body.

Symptomatic Differences between Osteoarthritis and Rheumatoid Arthritis

Osteoarthritis	Rheumatoid Arthritis
Usually affects the elderly	Can affect anyone, even children
Metabolic deficiencies or traumatic injuries are attributable origins	Unproven origin, but infections, particularly bacterial, have been indicated in many cases
Gradual onset of symptoms with mild pain and swelling; mild heat and redness in affected joints	Rapid onset with moderate to extreme pain and swelling; moderate to extreme heat and redness in affected joints
Stiffness from joint damage	Stiffness from swelling
Increased bone density	Loss of bone density

Source: Robert Bingham, M.D., *Fight Back Against Arthritis* (Desert Hot Springs, CA: Desert Arthritis Medical Clinic, 1994).

Food Allergies. Studies conducted by rheumatologists document the positive effect of removing food allergens from the diet of arthritis patients.[17] The top foods known to trigger rheumatoid symptoms include milk, yeast (both brewer's and baker's yeast), wheat, nightshade vegetables (tomatoes, eggplant, peppers, and potatoes), corn, and eggs. We've found that patients who eliminate these foods for three weeks (without other supportive treatments) and then reintroduce them one at a time will often develop their arthritis symptoms again, although they may have improved during the elimination period.

Fatty Acid Imbalance. Under healthy conditions, the chemical agents that cause inflammation are balanced in precise ratios with agents that suppress inflammation. In arthritis and autoimmune ailments, however, this ratio abnormally favors proinflammatory substances and results in too much inflammation. This imbalance is partially caused by diet because the raw ingredients needed to manufacture inflam-

 QUICK DEFINITION

Lectins are protein fragments of incompletely digested foods that bind with specific sugars on the surface of all cells of the body. They tend to stick like Velcro to the lining of the gastrointestinal tract, where they irritate the tissues and can destroy cell membranes. Most dietary lectins come from the indigestible fractions of plant products, often deriving from beans, grains, soy, and wheat. Lectins can lead to food allergies and toxic reactions at the mucosal membranes in the intestines. In particular, soybean and wheat lectins can produce an increase in permeability in the cells they bind to, often leading to cell death. Further, lectins can cause atrophying of the intestinal villi (the fingerlike projections that afford the intestines their absorptive surface area).

matory chemicals are typically derived from different types of fats. Prostaglandins, for example, are hormonelike substances involved in both causing and controlling inflammation. When a person's diet is rich in essential fatty acids, especially omega-3 fatty acids, prostaglandins that stop inflammation are manufactured in the body. On the other hand, eating large servings of commercial meat products or commercial baked goods made with hydrogenated oil introduces chemicals that the body converts into inflammation-causing prostaglandins and leukotrienes.

Patients with RA and other rheumatoid diseases have high levels of arachidonic acid in their tissues. A specific enzyme converts arachidonic acid into prostaglandins that worsen swelling and sensitize tissues to painful stimuli. Elevated concentrations of proinflammatory prostaglandins have been found in fluid and tissue samples taken from people with arthritis, especially RA.

Other Causes. Chronic exposure to certain chemicals, such as formaldehyde and benzene, can elicit symptoms similar to those of RA. Therefore, alternative health-care practitioners often evaluate the chemical load of patients with chronic pain. Due to exposure to a myriad of toxic environmental substances, including pesticides and herbicides in nonorganic foods, dry-cleaning fluids, and air and water pollution, as well as normal metabolic processes, the body is bombarded with free radicals. The body normally fights this bombardment by releasing antioxidants, which quench the effects of free radicals. However, chronic inflammation quickly consumes stores of antioxidants, leaving surrounding tissue vulnerable to attack.[18]

Causes of the Autoimmune Response

The underlying causes addressed above work in various combinations to trigger inflammation. Inflammation is actually a normal process in the body. It helps mend damaged cells, remove toxins, and attack invading microorganisms. During a normal inflammatory response, proinflammatory agents (leukotrienes and certain prostaglandins) dilate blood vessels, which facilitates the transportation of white blood cells to the injury. Increased blood flow causes swelling, redness, and heat. The second wave of proinflammatories (or chemotactic factors) are released to activate white blood cells so they can begin attacking pathogens and digesting immune complexes and damaged cells. White blood cells destroy pathogens by means of oxidizing chemicals that can also affect surrounding cells. As the disease-causing agents are destroyed and their cell fragments removed, the proinflammatory chemicals are soon suppressed by anti-inflammatory chemicals secreted by neighboring cells. The inflammatory response subsides: production of antibodies ceases, blood vessels return to normal size, and repair processes begin to mend damaged tissues.

But in patients with RA and other types of autoimmune disorders, this return to normalcy never occurs. The immune system resists attempts to suppress it and begins to produce antibodies that attack the body's own cells, called autoantibodies (meaning "against self"). The destruction of healthy cells can trigger a further autoimmune response. When cell membranes are torn apart, the cell's internal components leak out. Since the immune system is familiar only with the outer cell membranes, these internal cell components are viewed as foreign bodies and attacked.

We've already explored the causes of inflammation involved in RA—intestinal permeability, viral or bacterial infections, and toxicity. But these factors don't explain why the immune system seemingly loses control and begins to attack the body's normal cells. Several theories explain the immune system's chaotic and aggressive behavior.

Cell Wall Deficient Bacteria. Observation of live blood samples has identified an evolutionary trick of ordinary bacteria: They can change the shape of their cell wall to escape detection by the immune system. Known as "stealth pathogens" by microbiologists, these masked bacteria can then gain access to sensitive tissues and organs where the immune system has difficulty differentiating healthy cells from the disguised bacteria.

The cell wall, or membrane, composed of fats and proteins, regulates the passage of materials into and out of the cell. Stealth pathogens don't have cell walls, enabling them to assume the identity of the surrounding cells. "These organisms are clandestine, almost unrecognizable, and omnipresent," says Lida Holmes Mattman, Ph.D., professor emeritus in biology at Wayne State University. Dr. Mattman explains that these types of bacteria can exchange DNA with other cells, change shape, and increase their own growth rate. They can work their way into "all aspects of microbe participation in life" and create a myriad of new forms so that the body's immune system cannot recognize and efficiently eliminate them.[19]

In the case of RA, Philip Hoekstra, Ph.D., a student of Dr. Mattman's, has found that virtually all the patients he has studied have had significant amounts of the bacteria *Propionibacterium acnes*, a common bacteria that is often cell-wall deficient, which allows it to evade detection by the immune system. In our practice, we've observed what Dr. Hoekstra has described. After years of performing darkfield microscopic analysis on patients with arthritis, we've documented the presence of several microorganisms that look like a cross between bacillar, coccal, spirochetal, and fungal forms.

Dr. Mattman proved the causal relationship between *P. acnes* and RA in laboratory tests. She extracted bacteria from the synovial fluid of arthritis patients and injected it into chicken embryos. Soon after hatching, the chicks began exhibiting symptoms of RA. When she treated the chicks with antibiotics known to disable *P. acnes*, the disease disappeared. The *P. acnes* bacteria is passed from mother to fetus during pregnancy, and this may be responsible for the occurrence of RA in multiple generations. The prevalence of this bacteria in arthritis patients is not clear; however, some researchers suggest that the overuse of antibiotics may be a factor in encouraging its growth and increasing the number of new forms.

The autoimmune response is triggered when the immune system detects and attacks the camouflaged microorganisms. Nearby normal cells are damaged during the attack, then leak internal cellular material that isn't recognized by the immune system. As a result, the immune system initiates an attack against the healthy cells. This response becomes a self-perpetuating autoimmune cycle.

Homotoxins. One of the most comprehensive theories about the cause of the autoimmune response in RA was synthesized by Dr. Hans-Heinrich Reckeweg, a German physician who founded Heel, a company manufacturing homeopathic remedies, in 1936. Dr. Reckeweg theorized that the connective tissue is one of the most important detoxification pathways in the body, the area where the body neutralizes toxins that were not broken down by the liver or kidneys. Dr. Reckeweg and other researchers discovered that the connective tissue has a diurnal, or daily rhythm, similar to the ebb and flow of the ocean tides. At certain times in this 24-hour cycle, the connective tissue eliminates toxins from the body.

Beginning at 3 A.M., the acidic stage begins. Inflammation in the connective tissues increases, the lymphatic system swells, the metabolic rate increases, and body temperature rises. Dr. Reckeweg explained that this is when homotoxins (toxins that cause disease) are combusted and destroyed. Certain enzymes (such as histamine) cause the connective tissue to soften into a gelatinous state, which increases the pain and stiffness experienced by many arthritis sufferers in the morning. At 3 P.M., the cycle reverses and the alkaline stage becomes dominant. The connective tissue is gradually reorganized, and anti-inflammatory substances begin to take control. All results of the acidic stage are slowly reversed. In our clinical studies, we have observed that patients' pain and inflammation occur at predictable times—worsening of symptoms in the morning and improvement in the evening—coinciding with Dr. Reckeweg's theory.

Dr. Reckeweg felt that conventional medications (such as NSAIDs, cortisone, or antibiotics) inhibit the alkaline stage, during which tissues are reconstituted after the destruction of homotoxins. Thus, conventional medications trap homotoxins that are incompletely broken down inside the tissues. Dr. Reckeweg termed these "wild peptides," which are "foreign molecules of bacterial endotoxins, chemicals, and allopathic drugs, coupled with our own tissue albumin to create an alien protein."[20] The immune system then assaults these alien proteins with antibodies and aggressively hunts and destroys any similarly structured tissue in the body, and an autoimmune response is underway.

According to Dr. Reckeweg, autoimmune diseases, including arthritis, are the body's attempt to establish a state of balance, or homeostasis. Inflammation is the outward sign of the body's attempts to redissolve the tissues so it can free up and remove the homotoxins that have been trapped for eventual destruction. However, this process can be damaging if the cells' antioxidant levels are low, which is often the case in arthritis patients.[21]

Theory of Defective Immunoregulation. The theories above postulate that the immune system has lost control over itself while attacking foreign substances. In contrast, the theory of defective immunoregulation maintains that a faulty immune system, not invading microorganisms, produces an autoimmune response. The immune system, according to this theory, is so defective that it doesn't produce normal, healthy antibodies that can discriminate between cells. In addition, cells that control antibodies fail to stop the overzealous B-lymphocytes (cells that make antibodies), and the disease spirals out of control.

Rheumatoid Factor Theory. Rheumatoid factor (RF) is an immunoglobulin or antibody, usually of the IgM type. This specialized protein is programmed to attack IgG circulating immune complexes (CICs) or altered

IgG molecules. When RF attacks a CIC, it perceives it as being alien to the body, even though 50% of the molecule is foreign and 50% is your own protein (the antibody). The immune system then begins to attack the body's own tissues. RF is usually present in 70% of cases of rheumatoid arthritis, and it also appears in the blood of patients with tuberculosis, parasitic infections, leukemia, or other connective tissue disorders. RF is measured through a blood test and is often, but not always, high in patients who complain of joint pain and stiffness. A high RF level is one of the factors leading to a definitive diagnosis of RA[22]

Gout

Gout is caused by a buildup of uric acid (a waste product of the urine cycle), which deposits razor-sharp crystals in the joint spaces between bones. These daggerlike crystals often appear in the first joint of the big toe, but they also attack the wrists, knees, elbows, and ankles. Heat, swelling, and stiffness result. Gout usually strikes suddenly, with a rapid onset. A person once afflicted will often have recurring bouts, although isolated occurrences do happen. Raised bumps (caused by urate crystal deposits) can often be seen on the affected joints, as well as other areas of the body, notably the ear lobes. Gout is characterized by episodes of excruciating pain, redness, inflammation, severe discomfort upon moving the joints, and intermittent fever and fatigue.

The main cause of gout is high levels of uric acid (hyperuricemia) in body fluids. (However, not everyone with elevated uric acid develops gout.) This can occur due to genetic factors, biochemical abnormalities, underlying kidney disease, or poor diet. The body's fluids, including synovial fluid, become saturated with more uric acid than can be efficiently excreted through the kidneys, and uric acid crystallizes into urate crystals, which accumulate in the joints. We have often observed uric acid crystals floating in patients' blood samples while performing darkfield microscope examinations.

The needlelike crystals irritate surrounding tissues, and the body responds by sending in white blood cells, which flood the area and increase swelling and inflammation. Enzymes used by the white blood cells during the inflammatory response damage surrounding cartilage and cell membranes. Active neutrophils also release lactic acid, increasing acidity, which causes more crystals to form. As the white blood cells are destroyed, they release an alarm chemical that calls even more white blood cells to the area, and an inflammatory cascade ensues.

Although most people initiate a gout attack through poor lifestyle choices (obesity, rich foods, alcohol), 10% to 15% of gout patients have attacks due to metabolic problems, such as a deficiency of the enzyme (xanthine oxidase) that breaks down purines, or too much purine production by the body. Purines come from certain foods but are also normally present in the protein portion of our own body cells, such as DNA and RNA. Purines are broken down into uric acid, which is normally excreted through the urine. Purine content in body fluids is increased by obesity and consumption of alcohol (especially beer) and foods high in purines (milk; eggs; many types of beans, including soy; and meat products, especially liver and other organ meats, sausages and other processed meats, anchovies, crab, and shrimp).

Research has confirmed that alcohol increases the risk of gout, and beer stands out as the worst offender.[23] It's interesting to note that in the eighteenth century, port was stored in lead-lined casks, and probably caused low-level lead poisoning. Lead accumulates in the kidneys and depletes their ability to break down toxins, including uric acid. This may partially explain the high incidence of gout among port drinkers during that period of time.[24] Medications, including aspirin and diuretics, can cause gout by putting extra stress on the kidneys; 25% of new gout cases are caused by these drugs. Kidney stones and other kidney problems are present in 90% of gout sufferers because urate crystals also accumulate in the kidneys.

Less Prevalent Joint Diseases

There are a number of less-well-known types of joint or arthritic conditions, among them ankylosing spondylitis, psoriatic arthritis, infectious arthritis, and Lyme disease.

Ankylosing Spondylitis

Most common in young men, ankylosing spondylitis (AS) is an inflammatory disease that bends or fuses spinal vertebrae; over time, the spine stiffens. AS also inflames sacroiliac joints, where the spine meets the pelvis in the lower back. Symptoms include lower back pain, chest pain when inhaling (as the disease spreads upward), weight loss, fatigue, and lack of flexibility. In its advanced stage, AS causes the severe stooping posture sometimes observed in elderly men, the result of a permanently bent spine. Ankylosing spondylitis patients suffer increased stiffness and pain in their back, spine, and buttocks, particularly in their low back in the morning. Chronic inflammation in this region of the body leads to the development of bone bridges (osteophytes); eventually these can take an otherwise mobile joint and ankylose, or fuse, it. AS strikes one in 1,000 people under age 40 and is most common in males between the ages of 16 and 35. The disease is found almost exclusively in men who have the HLA-B27 gene; however, only 20% of men with that gene actually develop the illness. Researchers are now investigating whether certain infections trigger AS.

Psoriatic Arthritis

Psoriatic arthritis (PSA) occurs in about 10% of patients who have psoriasis, a skin disease that causes red, scaly patches, most frequently on the knees, neck, and elbows. Golden brown pitting in the fingernails is also a common symptom. The disease usually begins 10 to 20 years after the onset of psoriasis and includes swelling in many joints, particularly the end joints of the fingers and toes. While the disease is chronic, it's usually not disabling, although about 5% of PSA sufferers develop hand deformities.

We have also found that there are underlying factors that contribute to the onset of psoriasis. These include improper bowel and liver function as a result of an overgrowth of the yeast candida or infestations of other pathogenic organisms in the microflora of the bowels. Pathogenic microflora cause increased levels of toxins to enter the bloodstream. Research has revealed that patients with psoriasis or psoriatic arthritis have very high levels of circulating endotoxins (toxic substances resulting from the pathogenic bowel flora) as well as circulating immune complexes in the blood.[25] Studies have shown that the amount of essential fatty acids in the blood of patients with psoriasis and psoriatic arthritis is inadequate.[26] Copper toxicity is also a very important underlying pathologic problem in patients with psoriatic arthritis. High levels of copper decrease levels of zinc, which is important for skin health. Zinc has been found to be very low in patients with psoriasis.[27]

Arachidonic acid is a fatty acid present in animal products (shellfish, meats, and dairy products). In people with psoriasis, arachidonic acid is deposited into the cell membrane and, through the action of the enzyme lipoxygenase, is turned into inflammatory compounds that cause pain and redness.

Infectious Arthritis

Viruses, bacteria, and fungi can cause infectious arthritis, which most often inflames the knee joint and is characterized by fever and stiffness.

Conventional medicine has spent an enormous amount of time and research money searching for a particular microorganism as a cause of arthritis. As a result, many microorganisms have been linked to arthritis, but a direct causal relationship to any one species has never been established.[28] There are two basic kinds of infectious arthritis: septic arthritis, in which microorganisms directly infect the joints; and reactive arthritis, in which no microorganisms are found in the joints, but an inflammation reaction is triggered by microorganisms found elsewhere in the body. Lyme disease is yet another type of infectious arthritis.

In septic arthritis, the microorganisms directly invade the synovial membrane that surrounds the joint and the synovial fluid. Patients who suffer from chronic RA are more susceptible to the further complication of septic arthritis if they take oral corticosteroid drugs, have had cortisone injected directly into a joint, or have any weakness in their small blood vessels. These weakened vessels can be more easily invaded by opportunistic microorganisms. This kind of arthritis usually affects an isolated joint and is characterized by sudden onset, inflammation, swelling, and pain.

Reactive arthritis is an immunological disorder triggered by the presence of a systemic infection in the body. Immune complexes are formed, throwing the body into an autoimmune reaction. In reactive arthritis, there is no direct infestation of the joint by microorganisms, but the microbe itself or cell fragments of the microorganism are involved in triggering the immune system. Antibodies attach to the microbial substance and form circulating immune complexes, which leads to the development of arthritis.[29] Reactive arthritis, once initiated, may continue for years after the initial systemic infection clears up.[30] Reactive arthritis includes rheumatic fever and Reiter's syndrome, a type of arthritis that usually affects the eyes and urinary tract as well as the joints.

Lyme disease, first identified in 1976, was named after the town of

The Difficulty of Diagnosing Arthritis

The distinctions between different types of arthritis can at times become quite vague. Symptoms often overlap, and patients can have more than one type of arthritis. Here are a couple of common combination diagnoses.

- OA coupled with osteoporosis or less prevalent joint diseases, such as bursitis or gout
- Bursitis coupled with degenerative or intervertebral disk disease, infectious arthritis, gout, or OA

One type of arthritis can also develop into another type. For example, a patient may not recover completely from a joint infection or the infection may damage the blood supply to the joint, resulting in degenerative changes and OA. This makes it difficult to accurately diagnose the specific type of arthritis that may be affecting an individual.

Old Lyme, Connecticut, where the first cases appeared. Since its discovery, the number of cases has been steadily increasing. The Centers for Disease Control (CDC) reported more than 23,000 cases of Lyme disease in the United States in 2002.[31] Lyme disease is presumed to be caused by the spirochete bacterium *Borrelia burgdorferi* (similar to the spirochete that causes syphilis) and carried by a deer tick, or black-legged tick. The incubation period can be lengthy, with initial exposure commonly occurring during the summer and symptoms developing weeks or months later.

Lyme disease is a multisystem inflammatory disease affecting the skin in characteristic rashes at first, then spreading to the joints and nervous system later. The Lyme spirochetes have an affinity for nerve cells and, once they enter the nervous system, attack brain tissue and spinal cells. In our clinical experience, people with a long-term Lyme infection exhibit the blank expression, shuffling movement, and stiffness associated with syphilis. Symptoms are variable, including skin lesions or rashes, fatigue, flulike symptoms, sleeping difficulties, muscle pains and weakness, headache, back pain, fever, chills, nausea or vomiting, facial paralysis, enlargement of the lymph glands or spleen, irregular heartbeat, seizures, blurry vision, moodiness, memory loss, dementia, and joint pains similar to arthritis.

three

Diagnosing Arthritis

Patients who are eventually diagnosed with arthritis usually first come into their health-care practitioner's office complaining of joint pain and stiffness. Both conventional and holistic practitioners will perform several types of assessments to determine if the patient has arthritis and, if so, which kind. Most patients will not need every test listed in this chapter. Osteoarthritis, for instance, is fairly easy to diagnose from its symptoms, and X-rays can help diagnose the bone changes in later stages of OA. However, a positive diagnosis of rheumatoid arthritis requires more extensive laboratory tests. Gout, infectious arthritis, and Lyme disease all have specific tests as well.

An in-depth patient history and complete physical will help the practitioner determine the possibility of a genetic propensity toward arthritis. Most doctors will draw a sample of blood for analysis by the tests described below. Synovial fluid (transparent fluid secreted by membranes in joint cavi-

---

IN THIS CHAPTER

- Standard Laboratory Tests
- Alternative Medicine Diagnostic Tests
- Electrodermal Screening
- Digestive Function
- Liver Function
- Immune Function
- Hormonal Balance
- Allergies
- Nutrient Deficiencies
- Parasites
- Lyme Disease
- Heavy Metal Toxicity

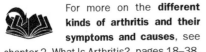
For more on the **different kinds of arthritis and their symptoms and causes**, see chapter 2, What Is Arthritis?, pages 18–38.

ties, bursas, and tendon sheaths) may also be drawn from joints for analysis. X-rays may be taken of the painful areas of the body. However, only in the more advanced stages of disease will bone changes be visible on X-rays, so they aren't a useful tool in early diagnosis. MRI (magnetic resonance imaging) can be more helpful in determining actual changes in cartilage, ligaments, tendons, and other soft tissues.

Standard Laboratory Tests

The different types of arthritis are often difficult to diagnose using only conventional tests. Patient symptoms and blood tests are most often used to attempt to confirm an arthritis diagnosis.

Osteoarthritis

OA is most often diagnosed by evaluating the patient's symptoms, which usually include pain in one or more joints combined with diminished joint mobility and grip strength. Diagnosis is confirmed by X-ray. The X-ray can reveal the degeneration of the cartilage that covers the end of the bone. However, the degree of pain a person experiences doesn't always correlate to the amount of bone changes seen on X-rays. A severely arthritic joint may cause no pain, while a mildly affected joint may be very stiff and painful.

Rheumatoid Arthritis

It's difficult to reach a conclusive diagnosis of RA when the disease is in its early stages. Usually the patient must have certain characteristic symptoms for at least six weeks to rule out the possibility of infectious arthritis. Tests on blood and synovial fluid may be performed to determine both the probability of RA and the extent of damage to joints and surrounding tissues that has already occurred at the time of diagnosis.

Blood tests can be used to assess inflammatory conditions and other indicators of RA. Here are some of the indicators most often tested for:

- Anemia: Anemia occurs when the number of red blood cells is lower than normal, causing diminished cellular oxygenation and slow toxin removal; 80% of RA patients are considered anemic. A soluble transferrin receptor and transferrin receptor–ferritin index test can help differentiate between iron deficiency anemia and anemia associated with chronic illness, such as RA.[1]

- Erythrocyte sedimentation rate (ESR): This test measures how quickly red blood cells settle to the bottom of a special tube. An elevated ESR indicates inflammation, and 90% of RA patients have elevated ESR.[2]

- Rheumatoid factor (RF): This antiglobulin antibody is usually present in 70% of cases of RA, but RF is not specific to this illness. An antiglobulin antibody is a specialized IgM immune protein that works against circulating immune complexes. An attack enhances the degree of joint inflammation, thus rendering joints more susceptible to damage by other immune cells.

- Elevated C-reactive protein: A nonspecific marker of inflammation, C-reactive protein is produced in the liver; it activates the immune system and increases white blood cell activity. It is often elevated in RA patients.

- Homocysteine: This amino acid is a normal by-product of protein metabolism; specifically, of the amino acid methionine, which is found in red meat and milk products. In the body, methionine undergoes a two-phase conversion, first being converted into homocysteine, then into cystationine, another amino acid. But in some individuals, the conversion stalls at the homocysteine phase and abnormally high levels of this amino acid begin to accumulate. Elevated homocysteine levels

Symptoms of Rheumatoid Arthritis

The diagnostic criteria for RA, as outlined by the American Rheumatism Association, requires that seven of the following symptoms be continuous for at least six weeks; failure to meet these criteria may mean that the disease is still in its early stages or that a different disease process may be in place:

1. Morning stiffness
2. Pain on motion or tenderness in at least one joint
3. Swelling (due to soft tissue thickening or fluid, not bony overgrowth alone) in at least one joint
4. Swelling of at least one other joint
5. Symmetric joint swelling (simultaneous involvement of the same joint on both sides of the body)
6. Nodules over a bony prominence; nodules are small rounded lumps of a mineral or mineral aggregate that typically appear on fingers, elbows, or knees
7. Changes revealed in X-rays typical of RA, including loss of bone calcium localized at the joints
8. Positive rheumatoid factor (confirmed by blood tests)
9. Synovial fluid with a high white blood cell count
10. Elevated sedimentation or C-reactive protein, a biological marker indicating inflammatory activity in the blood

are present in association with many diseases, including RA and heart disease.[3]

- Hyaluronic acid: Found in the skin and in ligaments of the joints, hyaluronic acid acts as a sponge, retaining water and moisture within these structures. Elevated levels of hyaluronic acid mean that the joint is retaining excess water. An elevated blood level of hyaluronic acid is actually more indicative than C-reactive protein or ESR for RA.[4]

- Antinuclear antibodies (ANAs): These antibodies, which attack the nucleus of a person's own cells, are often present in autoimmune diseases. Under a microscope, a blood sample will have a speckled pattern of ANAs if RA is present.[5]

- Genetic testing: Genetic testing screens for specific, physical patterns in a person's blood cells. The presence of the genetic markers HLA-DR4 and HLA-B27 indicates a predisposition for RA (HLA stands for *human leukocyte antigen*). The absence of protective genetic alleles (alternative forms of a gene) is also possible. Other markers include HLA-DMA*0103 and HLA-DMB*0104 alleles.[6]

- IL-2, IL-6, or IL-8: IL stands for *interleukin*, a type of compound that regulates the immune system. IL-2, IL-6, or IL-8 can be measured and indirectly indicate levels of tumor necrosis factor alpha (TNF-alpha). Elevated levels of TNF-alpha are often associated with autoimmune disease activity and chronic inflammation. Tests for interleukin levels can be used to monitor the progression of disease or the effects of immunomodulating medicines.

- IL-4: T-helper cells are subdivided into T-helper cells type 1 (Th1) and T-helper cells type 2 (Th2). IL-4 is a cytokine, a chemical that stimulates production of Th2, increasing inflammation. Arthritis sufferers tend to have high IL-4 and Th2. A health-care practitioner can measure the vigor of the Th2 response initially and also use IL-4 levels to monitor the effectiveness of therapies directed toward modulating or balancing the Th2 to Th1 ratio.

A physician can also use synovial fluid drawn from swollen joints to test for RA. If RA is present, the synovial fluid is usually thick and opaque, with a high white blood cell count and elevated rheumatoid factor. The fluid is cultured to determine whether bacteria or other microorganisms are present. The synovial fluid can also be examined microscopically for the presence of parasites and bacteria.

> From a holistic point of view, arthritis and other illnesses are an accumulation of problems that stem from layers of toxicity, malnutrition, and dysfunction.

Collagen is the fundamental component of the intracellular "glue," or connective tissue, that holds the cells of the body together. The amount of collagen that has been broken down and is present in the synovial fluids of patients with RA can help determine the progression of the disease. Elevated levels may indicate a breakdown in joint structure.[7]

Gout and Other Types of Arthritis

A diagnosis of gout is based on several factors. Blood levels of uric acid will be elevated (although many people who don't have gout have elevated blood levels of uric acid). Fluid taken from the affected joint is viewed under a microscope to determine whether uric acid crystals are present. A 24-hour urine collection is often performed when treating chronic gout to determine if the patient is producing too much uric acid or not excreting enough uric acid.

Conventional doctors sometimes use the drug colchicine diagnostically. Since this drug is specific for gout, relief of symptoms upon taking colchicine is considered a confirmation of the diagnosis of gout. However, colchicine can be quite toxic, causing nausea, cramps, vomiting, diarrhea, hair loss, fatigue, suppression of bone marrow production, anemia, leukopenia, bruising, numbness, and liver damage.

Streptozyme titer checks for the presence of antibodies to streptococcus bacteria (commonly referred to as strep), which may help diagnose infectious arthritis. Lyme titer checks for antibodies to *Borrelia burgdorferi*, the organism that causes Lyme disease. Unfortunately, this test has a low accuracy level, and many cases of Lyme disease remain undiagnosed and go untreated, which may lead to serious complications.

Alternative Medicine Diagnostic Tests

A holistic diagnostic approach to arthritis is less concerned with diagnosis and more interested in determining the underlying causes. We survey the body's organ systems to build a complete picture of the patient's illness. This helps us assess the phases of the body's dysfunction that precipitated the onset of arthritis. From a holistic point of view, arthritis and other illnesses are an accumulation of problems that stem from layers of toxicity, malnutrition, and dysfunction. This is why holistic doctors will investigate the functioning of a patient's digestive, immune, and detoxification systems. A psychosocial profile can help ascertain any mental and emotional stressors, which can contribute to the dysfunction of the endocrine glands and immune system, and the resultant illness. Personality and psychological profiles can reveal the negative or unresolved emotions that may perpetuate a cycle of illness. In some cases, a patient's joint pain may be the body's attempt to resolve mental suffering.

Of course, even in holistic medicine, serious bone and tissue deformities cannot be reversed. However, quality of life can be vastly improved, offering freedom from pain and increased mobility. Holistic physicians understand that pain and inflammation are due to a complex interplay of dynamic factors in the body and will use additional testing procedures to obtain a more individualized picture of the patient as well as the pathology.

Alternative Medicine Diagnostic Tests

- Electrodermal screening
- Digestive function tests
  —Comprehensive digestive stool analysis
  —Urine analysis
- Functional liver detoxification profile
- Immune system tests
  — Darkfield microscopic blood analysis
  — Herbal crystallization analysis
- Hormone tests
  —Adrenal stress index
  —RH (thyrotropin-releasing hormone) thyroid test
- Allergy tests
  —Applied kinesiology
  — EDS
  — IgG ELISA test
  —Blood typing
  —Skin testing
- Tests for nutrient deficiencies
  —Antioxidant profile
  —Functional intracellular analysis
  —Cell membrane lipid profile
  —Organic acid analysis
- Tests for parasites
- Tests for Lyme disease
- Tests for heavy metal toxicity
  —Hair trace mineral analysis
  —EDTA lead versenate 24-hour urine collection test

Electrodermal Screening

We use electrodermal screening (EDS) to determine where to start the protocol of intervention for an arthritis patient. Arthritis is a multifaceted illness, but we can't begin to change every aspect of the person's life at once—that would be too overwhelming. Instead, we use EDS testing to prioritize which system in the patient's body needs attention first.

By quickly pinpointing problems, EDS can indicate the degree of stress affecting an organ and prevent unnecessary guesswork testing. Specific

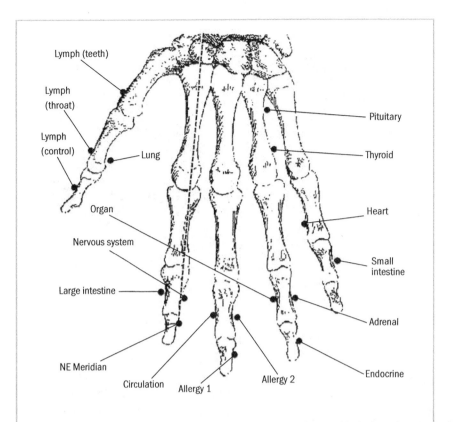

Lymph (teeth)

Lymph (throat)

Lymph (control)

Lung

Organ

Nervous system

Large intestine

NE Meridian

Circulation

Allergy 1

Allergy 2

Pituitary

Thyroid

Heart

Small intestine

Adrenal

Endocrine

Electrodermal screening probes specific points on the hands (see black dots above) to gather information about the health, function, or possible toxicity of organs and body systems. These points are associated with acupuncture meridians.

blood, urine, and stool analyses can then be ordered to confirm electrodermal results. For example, if EDS indicates that a person has a specific type of parasite, a stool analysis for that parasite eliminates trial-and-error testing for parasites. EDS can also help in selecting an individualized treatment protocol for each person based on their sensitivities to certain natural medicines or supplements.

In EDS, a blunt, noninvasive electric probe is placed at specific points on the patient's hands, face, or feet, corresponding to acupuncture points at the beginning or end of energy meridians. Minute electrical discharges from these points serve as information signals about the condition of the body's organs and systems. The key idea with EDS is that it is a data acquisition process in which a trained practitioner conducts an "interview" with the patient's organs and tissues, gathering informa-

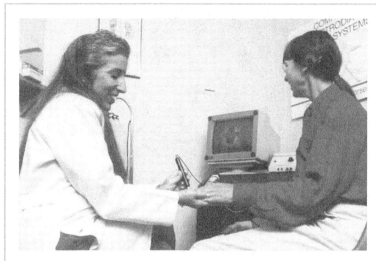

Ellen Kamhi performs electrodermal screening on a patient.

tion about the basic functional status of those systems and their energy pathways. As such, EDS is an investigational, not diagnostic, process because it requires the practitioner to be knowledgeable about acupuncture, physiology, and therapeutic substances in order to interpret the energy imbalances, establish their precise focus, and select the most appropriate therapeutic response. Nutrients are tested for each individual to develop an appropriate supplementation program.

 For more information on **digestive imbalances and arthritis**, see chapter 6, Eradicating Bacteria and Yeast, pages 115–133, and chapter 8, Alleviating Leaky Gut Syndrome, pages 149–165.

Digestive Function Tests

The health of the digestive system is of paramount importance in arthritis. Imbalances in the digestive system have far-reaching effects on the body and contribute to the development of many serious illnesses. The development of arthritic symptoms, such as joint pain and inflammation, can often be linked to chronic digestive inflammation.[8] Gastrointestinal problems such as irritable bowel syndrome, gas, bloating, diarrhea, or indigestion frequently lead to intestinal permeability, or leaky gut syndrome, in which the intestinal mucosa (lining) breaks down, allowing undigested food particles and other toxins into the bloodstream. Once in the bloodstream, toxins initiate a cascade effect that can ultimately weaken the immune system and put stress on the liver. Bacteria and parasites that escape through the permeable intestinal wall can gain access to vital organs and connective tissue. These pathogens play an important role in triggering the autoimmune response of RA. Synovial fluid taken from the joints of arthritis patients sometimes shows high levels of intestinal bacteria and parasites.[9] Malabsorption of nutrients also sets the stage for deficiencies of critical nutrients, like antioxidants, that quell joint inflammation and pain.

Since digestion has many phases (see "A Primer on Digestion," page 48), there are many abnormalities that can jeopardize the process. Stool and urine samples serve as a window into digestive inadequacies.

Comprehensive Digestive Stool Analysis. This broad spectrum analysis uses almost two dozen tests to review overall gastrointestinal health by investigating the patient's colonic environment, digestive abnormalities, and the integrity of the immune system.

Colonic environment: To give a better picture of the overall colonic environment, the stool analysis measures the following indicators of dysbiosis.

- Dysbiosis index: Intestinal dysbiosis refers to an imbalance of intestinal flora, including friendly bacteria, or probiotics (for example, *Lactobacillus acidophilus*), and harmful or unfriendly bacteria. At times, especially after the use of antibiotics, the balance of intestinal flora is skewed, allowing pathogenic bacteria to flourish. These harmful bacteria include *Pseudomonas aeruginosa*, *Proteus vulgaris*, and *Klebsiella pneumoniae*, which are particularly significant in arthritis. When the colonic environment favors unfriendly bacteria, the pathogenic bacteria begin to ferment, producing toxic by-products that interfere with intestinal pH, digestion and absorption, and the normal elimination cycle.

- Lactobacillus and bifidobacterium: These friendly bacteria are involved in vitamin synthesis, immune system support, and detoxification of procarcinogens (substances that become carcinogenic). Deficiencies of lactobacillus have been linked with a higher risk for many chronic diseases.

- *Candida:* The intestinal tract normally contains small amounts of *Candida albicans*, a yeastlike fungus, and other species of yeast. In some cases, wide use of antibiotics, birth control pills,

A Primer on Digestion

Digestion begins in the mouth—if you adequately chew your food—with digestive enzymes secreted by the salivary glands. From the mouth, food travels to the stomach, where more enzymes work to break down carbohydrates, fats, and proteins into their absorbable molecular components. In the stomach, food is also mixed with hydrochloric acid (HCl), which sterilizes the stomach so that bacteria can't grow. HCl also lowers the pH of the already somewhat digested food so that it is more acidic and ready to pass into the lower stomach for the next phase of digestion. Adequate HCl is required to activate pepsin, which digests protein in the lower stomach.

In the next stage of digestion, the partially digested food moves to the upper part of the small intestine, where bile and an alkalizing substance (bicarbonate) mediate the activity of digestive enzymes. Digestion continues in the next section of the intestine (jejunum) where sugar-digesting enzymes are secreted (if the jejunum is healthy). The majority of nutrients from digested food are absorbed into the blood from the small intestine. The large intestine's primary function is to absorb water (about 1 quart per day). This is also where intestinal microflora act upon soluble fiber, starch, and undigested carbohydrates to produce short-chain fatty acids, an energy source for colon cells. This undigested material is then stored until it can be excreted by the body through the anus.

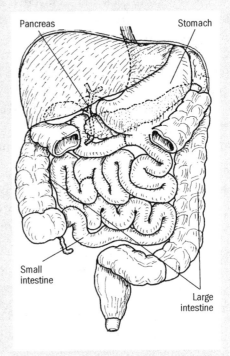

or a high-carbohydrate diet may cause an overgrowth of candida, a condition known as candidiasis. Overgrowth of *Candida albicans* and other intestinal yeasts has been linked to joint inflammation, food allergies, migraines, irritable bowel syndrome, indigestion, and asthma. The presence of candida is difficult to diagnose with standard medical tests.[10]

- Fecal pH: In this measure of the acid-alkaline balance in the colon, the preferred range is 6.0 (mildly acidic) to 7.2 (mildly alkaline). A fecal pH that is too alkaline suggests dysbiosis, as pathogenic bacteria thrive in an alkaline environment.

- Short-chain fatty acids (SCFAs): Elevated levels of any of the SCFAs may indicate poor nutrient absorption in the colon or bacterial overgrowth. Low levels suggest lack of dietary fiber, unbalanced metabolic processes, or dysbiosis. The key factor here is the ratio among SCFAs, which usually remains relatively constant in healthy individuals but can shift noticeably when metabolism becomes disordered.

- Beta-glucuronidase: Elevated levels of this enzyme produced by various bacteria in the colon may result from bacterial overgrowth and abnormal intestinal pH, too much dietary fat (especially from meat), or low levels of beneficial bacteria.

- Macroscopic aspects: Another indicator of intestinal health is the color of the stool. Yellow to green stools may indicate diarrhea and a bowel that has been sterilized by antibiotics. Black or red may reflect bleeding in the gastrointestinal tract. Tan or gray can indicate a blockage of the common bile duct. Mucus or pus can point to irritable bowel syndrome, polyps, diverticulitis, or intestinal wall inflammation. Occult (hidden) blood might result from eating too much red meat, hemorrhoids, or possibly colon cancer.

Digestive abnormalities: Maldigestion, or incomplete digestion, is a common problem for many Americans, especially people over 60. As people grow older (or due to an overgrowth of pathogenic bacteria), their production of HCl decreases, altering the stomach's pH and the release of digestive enzymes. Enzymes are necessary for digestion of carbohydrates, fats, and proteins, and without enzymes, these nutrients pass through the gastrointestinal tract undigested. Improper digestion affects the body's ability to absorb nutrients (resulting in malabsorption) and gives pathogenic bowel bacteria fodder, allowing them to multiply and crowd out the beneficial species. Different nutrients (fats, carbohydrates, and proteins) depend upon different digestive processes, and it's common for people to have malabsorption of one nutrient while adequately absorbing others. Stool analysis measures digestive abnormalities using the following markers to determine how well fats, carbohydrates, proteins, and other nutrients are being digested and absorbed.

- Triglycerides: Most dietary fats are triglycerides, a term that denotes their chemical structure. During digestion, lipase, a

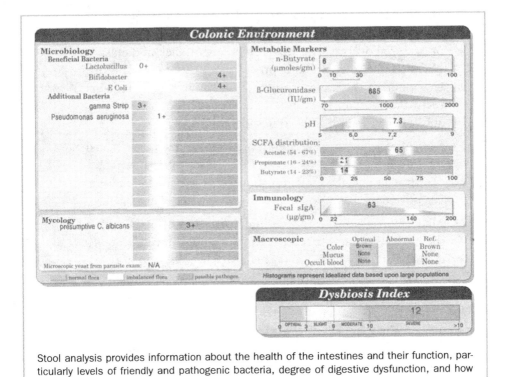

Colonic Environment

Microbiology

Beneficial Bacteria
- Lactobacillus 0+
- Bifidobacter 4+
- E Coli 4+

Additional Bacteria
- gamma Strep 3+
- Pseudomonas aeruginosa 1+

Mycology
- presumptive C. albicans 3+

Microscopic yeast from parasite exam: N/A

normal flora　imbalanced flora　possible pathogen

Metabolic Markers

n-Butyrate (μmoles/gm) 6 — 0 10 30 100

ß-Glucuronidase (IU/gm) 685 — 70 1000 2000

pH 7.3 — 5 6.0 7.2 9

SCFA distribution:
- Acetate (54 - 67%) 65 — 0 25 50 75 100
- Propionate (16 - 24%) 21
- Butyrate (14 - 23%) 14

Immunology

Fecal sIgA (μg/gm) 63 — 0 22 140 200

Macroscopic

	Optimal	Abnormal	Ref.
Color	Brown		Brown
Mucus	None		None
Occult blood	None		None

Histograms represent idealized data based upon large populations

Dysbiosis Index

12 — 0 OPTIMAL 3 SLIGHT 6 MODERATE 10 SEVERE >10

Stool analysis provides information about the health of the intestines and their function, particularly levels of friendly and pathogenic bacteria, degree of digestive dysfunction, and how well nutrients are being absorbed.

pancreatic enzyme, breaks down triglycerides into glycerol and free fatty acids. Elevated fecal triglyceride levels indicate incomplete fat digestion and possible problems in the pancreas.

- Chymotrypsin: Relative levels of this digestive enzyme, produced in the intestines, can indicate the patient's enzyme status and activity. Decreased levels mean the pancreas is not releasing enough enzymes and/or that the stomach is low on digestive acids, which are needed to activate chymotrypsin. Elevated levels suggest a rapid transit time (the speed at which fecal matter moves through the intestines). When material moves through the intestines too quickly, the body can't adequately absorb nutrients.

- Valerate and isobutyrate: These short-chain fatty acids are produced when intestinal bacteria ferment protein. Elevated levels indicate that the protein was not digested properly in the stomach and intestines. This can be due to many factors, including not enough time spent chewing, a diet too high in meat, a deficiency of hydrochloric acid, or a deficiency of pancreatic digestive enzymes.

- Meat and vegetable fibers: These are crude microscopic markers for digestive function. Elevated levels may indicate inadequate chewing, stomach acid, or digestive enzymes.

- Long-chain fatty acids (LCFAs): Under healthy conditions, LCFAs are absorbed directly by intestinal mucosa. Elevated levels reflect malabsorption of fats, a result of maldigestion or inflammation of the lining of the small intestine.

- Cholesterol: Cholesterol in the feces comes from either dietary fats or the breakdown of the cells lining the intestines. Generally, fecal cholesterol remains stable, regardless of dietary intake. Elevated levels of fecal cholesterol suggest malabsorption or irritation of the mucosal lining.

- Total fecal fat: Representing the sum of all fats, a high reading can indicate either maldigestion or malabsorption.

Integrity of the immune system: The largest part of the immune system is located just outside of the intestinal wall. Known as the secretory IgA, these antibodies act as sentries against escaping food particles or other inappropriate substances. A stool analysis can determine the level at which the secretory IgA is functioning. Low levels of fecal IgA indicate increased susceptibility to infection and food allergies, while high levels indicate normal activity or an active infectious process.

Urine Analysis. Many alternative health-care professionals rely on urine analysis (urinalysis) to assess a patient's digestive function and enzyme status. The urinalysis provides information on what a person cannot digest, absorb, or assimilate, along with any nutritional deficiencies the person might have. A urinalysis can also reveal kidney function, levels of bowel toxicity and pH, and how the body is handling proteins, fats, carbohydrates, vitamin C, and other essential nutrients. This test is prognostic rather than diagnostic, except for the identification of substances not normally found in the urine, such as glucose, which would indicate disease conditions (this is the focus of standard urine tests). In other words, it predicts what lies ahead if you don't clean up your diet and improve your digestion.

An individual's total urine output over a 24-hour period must be collected, not just periodic samples. This enables a physician to see how concentrations of various substances in a person's urine change over time. The fluctuations are then averaged to give a complete picture of digestive problems. Looking at a 24-hour urinalysis is a way of peeking at the blood. The health of the blood takes precedence in the body, and cells will sacrifice nutrients in the service of maintaining the blood's relatively narrow pH range of 7.35 to 7.45, as well as its supply of electrolytes, protein, and other nutrients. Thus, the blood takes what it needs from the cells to achieve its necessary balance, or homeostasis.

The following specific values are measured in urine analysis.

- Volume: Total urine output, either excessive (polyuria) or minimal (oliguria), in relation to the specific gravity (see below) indicates how well the kidneys are functioning.

- Indican (Obermeyer test): Indican, which comes from putrefying proteins in the large intestine, is extremely toxic and may cause inflammation, among other symptoms. Indican levels in the urine indicate the degree of putrefaction, gas, and fermentation in the intestines. The higher the level, the greater the toxicity or inflammation in the digestive tract.

- Calcium phosphate: In this measure of the status of carbohydrate digestion, a reading of 0.5 is normal.

- pH: This value indicates how acidic or alkaline the urine is on a scale of 0 to 14.0, with urine pH usually ranging from 4.8 to 8.0 and with 7.0 being neutral.

- Chloride: These are salt residues in the urine, and the values here give information on salt intake and assimilation. Too much or too little natural salt intake can influence inflammation in arthritis.

- Specific (SP) gravity: In this measure of the weight of total dissolved substances in the urine against an equal amount of water, a normal reading of 1.020 means that the urine is 20% heavier than water. Specific gravity shows the general water content (hydration) of the body. Values typically range from 1.005 to 1.030; a high reading indicates high concentrations of dissolved substances and possible kidney stress. Low levels may indicate that the body is retaining too much fluid.

- Total sediment analysis: This indicates the amount of dissolved organic and mineral substances remaining in the urine after digestion. The three sediment categories are calcium phosphate,

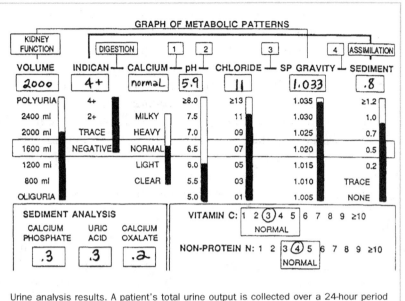

Urine analysis results. A patient's total urine output is collected over a 24-hour period and analyzed in a laboratory for the status of key biochemical factors.

uric acid, and calcium oxalate, and an optimal total reading for the three sediment categories is 0.5. High sediment readings may indicate the accumulation of sediment crystals in body fluids. These crystals are ultimately deposited in joint tissues, leading to pain and inflammation. Calcium phosphate indicates the status of carbohydrate digestion. Uric acid is a by-product of the breakdown of purines (a kind of protein), mostly excreted by the kidneys; a high reading of uric acid may indicate gout. Calcium oxalate indicates the status of fat digestion; a reading of 0 signifies optimum fat digestion.

- Vitamin C: Levels of vitamin C indicate body reserves of this key nutrient; a reading of 1.0 is high, 2.0 to 5.0 is normal, and 6.0 to 10.0 is deficient.

Functional Liver Detoxification Profile

The liver is the body's main filter of blood and lymphatic fluid; it neutralizes and eliminates cholesterol, metabolic wastes, and antigens (foreign substances that provoke an immune response). But abnormalities in the digestive system (such as intestinal permeability) or exposure to toxic chemicals can overburden the liver and its detoxification functions.

This can lead to an increase in production of free radicals and accumulation of toxins in the bloodstream, organ tissues, and connective tissues. Undischarged toxins can contribute to autoimmune reactions associated with RA.

This test can identify abnormal liver function earlier than standard liver tests, which measure only levels of enzymes. Early detection of liver dysfunction can prevent irreversible damage to the liver. The liver detoxification profile tests the liver's ability to detoxify various substances. The patient swallows tablets of aspirin, acetaminophen (Tylenol), and caffeine, all common substances detoxified by the liver. Then urine and saliva samples are collected at specific time intervals and sent to a laboratory for analysis. In addition to revealing the liver's ability to detoxify the body, the test also indicates where specific irregularities are occurring in the detoxification system. In addition, blood can be drawn and examined for the presence of free radical metabolites and antioxidants, especially glutathione, a key component in liver detoxification. This can help guide the practitioner on the correct course of action for the individual patient.

Immune System Tests

Alternative health-care practitioners use two tests to assess overall immune system function: darkfield microscopic blood analysis and herbal crystallization analysis.

Darkfield Microscopic Blood Analysis. Darkfield microscopic blood analysis, or darkfield microscopy, is a way of studying living whole blood cells under a specially adapted microscope that projects the dynamic image, magnified 1,400 times, onto a video screen. For arthritis patients, darkfield testing can be particularly useful for viewing the distortions of red blood cells, which can indicate fatty acid deficiencies. This technique also reveals crystalline substances that can lead to joint pain and inflammation. Immune function can be analyzed by looking at the size, shape, and motility of the white blood cells. Allergic status can be ascertained by the activity of the basophils (white blood cells that release histamines). Darkfield analysis is a particularly useful tool because it helps patients visualize what's happening in their blood during the disease process; it also gives them immediate feedback on their efforts to improve their health.

Herbal Crystallization Analysis. Austrian philosopher and scientist Rudolf Steiner, Ph.D., noticed that by looking at crystallized saliva samples, he

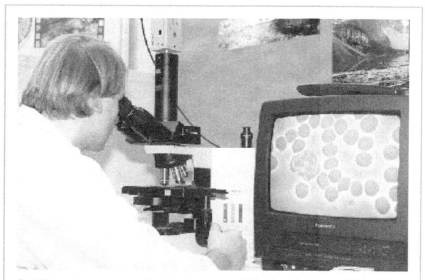

Darkfield microscopy reveals distortions of red blood cells (which indicate nutritional status), possible undesirable bacterial or fungal life-forms, and blood ecology patterns indicative of health or illness.

could recognize specific states of illness and disease and also determine which herbal and homeopathic treatments would be most useful for a given patient. The herbal crystallization analysis test is a simple saliva test wherein a sample is analyzed under a microscope and compared with known herbal patterns. It reveals exactly which herbs the body may require and in what amounts. The result is a personalized combination of herbs to help enhance the vitality and well-being of the individual. Botanist George Benner, inspired by Steiner's work, delineated over 800 species-specific herbal crystal patterns in the 1980s. He was surprised to find that the crystalline pattern in a person's saliva was a clue to the herbs they need. His first discovery involved a colleague whose saliva crystallized in the pattern of juniper berries, an herb known to tonify the kidneys. Upon questioning him, Benner learned that the man had been taking diuretics for weak kidneys.

The saliva sample is taken in a practitioner's office and the dried saliva sample (on a slide) is mailed to a laboratory for analysis. The results are returned to the practitioner within two weeks. Several patterns usually appear on the slide, and all are evaluated for levels of importance or need. After receiving the results of an herbal crystallization analysis, we prepare an herbal formula mixed in the exact proportions indicated by the test. Our patients usually respond excellently to these individualized herbal mixtures.

Hormone Tests

Hormone imbalances are commonly associated with arthritis. The stress hormones DHEA, cortisol (SEE QUICK DEFINITION, page 57), and adrenaline are frequently implicated in symptoms of fatigue and muscle and joint pain. These and other hormones are secreted by the adrenal glands (located above the kidneys), which play a central role in maintaining the body's energy levels. Abnormal rhythms in the adrenals' cyclical release of hormones are known to compromise tissue healing. Reduced tissue repair and increased tissue breakdown leads to muscle and joint injury, chronic pain, and arthritis. In hypothyroidism, an underactive thyroid causes the adrenal glands to work overtime to compensate for the malfunctioning of the thyroid gland. (For more on hypothyroidism, see "The Thyroid," page 58).

Adrenal Stress Index. Simple and noninvasive, the adrenal stress index (ASI) can pinpoint whether an imbalance in the production of hormones by the adrenals may be contributing to arthritis. The adrenal glands don't secrete hormones at a constant level throughout the day; instead, hormones are released in a cyclical pattern, with the highest volume in the morning and the lowest at night, following a 24-hour cycle (circadian rhythm). For the ASI, four saliva samples are taken at intervals throughout the day to plot the adrenal rhythm and determine if the main adrenal hormones (DHEA, cortisol, and adrenaline) are being secreted in proper amounts and ratios and at the appropriate times.

TRH (Thyrotrophin-Releasing Hormone) Thyroid Test. Conventional testing often misses malfunction of the thyroid gland because the tests aren't sensitive enough to identify subclinical hypothyroidism, but the TRH test is often able to detect even slightly lowered hormone levels. The TRH test measures abnormal function levels, while standard blood tests only measure extreme pathology. Although this test is slightly cumbersome and time-consuming, it's important for correctly evaluating thyroid function. This test can also be used to monitor the effectiveness of thyroid hormone supplementation.

First, through a simple blood test, the health-care practitioner measures the patient's level of thyroid-stimulating hormone (TSH), an indicator of thyroid functioning. The practitioner then gives the patient an injection of TRH (a completely harmless synthetic hormone), which stimulates the pituitary gland to produce TSH. After 25 minutes, blood is drawn again to remeasure TSH levels. The results can determine if the thyroid gland is functioning properly. In arthritis and other degenerative diseases, the thyroid is usually underactive, even if conventional testing doesn't indicate that this is the case.

A simple at-home temperature test can also be used to determine thyroid function. A basal thermometer (available in most drugstores), several small disposable cups, and graph paper are the only materials needed. In the morning, catch some urine in a cup, place the thermometer in the urine, and record the temperature on the graph paper; repeat the test every day for one month. At the end of the month, calculate your average daily temperature. An average temperature of less than 97.8°F usually indicates an underactive thyroid, although it can indicate low adrenal function as well.

Allergy Tests

Unhealthy eating habits and food sensitivities (allergies) are primary factors in joint pain.[11] The gold standard of food and allergy testing is accomplished by fasting and then challenging the body by reintroducing one new food at a time. The patient completely eliminates the suspected food allergen, such as wheat, for two weeks. They then eat the substance on the challenge day and record any reactions over the next two to three days. Although quite accurate and inexpensive, this method may be impractical due to time considerations, as each suspected food must

Cortisol is a hormone secreted by the adrenal glands, which are located atop the kidneys. Cortisol secretion (as well as secretion of the adrenal gland's other hormones, DHEA, adrenaline, and aldosterone) occurs in daily cycles, peaking in the morning and having the lowest values at night. Cortisol promotes protein-building, regulates insulin and glycogen synthesis, and helps produce prostaglandins. Under conditions of stress, high amounts of cortisol are released; chronic excess secretion is associated with obesity and suppressed thyroid function. Imbalances in cortisol secretion are linked with low energy, muscle dysfunction, impaired bone repair, thyroid dysfunction, immune system depression, sleep disorders, poor skin regeneration, and decreased growth hormone uptake.

DHEA (dehydroepiandrosterone) is naturally produced by the human adrenal glands and gonads, with optimal levels occurring around age 20 for women and age 25 for men. After those ages, DHEA levels gradually decline, so a person 80 years old produces only a fraction of the DHEA they did when they were 20. Functioning as an antioxidant, hormone regulator, and the building block from which estrogen and testosterone are produced, DHEA is vital to health. Low DHEA levels have been associated with cancer, diabetes, multiple sclerosis, hypertension, obesity, AIDS, heart disease, Alzheimer's, and immune dysfunction illnesses. No serious side effects have been reported to date, although acne, oily skin, facial hair growth on women, deepening of the voice, irritability, insomnia, and fatigue have been reported with high doses of DHEA. It is recommended that DHEA levels are tested and evaluated by a health-care practitioner before taking a DHEA supplement.

The Thyroid

The thyroid gland, the largest of the body's seven endocrine glands, is located just below the larynx in the throat. The thyroid is the body's metabolic thermostat, controlling body temperature, energy use, and, for children, the body's growth rate. It affects the function of all body processes and organs.

Hypothyroidism is a condition of low or underactive thyroid gland function that can produce numerous symptoms. Among the 47 clinically recognized symptoms are fatigue, depression, lethargy, weakness, weight gain, low body temperature, chills, cold extremities, general oversensitivity to cold, infertility, rheumatic pain, menstrual disorders (excessive flow, cramps), repeated infections, colds, upper respiratory infections, skin problems (eczema; psoria-

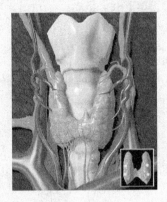

sis; acne; skin pallor; and dry, coarse, scaly skin), memory disturbances, difficulty concentrating, paranoia, migraines, muscle aches and weakness, anemia, constipation, brittle nails, and poor vision.

be challenged separately. Other effective and more convenient tests for identifying allergens include applied kinesiology, electrodermal screening, the IgG ELISA test, blood typing, and skin tests. Although most of these tests aren't recognized by mainstream medicine, many holistic practitioners and their patients find that they can help provide an individualized protocol that promotes healing.

Applied Kinesiology. Alternative health-care providers sometimes use the basic techniques of applied kinesiology (SEE QUICK DEFINITION) to test for food allergies. To isolate the allergy-inducing substances, we ask our patients to come into the office with small samples of food items that are regularly part of their diet. While holding one food sample in their hand and pressing it against the parotid gland in their cheek, pressure is applied to a specific muscle. If the muscle can resist the pressure, it indicates that the sample does not cause a sensitivity reaction, but if the muscle cannot withstand the

 Applied kinesiology, developed by Detroit chiropractor George Goodheart, is the study of the relationship between muscle dysfunction (weakness) and related organ or gland dysfunction. Applied kinesiology uses a simple strength resistance test on a specific indicator muscle related to the organ or part of the body being tested. For example, the deltoid muscle in the shoulder has a relationship to the lungs and therefore is a good indicator of any problems there.

applied pressure, the tested substance is suspected of causing a sensitivity in that individual. We continue this process until the most common foods in the patient's diet have been tested. This technique is so easy and noninvasive that we teach it to our patients, so they can test themselves at home. Although the results aren't always precise, it gives patients a feeling of control over their food allergies. Also, patients often report that by avoiding the foods found to be suspicious, they experience a sometimes dramatic decrease in joint pain.

Electrodermal Screening. Electrodermal screening (EDS) can be a useful tool to help track down potential allergens, including foods and environmental substances.

IgG ELISA Test. Conventional allergy tests usually measure the presence of one particular antibody—immunoglobulin E (IgE; SEE QUICK DEFINITION). IgE allergies cause immediate reactions that patients can usually recognize soon after eating the offending food. However, some allergies are more difficult to identify because they result in delayed reactions occurring 48 to 72 hours after ingestion of the offending food. Delayed food allergies involve another type of antibody—IgG. The IgG ELISA test analyzes a blood sample for the presence of IgG antibodies. (ELISA stands for enzyme-linked immunosorbent assay.) When patients have a high IgG response to a certain food substance, their immune system becomes activated when that substance is present. Antibodies are released and attach to the allergen, forming a CIC (circulating immune complex). This can lead to inflammation and pain, especially in people with a compromised immune system, such as those who suffer from autoimmune illnesses like RA or irritable bowel syndrome. Studies have shown that patients who avoid those foods to which they have a high IgG response experience relief from both physical and psychological symptoms.[12]

 Immunoglobulins fall into five classes of specially designed antibodies produced in the spleen, bone marrow, or lymph tissue and are involved in the immune system's defense response to foreign substances. The main types of immunoglobulins, grouped according to their concentration in the blood, are IgG (80%), IgA (10%-15%), IgM (5%-10%), IgD (less than 0.1%), and IgE (less than 0.001%).

Blood Typing. A simple blood test, also referred to as a lectin serotype test, determines a patient's blood type (A, B, AB, or O). Peter D'Adamo, N.D., developed a theory that each blood type tends to be more or less compatible with specific foods. After determining a patient's blood type, which correlates with specific dietary lectins, a patient can choose to avoid those foods that may aggravate their symptoms. Many people report great improvement when they follow these dietary suggestions, and there are no adverse effects to giving it a try.

Skin Testing. There are two types of skin tests used to determine allergies to molds, dusts, pollen, and other environmental factors. Serial end-point titration (SET), also called the Lee-Miller neutralization test, is far more accurate than the commonly used scratch test. During a SET test, a diluted form of a potential allergen is injected just under the skin. The body immediately reacts to the introduction of this foreign substance by forming a wheal about 4 mm in diameter. After 10 minutes, another measurement is taken. The wheal will grow according to the severity of the immune reaction. A 5 mm diameter wheal indicates no allergic reaction, while a 7 mm wheal (or larger) indicates an allergic response. If the test shows a positive result, the process is repeated with increasingly diluted forms of the same allergen to evaluate the degree of sensitivity. After the offending foods or environmental allergens are determined, a formula is created specifically for the patient. Each allergic substance is combined in a vial in the exact concentration needed to help neutralize the allergic effect. The patient still needs to avoid those foods to which they are highly allergic, but injections of the formula help rebuild the immune system and lessen the overall allergic response.

Tests for Nutrient Deficiencies

Deficiencies and imbalances of various vitamins and other nutrients are well documented in arthritis patients.[13] Specifically, arthritis patients tend to be deficient in vitamins A and E, beta-carotene, and essential fatty acids. Deficiencies can be due to poor diet, stress, impaired digestion, environmental toxins, or a combination of these factors.

Antioxidant Profile. Practitioners can order an evaluation of key antioxidants, such as vitamins A and E, carotenoids, coenzyme Q_{10}, iron, and water-soluble antioxidants (vitamin C, uric acid, bilirubin), to determine if the patient is getting the right antioxidants in the correct amounts.

Functional Intracellular Analysis. Functional intracellular analysis (FIA) is a group of tests that measure the cellular function of key vitamins, minerals, antioxidants, amino acids, fatty acids, and metabolites (choline, inositol). Rather than simply measuring the levels of micronutrients in the blood (which may or may not provide useful information about actual cell metabolism), FIA measures how these micronutrients are actually functioning within the activities of living white blood cells. More specifically, FIA assesses the amount of cell growth for metabolically active lymphocytes, a type of white blood cell, as a way of identifying micronutrient deficiencies

 For more information on **nutrients for arthritis relief**, see chapter 13, Supplements for Arthritis, pages 257–294.

known to interfere with growth or immune function in the cell. These tests also assess the status of carbohydrate metabolism in terms of insulin function and fructose intolerance.

Cell Membrane Lipid Profile. The correct formation of cell membranes is dependent upon essential fatty acids, and the cell membrane lipid profile, a blood test, takes advantage of this, screening for adequate levels of essential fatty acids by analyzing red blood cell membranes. The test measures levels of omega-3 and omega-6 fatty acids that inhibit inflammation as well as toxic proinflammatory fatty acids. Fatty acid content in the body is extremely important in arthritis and other inflammatory processes. Dietary supplementation to correct fatty acid imbalances can be accurately monitored through this profile, as well.

Organic Acid Analysis. The levels at which organic acids appear in the blood or urine helps the practitioner determine if the energy "engine," called the Krebs cycle, is functioning properly. Since certain organic acids are required in specific amounts to regulate the rate and activity of the many chemical reactions carried out within the Krebs cycle, low or high levels of a particular organic acid suggest a deficiency in a specific amino acid, vitamin, or mineral needed for its corresponding biochemical reaction. This information can be useful in developing therapeutic programs for nutritional support and in avoiding problem foods.

Tests for Parasites

The presence of parasites in the human body is a little-appreciated but major health problem, and is closely monitored by the Centers for Disease Control.[14] Many U.S. residents assume they're vulnerable to parasites only when traveling in tropical countries, but the United States has an undiagnosed parasite epidemic.

Parasites tend to reside in the intestines, but in various stages of their life cycle they can migrate to the blood, lymph, heart, liver, and other vital organs. Parasites are a very common problem in people with arthritis.

Infestations by some types of parasites cause symptoms strikingly similar to arthritis, such as inflammation and pain in joints and destruction of cartilage. Parasites can destroy cells faster than they can be regenerated, and over time they can exhaust the immune system.

If you suspect you have an intestinal parasite (symptoms include bloating, skin itching and rashes, and digestive issues), make sure the testing facility follows the guidelines set by the U.S. Centers for Disease Control in the *Manual of Clinical Microbiology*.[15] A simple stool test is not sufficient to determine the presence of parasites. It should be used along with a more specific test, such as immunofluorescent staining. This technique uses parasite-specific antibodies tagged with fluorescent dyes that make them highly visible under the microscope. As they attack specific parasites, the antibodies will show up only where there is a parasite presence. Darkfield microscopy can also be used to analyze a blood sample for long tubules. The presence of such tubules typically correlates with an infestation of parasites, although it doesn't determine the extent of infestation or the exact species of parasite that may be present.

Tests for Lyme Disease

Lyme disease, caused by the *Borrelia burgdorferi* spirochete, is very challenging to diagnose. Several tests are used, but none of them are definitive. Many people who suffer from arthritis and other symptoms are infected with this organism but never get a positive result from tests for Lyme disease. Practitioners are encouraged to take a full history and not to rule out Lyme disease due to lack of laboratory evidence.

Most tests for Lyme disease use either direct detection of the organism or measurement of antibodies, the latter indicating the body's response to infestation. Direct detection employs culturing, staining, and antigen tests. These are the most common tests currently in use:

- Indirect fluorescent antibody (IFA): Fluorescent dye is added to a slide containing a blood sample and a dead *B. burgdorferi* specimen. The slide is then viewed under a fluorescent or ultraviolet light. If a green color appears, the test is considered positive. Although considered to be very inaccurate, it's still used by conventional medical practitioners.

- Enzyme-linked immunosorbent assay (ELISA): This test uses enzymes to detect *B. burgdorferi* antibodies.

- Western blot test: In this test, a strand of *B. burgdorferi* DNA is fragmented using a detergent. The resulting mixture is applied to a strip of gelatinous material, which is zapped by an electrical charge. This causes the *B. burgdorferi* specimen to further fragment and separate according to weight. The various *B. burgdorferi* antigens are then exposed to the patient's serum, and any antibodies present in the serum bind with the antigens, constituting a positive result.

- Lyme dot blot assay (LDA): This test detects Lyme antigens shed in the urine. The patient first must follow a vigorous antiparasite protocol for one week to draw out the spirochetes, then collect their urine for several days. A positive result indicates that the Lyme antigen was found in the urine sample and is considered "presumptive positive" until confirmed by another method.

- Rapid identification of *B. burgdorferi* (RIBb): A highly purified fluorescent antibody stain specific for *B. burgdorferi* is used to detect the organism in a blood sample. Although this test appears to be much more accurate than other tests, it currently isn't recognized by the FDA.

- Other tests include the borreliacidal antibody test (BAT), immune complex test, PreVue test, and C6 peptide test.

Tests for Heavy Metal Toxicity

Chronic low-level exposure to a variety of toxic heavy metals (such as aluminum, lead, copper, and mercury) poses serious health dangers to the body. These toxins are commonly found in our food, water, and air, as well as in auto exhaust, tobacco smoke, mercury fillings, and many of the building materials and fabrics in our work and living environments. Exposure to toxic materials and accumulation of them in the body can wreak havoc on a person's immune system function and their level of wellness. Other toxic substances such as benzene, PCBs (polychlorinated biphenyls), PBBs (polybrominated biphenyls), and organic pesticide residues, among others, are highly implicated as a possible cause of arthritis.[16]

High levels of copper, mercury, cadmium, and aluminum are found in many arthritis patients. Excess copper along with iron depletes vitamin C (which is needed to build connective tissue) and zinc (an antioxidant important for protein and cartilage synthesis). Copper also creates free radicals that attack and erode joint cartilage.[17] Physical and emotional stress, as well as adrenal exhaustion and thyroid imbalances, have been linked to toxic levels of copper.[18]

Imbalances in important minerals (such as boron, selenium, manganese, molybdenum, zinc, and calcium) can result from heavy metal toxicity. Often the ratio of one mineral to another is even more important than the levels of the individual minerals. For example, sodium and potassium must remain in strict balance in the body to ensure proper functioning of the adrenal glands. When sodium levels are higher than potassium, the body becomes more inclined toward inflammation. Other problems occur when potassium is at a higher level than sodium. This imbalance typically indicates a degenerative condition accompanied by adrenal exhaustion due to high levels of cortisol (an adrenal stress hormone). In the first stages of arthritis, many patients exhibit high sodium to potassium ratios. But as the disease progresses, and especially after prolonged use of conventional cortisone treatments, they will exhibit low sodium to potassium ratios.

Calcium may be displaced by heavy metals (such as aluminum and copper) and begin accumulating in muscles, tendons, and ligaments rather than in bones. This leads to hardening of affected areas in the muscles and joints, which can alter the way the joint moves, leading to arthritis. Calcium can also be lost due to deficiencies of magnesium, manganese, and boron. Accumulation of calcium in the muscles due to displacement can be one of the causative factors in fibromayalgia and other painful conditions.

Testing for heavy metal toxicity can identify which metals are present and in what amounts. On the basis of this information, a practitioner can develop an individualized detoxification and nutritional prescription program to eliminate the toxic metals from the patient's system and to restore depleted essential nutrients.

Hair Trace Mineral Analysis. Hair trace mineral analysis measures the levels of critical minerals and toxic metals in the body's tissues. The U.S. Environmental Protection Agency states that hair analysis is an accurate, inexpensive screening tool for heavy metal toxicity, and this technique is often used to assess levels of heavy metals.[19] Although hair is technically dead, the minerals present in the hair cell during its formation are locked within the hair. Both minerals and toxic metals exist in higher concentrations in the hair than in the blood, making them easier to measure through analysis of hair than blood.

Hair analysis provides an average reading covering a several-month period; it gives a larger picture of the body's metabolic changes over time. A 1-gram sample of hair is cut and sent to the laboratory by the health-care practitioner. (The hair can't be dyed, permed, bleached, or treated; pubic hair can be substituted.) The laboratory burns the hair, then views and quantifies the elements present by means of atomic spectroscopy. The results are then returned to the practitioner for interpretation.

EDTA Lead Versenate 24-Hour Urine Collection Test. In the EDTA lead versenate test, which must be administered by a physician, EDTA (ethylenediaminetetraacetic acid), a chemical that chelates or binds with heavy metals, is administered intravenously. EDTA pulls heavy metals out of the patient's system. The patient's urine is then collected over a 24-hour period and analyzed by a laboratory for proportions of heavy metals present in the urine.

DMSA (Dimercapto Succinic Acid) is another agent utilized for provocation of heavy metals; it is administered orally based on a patient's weight, followed by collection and analysis of the patient's urine.

four

General Detoxification

Arthritis isn't usually caused by a lone factor. More often it results from a gradual degeneration of internal organs and tissues brought about by a variety of stressors and imbalances, including environmental pollutants and dietary factors. Toxic chemicals that accumulate in the body contribute significantly to this problem, impairing the function of organs and related systems that are involved in neutralizing harmful substances (intestines, liver, kidneys, skin, connective tissue, and the lymphatic and respiratory systems). When these organs are overloaded and working improperly, the toxins they normally process are not fully eliminated from the body, leaving a toxic residue. This "undischarged" toxicity can cause damage directly related to arthritis, such as joint degeneration and inflammation. It may, in fact, be one of the prime contributors to arthritis.

Detoxification protocols are designed to flush out toxins circulating in the bloodstream, embedded in soft tissues, and clogging important organs. These therapies can target the body in general or specific organs (the latter is covered in the next chapter). The most effective general detoxification program includes physician-supervised fasts. We have seen patients make remarkable progress in reversing all types of arthritis following an individualized fasting program. Fasting and similar therapies cleanse the body of detrimental substances, heal the gastro-intestinal tract, alleviate allergies, and help quell excessive inflammation.

Therapies for General Detoxification

- Arthritis diet
- Fasting
- Juicing
- "Green" foods

Success Story: Detoxifying Relieves Painful Hips

Maggie, 48, complained of pain in both hips. She was diagnosed with OA by her orthopedic physician and was advised to stop exercising and start taking anti-inflammatory medications. Her doctor also said there was no other treatment for OA and that Maggie could expect her condition to progressively grow worse. Maggie, not willing to accept this, came to us looking for another option.

In our initial exam we found that, in addition to OA, Maggie had chemical sensitivities, seasonal allergies, and occasional symptoms of PMS (premenstrual syndrome). Examination of her blood using a darkfield microscope revealed a high level of spicules, small particles that can indicate liver dysfunction, and elevated levels of red and yellow crystals, metabolic by-products that correlate with joint pain. Her white blood cells were overactive, something often seen in autoimmune conditions (wherein the immune system attacks the body's own tissues). We also saw increased numbers of basophils, an immune cell associated with allergic reactions, and eosinophils, white blood cells that may indicate a parasite infestation. In addition, she had an elevated level of candida yeast.

A blood test, which showed elevated levels of anticandida antibodies, confirmed the yeast infection. Maggie's blood test also revealed several other factors that were contributing to her arthritis. We found low magnesium and high protein levels, as well as a slightly elevated cholesterol count of 220 (normal is 135-200) and triglycerides. These results indicated that Maggie's diet needed to be improved dramatically. An organic, mostly vegetarian diet high in omega-3 fatty acids could decrease her cholesterol and triglycerides and give her higher levels of minerals, such as magnesium, needed to help reverse her arthritis.

> Arthritis isn't usually caused by a lone factor. More often it results from a gradual degeneration of internal organs and tissues brought about by a variety of stressors and imbalances, including environmental pollutants and dietary factors.

Elevated levels of Epstein-Barr antibodies were also detected, indicating a past infection with this virus.

A 24-hour urinalysis revealed that Maggie's creatinine clearance was low at 41 (normal range is 80–110). The creatinine clearance test shows the patient's level of kidney function, and this result clearly indicated that Maggie's kidneys were underfunctioning. The urinalysis also showed some heavy metal toxicity, with high levels of aluminum and copper. A food allergy test (IgG ELISA) revealed a multitude of food sensitivities. Maggie was allergic to barley, buckwheat, rice, cabbage, carrots, cauliflower, celery, cucumber, lettuce, onion, squash, string beans, tomatoes, cantaloupe, grapefruit, oranges, peaches, pineapple, plums, kidney beans, lentils, peanuts (high sensitivity), black pepper, chocolate, coffee, and licorice.

 For more information on the **24-hour urinalysis** and the **IgG ELISA food allergy tests**, see chapter 3, Diagnosing Arthritis, pages 39–65.

Odd as it may sound, Maggie was actually delighted that we had run so many tests while investigating the source of her hip pain, particularly since her conventional physician had simply X-rayed her hips and put her on medications. All of these tests told us something that a simple X-ray could not—that Maggie's joint degeneration had multiple causes we needed to address.

Our initial treatment was designed to detoxify Maggie's colon and large intestine. We started her on a cleansing product that combines apple pectin, flaxseed powder, and psyllium (all fiber sources for intestinal cleansing), along with herbal cleansers such as red clover, dandelion, yellow dock, burdock root, fenugreek seed, ginger, and cascara sagrada. We also started her on supplements of the "good" fats, especially omega-3 fatty acids, including flaxseed oil and powder, and vegetable and fish oils.

Maggie also began a rotational diet to alleviate her food allergies; this involved total avoidance of her most highly allergenic foods and eating lower-level allergenic foods only once every four days. For extra support, she took a multivitamin-multimineral formula along with extra vitamin E (400 IU) and an acidophilus (beneficial intestinal bacteria) supplement to help address her yeast infection. To help revitalize her liver, we suggested a garlic and glutathione formula. For her hip degeneration she was given a combination of microcrystalline hydroxyapatite, calcium, magnesium, boron, and vitamin D, along with glucosamine sulfate.

After two weeks on this dietary and supplement program, Maggie reported that her joint pain had improved to some degree. We advised her to begin an exercise program, being careful to avoid any exercises that put direct stress on her hip joints. She began a yoga stretching and breathing program, along with swimming at her local pool once a week. She also started getting weekly physical therapy in the form of chiropractic adjustments and massage. After two more weeks, she reported that her hip pain had definitely lessened.

A stool analysis had revealed that Maggie had a parasite infection, including cysts of *Giardia lamblia*. The test had also indicated that her liver's ability to detoxify her body was compromised. We were already addressing her liver function with glutathione supplements, and we decided to postpone parasite treatments because it would have been too stressful to her body at the time.

To further alleviate her allergies, we started her on a special desensitization program. We prepared a vial of her allergenic substances in dilution, which she was instructed to inject every other day. This is different from getting a conventional allergy shot; it's an individualized treatment to address the patient's specific allergies.

After six months, we repeated the initial tests. The darkfield tests showed reduced levels of red and yellow crystals (correlating with Maggie's report of decreased joint pain), the movement and number of her white blood cells now appeared normal, and the visible yeast forms were greatly reduced in number. At this point, we began to deal with her parasite infection, using homeopathic preparations as well as herbal preparations containing the antiparasitic substances *Artemisia annua* and citrus seed extract.

After five days, Maggie called to say that both her hips were very tender to the touch and that other joints in her body were also sore. The exacerbation of symptoms is not unusual while going through a detoxification program. It's a sign, in fact, that the program is working and the body is trying to rid itself of toxins. To deal with these uncomfortable symptoms, we encouraged Maggie to see a colon therapist for colonics to help speed the cleansing of her system. We advised her to drink more vegetable juice containing yellow dock root, ginger, escarole, kale, and other bitters, along with a bit of carrot to offset the bitter taste. (Maggie had to limit carrots due to her sensitivities.)

Two weeks later, Maggie said that the exacerbation of her symptoms was completely resolved. In fact, she said that her yoga stretches seemed easier than before the parasite cleanse. After remaining on a basic program for several years, Maggie has reported that all symptoms of her OA are completely gone, and she has also maintained normal levels of cholesterol and triglycerides.

The Toxic Load

An analogy may help exemplify the negative cumulative effects of undischarged toxicity: Our organs of detoxification accumulate toxins like a barrel collecting rainwater. If the amount of toxins being absorbed exceeds the amount of toxins eliminated, the barrel eventually overflows. Once that happens, toxic substances circulate throughout the system, progressively damaging organs and tissues and creating numerous acute or chronic problems, much as the overflowing rainwater may damage the foundation of a house. This can lead to allergies, immune system breakdown, and chronic degenerative conditions such as arthritis.

Our bodies are designed to handle a certain level of toxins, but stress, environmental pollution, and poor dietary choices can overtax the system. Biopsies of fat samples taken from patients found over 300 foreign chemicals, concentrated most notably in the brain, the nervous system, and breast milk.[1] Another study discovered 167 pollutants in the blood and urine of people tested, including an average of 56 carcinogens in each person.[2]

The Loading Theory

Serafina Corsello, M.D., formulated the loading theory, which states that multiple stressors weigh down the immune system and eventually throw it out of balance. This cumulative load of stressors, rather than just a single factor, creates an illness. People don't "get" most diseases—they develop them. Among the typical stressors are toxic metals (mercury leaching from dental fillings, copper, and aluminum), petrochemical residues (from pesticides and fertilizers), chemical pollutants in the water and air, electromagnetic pollution (from power lines), undiagnosed food allergies, nutritional deficiencies, biochemical imbalances, insufficient exercise, emotional stress (family, job, and personal), and inappropriate foods (trans-fatty acids [SEE QUICK DEFINITION] in many cooking oils and convenience foods). These factors impinge on the immune system's natural ability to resist the downhill slide into illness. Dr. Corsello explains that these stressors may be accumulating for years, over a lifetime, before they send the system into disrepair. One injurious effect these factors have is to lower the body's threshold of resistance to illness.

 A **trans-fatty acid** (TFA) is a chemically and structurally altered hydrogenated vegetable oil (such as margarine). It is estimated that Americans consume over 600 million pounds of TFAs annually in the form of frying fats. TFAs can increase the risk of heart disease by 27% when consumed as at least 12% of total fat intake. The FDA has ordered all food manufacturers to list the amount of TFAs on all products. You will find trans fat listed on the Nutrition Facts panel directly under the line for saturated fat.[3]

An **antioxidant** (meaning "against oxidation") is a substance that protects living cells from harmful free radicals. Antioxidants react with oxygen breakdown products and neutralize them before damage occurs. Many vitamins and minerals act as antioxidants, including vitamins A, C, and E, beta-carotene, and selenium. Many herbal products are high in antioxidants as well, such as green tea, grape seeds, and milk thistle.

How Toxins Become Harmful

While our emotional and physiological systems are remarkably resilient and adaptable, they need to be maintained to adequately defend against outside contamination. Factors increasingly common in modern life—the barrage of psychological stress, environmental pollution, junk food, a sedentary lifestyle, and chronic constipation—can allow toxins to accumulate to dangerous levels. The constant circulation of toxins in the body taxes the immune system, and this can lead to a deregulation of the immune response as well as contribute to the development of acute and chronic illnesses, including arthritis.

The Damaging Effects of Free Radicals

Having one or more unpaired electrons, free radicals are highly reactive molecules that aggressively attack cell membranes. This attack initiates the process of oxidation, the same process that causes iron to rust and the exposed surfaces of sliced apples to turn brown. Inside our bodies, oxidation creates the same sort of deterioration. To counter these effects, our bodies release antioxidants, which bind with free radicals and eliminate them before they have a chance to attack healthy cells. Toxins,

Factors increasingly common in modern life—the barrage of psychological stress, environmental pollution, junk food, a sedentary lifestyle, and chronic constipation—can allow toxins to accumulate to dangerous levels. The constant circulation of toxins in the body taxes the immune system, and this can lead to a deregulation of the immune response as well as contribute to the development of acute and chronic illnesses, including arthritis.

however, impede this process by creating too many free radicals, which quickly deplete the body's reserve of antioxidant nutrients.

Sources of Toxins

Every day we are exposed to toxins, from pesticide residues and chemicals in food, mercury amalgam dental fillings, biological contaminants such as pollen and parasites, and genetically altered foods, among other sources. Even normal metabolic processes produce toxins that can prove harmful if out of balance.

Toxins in the Environment

Toxins emanate from a variety of noxious sources, mixing together in our bodies to form a chemical cocktail of industrial by-products, pesticides, herbicides, household contaminants (found in cleaners, paints, plastics, and solvents), and biological contaminants (pollens, molds, dust mites, and parasites). In addition, processed or genetically altered foods, alcohol, tap water (which usually contains heavy metals), and other chemicals, such as newspaper print, add to a potentially dangerous mixture.

Physicians use the term sick building syndrome (SBS) to refer to a host of symptoms produced by low-grade toxic environmental conditions in living or office spaces. SBS symptoms include headaches, memory loss, fatigue, infections, irritability, impaired balance, and respiratory, eye, and skin diseases.[4] All of these suppress the immune system, rendering those afflicted susceptible to long-term chronic illness.

Office workers are exposed to toxic air that's continuously recycled throughout sealed buildings.[5] Considering that most people in industrialized nations spend more than 90% of their time indoors, indoor pollutants can cause chronic exposure to toxic substances. In many cases, ventilation systems are poorly designed and inadequate.[6] The combined influence of toxic fumes produced by construction materials and bio-electromagnetic pollution can result in seemingly inexplicable illnesses that affect neurological and biochemical processes.

Xenobiotics, or environmental estrogens (SEE QUICK DEFINITION), have been linked to endocrine disruption and to severe breakdown of the integrity of the digestive system, which can lead to arthritis.[7] Each year, an estimated 1,000 new synthetic chemicals enter the world market, swelling the planetary total to well over 100,000. All of these are completely foreign and potentially harmful to the human body, especially the function of the digestive system and endocrine glands (SEE QUICK DEFINITION). Evidence is accumulating that these chemicals, even at very low concentrations and exposures, cause "hormone havoc"—autoimmune diseases, clinical depression, and reproductive system disorders—among other problems.

Toxins can enter the body in ways other than breathing or swallowing—in particular, they may enter through the skin's pores. (Those same pores, of course, also facilitate the elimination of toxic chemicals.) One example is tap water. In the United States, tap water commonly contains chlorine, aluminum, pesticides, lead, copper, and other toxic substances.[8] Approximately 70% of the toxins from tap water enter the body through the skin; the remaining 30% enter via ingestion.

Environmental estrogens are foreign compounds and/or chemical toxins that mimic the effects of estrogen in the body. Environmental estrogens, also called xenobiotics or xenoestrogens, are present primarily in man-made chemicals (greenhouse gases, herbicides, and pesticides such as DDT) and industrial by-products (from the manufacture of plastics and paper, as well as from the incineration of hazardous wastes).

Endocrine glands, including the testicles, ovaries, pancreas, adrenals, thyroid, parathyroid, and pituitary, are central to the regulation and normalization of all the body's complex, interconnected systems, from metabolism and heat production to spermatogenesis and uterine preparations for pregnancy.

Harmful Metals and Chemicals

Conventional dental amalgams or "silver" fillings are actually made of tin, copper, silver, nickel, zinc, and the toxic metal mercury. These fillings disintegrate over time and have been shown in some instances to release toxic metals into the body. Mercury toxicity effects bones, joints, the central nervous system, and the brain.[9] Symptoms of mercury toxicity include some of the hallmarks of arthritis, such as joint aches and pains, as well as immune dysfunction. Mercury and other toxic metals increase free radicals, which attack cell membranes and initiate swelling and inflammation.

Copper-lined pipes in plumbing systems can be another source of toxicity. A greenish brown ring around the tub, sink, or toilet can indicate that your water is contaminated with copper, which is toxic at high levels. High copper intake has been found to interfere with the formation of healthy fats, increase free radical damage, and interfere with kidney function, all of which can have a negative impact on arthritis.[10]

High copper levels in the body can also cause calcium deposits to accumulate in muscle tissue, which may contribute to fibromyalgia, other muscle pain syndromes, and the formation of bone spurs, or osteophytes. Arthritis patients often have a high copper level in their tissues.[11] People who drink unfiltered water, as well as welders, metal and construction workers, plumbers, and auto mechanics can be exposed to potentially toxic levels of copper. Other sources include birth control pills, intrauterine devices, and many fungicides and pesticides—all of which contain copper as a main ingredient. A thorough analysis from a health-care practitioner, including nutritional and heavy metal assessment, can determine whether copper detoxification or possibly even supplementation is needed if copper levels are deficient rather than too high. Chemicals found in dry-cleaning fluids (trichloroethylene), paint solvents (toluene), municipal water supplies (phenol and chlorine), carpets and flooring (formaldehyde), and some imported produce (DDT pesticide residues) are also potentially harmful, depending on your level of susceptibility. Studies have proven that these chemicals can interfere with proper nerve and muscle function, cause skeletal and muscular changes, and interfere with reproductive function.[12] Often only a very small dose of these toxic agents is required to produce injurious effects, especially in hypersensitive individuals.

 See chapter 3, Diagnosing Arthritis, pages 39–65, for information about the following tests for determining possible mercury toxicity: **hair trace mineral analysis** and the **EDTA lead versenate 24-hour urine collection test** (checks for mercury, along with lead, cadmium, aluminum, and copper). Copper is potentially dangerous at high levels, but an appropriate amount benefits the body by assisting in the repair of connective tissue. See chapter 13, Supplements for Arthritis, pages 257–294, for more information about **supplementing with copper**.

Inner Toxins

Environmental toxins are only one layer of the toxic load that our bodies must process. Endobiotics—toxins produced within the body—are also potentially dangerous if not efficiently eliminated. Endobiotics include uric and lactic acid, homocysteine, nitric oxide, intestinal toxins, and cellular debris from dead microorganisms. These normal by-products of metabolic processes are typically broken down by the liver and excreted from the body. But in someone with a compromised immune system, they tend to accumulate in the blood, where they burden the detoxification pathways or initiate an allergic reaction. The immune system views these substances as a threat and sends antibodies (SEE QUICK DEFINITION) to bind with the antigen, forming circulating immune complexes. If too many immune complexes accumulate, the kidneys can't excrete enough of them via the urine, in which case they are stored in soft tissues, triggering inflammation, bringing stress to the immune system, and potentially leading to arthritic conditions.

For example, arginine and ornithine (important amino acids) enter the body as part of a normal diet, but if they are not digested properly, they undergo unfavorable chemical changes. Orni-

An **antibody** is a protein molecule made from amino acids by white blood cells in the lymph tissue and set in motion by the immune system against a specific foreign protein, or antigen. Antibodies, also referred to as immunoglobulins, may be found in the blood, lymph, saliva, and gastrointestinal and urinary tracts, usually within three days after the first encounter with an antigen. The antibody binds tightly with the antigen as a preliminary step in removing it from the system or destroying it.

thine is converted by bowel bacteria into a toxic substance called putrescine, which in turn degrades into polyamines, such as spermadine, spermine, and cadaverine (literally meaning "the essence of dead cadavers"). Levels of putrescine and cadaverine tend to be high in individuals with psoriasis, psoriatic arthritis, and other forms of arthritis.

Basic Detoxification Strategies

A detoxification program should be tailored to the individual's specific condition, including disease state, toxic burden, and the functional capacity of their major detoxifying organs (intestines, liver, and lymphatic system, among others). People with arthritis are often too toxic or too deficient in functional capacity to attempt to aggressively and rapidly rid the body of toxins (see "Testing Your Detoxification Capabilities," page 76). The process must progress at a rate that the body can handle without causing greater injury.

During detoxification, many people experience a healing crisis, a brief worsening of symptoms immediately followed by significant improvement. Although the healing crisis is uncomfortable, it usually indicates

Testing Your Detoxification Capabilities

Determining how efficiently the body can detoxify itself is especially useful for those suffering from arthritis. Here are two laboratory tests that can help.

Functional liver detoxification profile: A liver that is unable to adequately detoxify your body's store of toxins and waste products may contribute significantly to the emergence and continuation of arthritis. Excess free radicals and by-products of incomplete metabolism resulting from poor detoxification can create problems in the cells. Specifically, they can interfere with the movement of substances across the cell membrane and induce damage to the mitochondria, the cells' "energy factories." The detoxification profile helps to identify places where your system's ability to detoxify is impaired. It assesses the liver's ability to convert potentially dangerous toxins into harmless substances that can then be eliminated by the body. This conversion process occurs in two major chemical reactions referred to as phase I and phase II. The detoxification profile determines the presence of enzymes needed to start the conversion process and the rate at which phase I and phase II detoxification are operating.

Oxidative stress profile: When your ability to detoxify is impaired or you're deficient in antioxidants, free radicals run unchallenged throughout your body, damaging cells. They tend to affect the immune, endocrine, and nervous systems, damaging mitochondria, interrupting communication among cells, and depleting key nutrients and antioxidants. This is called oxidative stress. The oxidative stress profile assesses the degree of free radical damage in the body and measures the body's levels of glutathione, an amino acid complex central to detoxification.

that toxins are being effectively removed from the body. However, a health-care professional should be alerted when symptoms worsen during detoxification to avoid complications or injury. Efforts must be made to increase production or consumption of antioxidants through fruits, vegetables, and supplements prior to any detoxification program to avert or diminish a healing crisis.

Before getting started on a detoxification program, it's important to make fundamental lifestyle and dietary changes so that you don't introduce more toxins for your body to process. Some basic steps you can take to reduce your toxic load follow.

Use only organically raised foods. Take this recommendation as a mandatory general guideline when making food choices. Eat foods that are certified as having been grown organically. They will be free of the contaminants, synthetic pesticides and herbicides, hormones, preservatives, dyes, artificial colorings, and antibiotics found in conventionally raised foods. Many health food stores offer organic produce and meat, as do some farmers' markets and even some conventional grocery stores.

Get the poisons off your vegetables. Since the U.S. Food and Drug Administration tests only about 1% of produce for pesticide residues, cleaning your food is the only way to ensure that you aren't eating agricultural poisons. Even organic foods may have residues of potentially harmful substances. Consider using naturally derived produce washes, now available to consumers concerned about preventing food-borne illnesses.

Maintain a household free of toxic chemicals. Remove chemical contaminants and toxic household cleansers from your home, or at least limit your exposure to them. Instead, use natural cleaning products, such as distilled white vinegar, baking soda, borax, lemon juice, citrus cleaners (not petroleum-based), castile soaps, and environmentally-safe commercial products. These products are available in many health food stores or by mail-order; increasingly, they're even available in standard supermarkets.

Breathe clean air. Since the average American spends most of their time indoors, indoor air quality is crucial. Unfortunately, indoor air ranks near the top of the list of polluted environments. Toxic substances such as pollens, dust mites, mold spores, tobacco smoke residues, benzene, chloroform, chemical gases, and formaldehyde are now commonly found in tightly sealed indoor environments. Whenever possible, open windows in your house, even if for only part of the day. In nature, a thunderstorm can clean up the stagnant air in a local environment by way of ionization and ozone release. Commercial air filters are available that produce ions and low levels of ozone (O_3), creating air that's refreshed as after a thunderstorm. Common houseplants can also be used as filters to remove pollution from indoor air, an idea that first came out of NASA space research in the 1970s. Scientists discovered that not only do plants recycle oxygen, they remove air pollutants too.[13] Common plants that are especially effective include English ivy, spider plants, peace lily, snake plant, pothos, philodendrons, palms, mums, and ferns.

 Any detoxification effort should always be planned and carried out under professional supervision. Alcoholics, diabetics, people with eating disorders, those recovering from substance abuse, people who are underweight or physically weak, and those who have an underactive thyroid or hypoglycemic condition are urged not to detoxify without consulting a licensed health-care professional.

Filter your household water. Tap water is a major source of toxic chemicals that the liver is required to process. The practical solution is to get a water filter for your home and office, a cost-effective alternative to using commercially purified and bottled water.

Therapies for General Detoxification

Detoxification strategies can help arthritis patients reverse the accumulation of toxins that otherwise promote the destruction of joint tissues and contribute to other degenerative conditions. You can choose from several different methods of detoxification, including fasting, drinking fresh juices, and following specific diets. Related therapies for detoxification are colon- and bowel-cleansing treatments, renal (kidney) cleansing, homeopathic remedies, bodywork, lymphatic drainage, aromatherapy, antioxidant support, and nutritional and herbal support to bolster the organs of detoxification. Any program of detoxification must also address the mind to foster positive thoughts and feelings. The mind-body connection must not be overlooked in arthritis, because stress releases hormones that directly and adversely affect the immune system.

The first step in most detoxification protocols is a general body cleanse, utilizing such methods as eating nutrient-specific diets, fasting, and consuming fresh juices. These methods are the cornerstone of detoxification therapy and are critical for the successful treatment of arthritis. Avoiding solid foods and ingesting only liquids or teas allows the body to focus on cleansing, breaking down circulating toxins, and decreasing their adverse effects.

Researchers have documented decreased joint stiffness in patients with arthritis after a program of fasting and a follow-up arthritis-friendly vegetarian diet.[14] Biological indicators of inflammation tend to decrease after a fast. These indicators include SED rate, C-reactive protein, and proinflammatory immune cells, such as leukotrienes and eosinophils.[15] In addition, patients report a substantial improvement in symptoms and an overall cessation or reduction of the inflammatory response. Fasting and similar therapies are also credited with improving energy levels, reducing allergies and acne, aiding in weight loss, and sharpening mental acuity.

The Arthritis Diet

An overwhelming number of arthritis sufferers will experience partial to complete relief of symptoms after a month of strict adherence to a primarily vegetarian, arthritis-friendly diet. The diet eliminates refined, canned, and processed foods, hydrogenated oils and rancid fats, alcohol, caffeine, refined sugars, most animal products, and any foods that cause food allergies and toxic reactions. Additional foods to avoid include yeast, wheat and other high-gluten grains, cow's milk and dairy products,

> Detoxification strategies can help arthritis patients reverse the accumulation of toxins that otherwise promote the destruction of joint tissues and contribute to other degenerative conditions.

refined or concentrated natural sugars (even fruit juices), corn, and night-shade vegetables (tomatoes, peppers, eggplant, and potatoes). Organic vegetables and fruits should be incorporated into the diet daily. We've found that arthritis patients suffer relapses of symptoms when they deviate from this diet. Typically, we prescribe the arthritis diet for one month, during which time we carefully monitor the patient for nutritional status, inflammatory markers, and digestive function. Based on the results of these tests, the diet can be tailored to meet the individual's needs.

Fasting

Each cell needs a constant supply of nourishment in the form of oxygen, proteins, glucose, amino acids, fatty acids, vitamins, minerals, and trace elements. Equally important to the cells is waste removal. Metabolic wastes are poisonous and must be carried away from the cells by the lymphatic system, the "garbage disposal" of the cells. When nutritional deficiencies, sluggish metabolism, lymphatic stagnation, and environmental and internal toxins have choked the cells, fasting is a necessity. True fasting is done by consuming only filtered water and/or herbal teas, with zero caloric intake. Fasting on water causes rapid release of toxins from the body, where they have been buried in the fat for long periods of time.

Incorporating vegetable or fruit juices and "green" foods into a fasting regime is less aggressive than a true, water-only fast and is better tolerated by most people with borderline hypoglycemia (low blood sugar). In fact, for many people, fasting on water can create health problems if their body isn't adequately prepared for this shock. While we feel water fasting is the best method of detoxification, especially for arthritis, it should be done only under the guidance of a health-care practitioner who has experience in supervising fasts of this type. We recommend that water fasts always follow a healing, nutrient-dense detoxification diet emphasizing a wide

 For more on **stress and arthritis**, see chapter 11, Mind-Body Approaches to Arthritis, pages 200–224.

range of antioxidants and lipotropic nutrients. Such a diet supports the kidneys and other eliminative organs, which is important because toxins can reach high concentrations in the stool, lymph, blood, urine, and breath during fasting.

Preparing for the Fast. Fasting traditionally starts at the beginning of a new season (typically autumn or spring) but can be undertaken at any point during the year. For several weeks before a fast, follow the arthritis diet (see chapter 12, The Arthritis Diet) and incorporate into your daily diet two glasses of Rainbow Feather Veggie Juice, six or more cups of Detox Tea, and the supplements recommended below.

 For the full program of the **arthritis-friendly diet**, see chapter 12, The Arthritis Diet, pages 225–256.

▩ Rainbow Feather Veggie Juice

$1/2$ beet root
3 to 5 beet greens
1 cucumber
$1/2$-inch slice ginger
1 to 3 carrots
2 stalks celery
$1/2$ fennel stalk
1 bunch parsley and/or cilantro
2- to 4-inch piece burdock and/or yellow dock root
1 lemon, juiced
1 tablespoon spirulina, chlorella, or any of the organic "green" food combinations available in health food stores

Use organic vegetables only. Juice the beet, greens, cucumber, ginger, carrots, celery, fennel, parsley, and burdock in a juicer. Add the lemon juice and spirulina and dilute by 50% with filtered or purified water.

▩ Detox tea

Mix together equal parts of dandelion, burdock, red clover, peppermint, and green tea. Use 1 tablespoon of this blend per cup of tea. To prepare, bring filtered water to a boil and pour over the tea blend. Allow the blend to steep for 5 minutes, then pour the tea through a strainer. Drink six or more cups of the tea per day for one month prior to a fasting period.

Mucus-Cleansing Diet

Mucus is created by the body to trap toxins or disease-causing organisms circulating in the sinus cavity and gastrointestinal tract. Certain foods can also trigger the release of mucus and may lead to buildup that causes waste elimination and other processes to stagnate. The mucus-cleansing diet consists of foods and beverages that help thin and dislodge mucus. This diet should be followed for three to five days to be effective for conditions such as obstinate sinusitis, asthma, hay fever, or other allergies. It is also very beneficial for arthritis and to prepare for a fast.

An excellent combination to start with is The Lemonade Special, which contains a freshly juiced lemon. Lemons help loosen mucus and cleanse the liver. Those with candida infections should use stevia rather than honey.

1. Place the juice from a freshly squeezed whole organic lemon into a 1-quart glass jar.

2. Fill the jar with filtered water.

3. Add 1 teaspoon of raw honey (or substitute the herb stevia, a natural sweetener).

4. Add a pinch of ground cayenne pepper (or a little fresh grated horseradish).

5. Make an 8- to 12-ounce glass in the morning and continue to drink it throughout the day. Take a few gulps at least once per hour. If you finish the first 8- to 12-ounces, prepare another batch. You should finish two to four full glasses of the combination per day.

Also drink water, another great mucus cleanser, throughout the day, as well an herbal tea consisting of peppermint, spearmint, fenugreek, eucalyptus, ginger, and licorice. These herbs have mucus-removing properties and can be mixed in equal proportions for a tea that should be consumed five or more times a day.

You can also enjoy a potassium-rich broth throughout the day. Simmer about 1 cup each of chopped celery, carrots, beets, onions, parsley, kale, and parsnips (use only organically grown produce) and 4 cloves of garlic in two quarts of filtered water for 45 minutes. You can add sea salt and/or Bragg Liquid Aminos (containing soybeans and filtered water) to enhance the flavor. Strain the stock and store it in the refrigerator, consuming it within a day or two. Steamed carrots, mustard greens, onions, and garlic should be eaten throughout the day as an accompaniment. Horseradish (fresh, not pickled) can be grated on top.

Daily supplements. It's also important to boost your nutritional reserves with supplements before beginning a fast. For one month prior to starting the fast, take the following supplements:

- Multivitamin-multimineral without copper: two to three tablets with each meal

- Multiple antioxidant: two to three tablets with each meal

- Lipotropic factors, which suppport detoxification: three tablets, two times a day

- Bioflavonoids: liquid form preferred, one tablespoon per day

The 15-Day Fast. It's best to ease into this fast over a three-day period. The fast itself lasts for five days. Then we recommend a full week to slowly reintroduce healthy foods back into your diet.

Day 1. Eliminate beans and whole grains. Eat only fruits, vegetables (raw or cooked), tofu, nuts and seeds, and juices. Always dilute juices by 50% to 75% with purified water. Drink at least eight glasses of water. Drink the detox tea described above and use stevia to sweeten it if you wish. Take the nutritional supplements discussed above for the duration of the fast.

Day 2. Consume only fruits and raw or steamed vegetables. Eliminate tofu, nuts, and seeds. Limit portions to decrease the capacity of your stomach.

Day 3. Eat only raw vegetables and fruits and chew them thoroughly.

Days 4 through 8. Eliminate all solid foods. Drink unlimited quantities of warm herb tea throughout the day. Consume liberal quantities of water, which will dilute body fluids and flush the lymphatic, circulatory, and urinary systems; urine must stay diluted to avoid damaging your kidneys. Water should be filtered through a solid-block carbon filter or through reverse osmosis and then a solid-block carbon filter. Distilled water is not acceptable, as it is an active dipolar molecule that aggressively pulls plastic molecules from plastic containers and is usually high in toxins.

Take the following supplements to support your organs of detoxification and minimize any temporary worsening of symptoms (healing crisis): the antioxidants milk thistle (80% standardized silymarin, 450 mg, three times a day) and artichoke root (5% standardized cynarin, 300 mg, three times a day); and the amino acids SAMe (S-adenosylmethionine, 500 mg, twice daily), NAC (N-acetylcysteine, 500 mg, twice daily), glutathione (150 mg, twice daily), and L-glutamine (4 grams daily). L-glutamine is an amino acid that supports regeneration of the gastrointestinal barrier and is particularly useful during a fast.

CAUTION When calories are restricted, toxins embedded in fatty tissues are liberated and can be flushed out of the body. Care must be taken to decide how rapidly to mobilize the pollutants in the body. It is imperative to consult with a health-care practitioner before starting any detoxification therapy.

Day 9. Take a full week to ease into your healthy diet again. On the first day of eating solids, consume only one light meal of steamed or baked vegetables such as squash, sweet potatoes, or carrots. Eat only one type of vegetable; don't mix them. With your meal, take one to three capsules of digestive enzymes or bromelain (an enzyme from pineapples) to help support your digestive system, which has now been inactive for an extended time.

Day 10. Now you may supplement your diet with more varieties of cooked foods and a raw salad (with a dressing of flaxseed oil, lemon juice, and sea salt). Look for reactions to foods as you reintroduce them into your diet. Work with a health-care practitioner to determine the extent of your hidden food allergies and sensitivities.

Days 11 through 13. Reintroduce into your diet easily digestible proteins, such as organic tofu, and whole grains, such as brown rice, millet, quinoa, amaranth, and buckwheat. Avoid high-gluten foods, such as wheat, spelt, rye, barley, and oats.

Days 14 through 15. Now you can return to following the arthritis diet. At this point, you have successfully completed the fast.

Activity during the fast. During a fast, it's important to get enough rest and to conserve your energy. Vigorous exercise is discouraged because it increases your physiological need for glucose, which will come from either fat or muscle protein if you push yourself too hard. Light aerobic exercise, such as walking or swimming is fine, and stretching, yoga, and tai chi are encouraged. Stress, whether physical or psychological, hampers your healing and even promotes toxemia by producing stress hormones and free radicals. Focus on reducing any negative emotions through creative endeavors, such as meditating or writing in a journal. Good strategies to deal with potential food obsessions or excessive hunger during fasting are light exercise, sleep, or avoidance of situations where food is prominent. Avoid being around food as much as possible, and have someone else prepare meals for the family if this is one of your responsibilities. Many people find that food cravings abate after the first couple of days of fasting. We recommend taking time off from your job or normal routine during the fast.

Bathing and bowel detoxification while fasting. About one-third of all body impurities are eliminated through the skin, commonly referred to as the "third kidney." During a fast, your sweat and sebaceous secretions will contain higher concentrations of fat-soluble pollutants,

 For information on **detoxifying baths**, see the hydrotherapy section in chapter 14, Exercises and Physical Therapies, pages 295–320.

Shorter Fasts

Two-day fast: For two days, drink the Rainbow Feather Veggie Juice (see the recipe on page 80), whey-, rice-, or soy-based protein powder shakes (two a day), and the detox tea (see page 80). Select a protein powder that has *very few* ingredients. They vary greatly; read the label and take special note of the section titled "other ingredients."

Three- to five-day fast: Follow the guidelines for the two-day fast, adding an organic vegetable soup prepared with the following ingredients: 1 cabbage, 4 leaves of kale, 2 carrots, 1 onion, 2 cloves garlic, 1 bunch of parsley, 2 stalks of celery. Cut the vegetables into bite-size pieces and place them in a soup pot with 1 gallon of filtered water. Simmer for 1 hour, then add Bragg Liquid Aminos (available in most health food stores) to taste. You may eat a bowl of this soup as many times a day as you choose.

Three- to five-day mono diet: For those who find it difficult to complete a liquid fast, try eating only one type of nonallergenic food for several days. The proper food to consume on your mono diet can be chosen by you and your health-care professional. Good choices include pears, brown rice, apples, squash, and carrots (if hypoglycemia is not a problem). The food can be prepared raw, boiled, steamed, or baked. At least 2 quarts of filtered water and/or herb tea should be consumed daily during the mono diet. The mono diet is typically followed for three to five days. Break the mono diet by slowly reintroducing foods allowed on the arthritis diet.

heavy metals, and salts. Shower or bathe three times per day during the fast to prevent reabsorbing these toxins. Adding Epsom salts, baking soda, sea salt, diluted hydrogen peroxide, ginger root, bentonite clay, and/or burdock root to the bath will help remove toxins more quickly. To encourage drainage of lymphatic fluid through your skin, use a loofah sponge or soft brush on dry skin. Taking showers or baths in which the temperature of the water alternates between hot and cold aids in detoxification and flushes the lymphatic system. Fat-soluble toxins present in your body, made up primarily of bile formed by the liver, will be flushed out through the stool. The stool of an individual fasting typically contains more toxins than normal. For this reason, it's important to avoid constipation and to encourage elimination through colonics, enemas, and herbal support (see chapter 5, Detoxifying Specific Organs, for recommendations).

Experiences during a fast. People report a spectrum of feelings as they proceed through a fast. Most experience physiological and psychological withdrawal effects during the first three days and, in some cases, for longer periods. The more prepared your body is, the fewer and less intense the side effects. Transient headaches, energy fluctuations, hypoglycemia, halitosis (bad breath), increased body odor, constipation, nausea, rectal mucus discharge, acne, and a temporary aggravation of many conditions are common. Serious side effects are very rare (especially in those who have adhered to the prefasting program previously outlined) and usually occur when people who should be under medical supervision undertake long fasts. Symptoms can include fainting or dizziness, dangerously low blood pressure, cardiac arrhythmias, severe vomiting or diarrhea, renal problems, and gout. As we've emphasized before, it's important to consult with a practitioner who's knowledgeable about fasting before you undertake this vital aspect of detoxification.

Support Therapies for Detoxification

Specific nutrients, particularly the "green" foods, along with fresh juices can help support the body nutritionally during an intensive fast. They're also useful for promoting cleansing on a daily basis.

Juicing. Many people attempt to fast on juice. While juice fasts have positive benefits, the carbohydrates in the juice decrease the rate of toxin removal. Consuming fresh juices can, however, prepare your body for fasting and should become a part of your daily diet. Fresh juices are a simple way to obtain the 8 to 10 daily servings of fruits and vegetables recommended by the National Cancer Society, National Cancer Institute, and the American Heart Association. Juices help repair damaged body tissues, due to their high concentration of vitamins, minerals, natural sugars, intact enzymes, and phytonutrients (plant compounds with health-protecting qualities). They are easily digested, and their nutrients are in a form that can be quickly utilized by the body.

- Juiced watermelon with rind helps cleanse the kidneys and decrease joint pain.
- Cherries are especially helpful for gout, due to their anti-inflammatory properties.

Tips for Juicing

- Use only organic, nonirradiated fruits and vegetables.
- If organic produce isn't available, wash off pesticide residues using fruit and vegetable washes.
- Always peel away the skins of citrus fruits before juicing (except lemons and limes), but retain as much of the white layer between the peel and fruit as possible, because it contains vitamin C and bioflavonoids.
- Remove pits, stones, and hard seeds from fruits such as cherries, plums, and mangoes.
- Juice the stems and leaves of most produce, such as beets, grapes, and apples, but remove the greens of carrots and rhubarb.
- Fruits with a low water content, such as papayas, mangoes, avocados, and bananas, won't juice well, but they can be prepared in a blender as smoothies.

- Okra and cabbage contain the amino acid glutamine, which helps repair the intestinal lining. (When the intestinal lining loses integrity, it allows inflammation-provoking substances to escape into the bloodstream and body tissues.)

- Pineapple and papaya contain natural plant enzymes that, when taken on an empty stomach, digest the protein layers of circulating immune complexes (antibody and antigen compounds), which also play a role in causing inflammation. Use only organic and non-irradiated fruit and add a little ginger to your pineapple juice for extra enzyme power and to soothe any gastrointestinal irritation.

"Green" Foods. "Green" foods (blue-green algae, chlorella, spirulina, wheatgrass, and barley grass) act as powerful antioxidants, support the liver, and aid in detoxification.[16] They're popular in juiced drinks available at most health food stores, or they can be juiced at home. Green foods are rich in vitamins, minerals, and chlorophyll, the green pigment found in most plants. Chlorophyll has long been used as a healing agent and is well-known for its antiaging properties. It helps heal wounds of the skin and internal membranes, stimulates the growth of new cells, and hinders the growth of bacteria. Important in detoxifying, chlorophyll also promotes bowel regularity. We recommend a mixture of these green foods as an excellent nutrient-building food before a water fast or in preparation for a mono diet.

Blue-green algae *(Aphanizomenon flos-aquae).* This single-cell freshwater microalgae plant is used for increasing physical and mental strength and stamina. Blue-green algae is a source of eight essential amino acids and is high in trace elements, vitamin A and carotenoids, and vitamin B_{12}.

Chlorella *(Chlorella pyreniodosa).* This freshwater single-cell green algae is more popular than vitamin C in Japan. Chlorella is approximately 60% protein, including all the essential amino acids, and contains high levels of carotenoids and chlorophyll, important detoxifying agents. It has very high levels of RNA and DNA, which support tissue repair and healing. An antioxidant, chlorella also helps remove heavy metals (cadmium, mercury, lead, and aluminum) and pesticides (DDT and chlordane) from the body. Chlorella absorbs toxins from the intestines, helps relieve chronic constipation, and promotes the growth of healthy intestinal flora.

Chlorella is excellent for reversing the damage of NSAIDs (non-steroidal anti-inflammatory drugs) on the intestinal lining.

Spirulina. This specific type of blue-green algae contains eight times more protein than tofu, five times more calcium than cow's milk (in a more easily absorbed form), and is higher than most vegetables in amino acids. Spirulina is important in reversing adrenal and thyroid exhaustion and battling depression and mood swings; it's also excellent for weight control because it acts as an appetite suppressor. Spirulina chelates (binds with) heavy metals and helps remove them from the body.

Wheatgrass. Well-known for its ability to cleanse and detoxify, wheatgrass is available in two forms. The variety of wheatgrass grown indoors for juicing is a good source of chlorophyll and is used as a purifying tonic. Dehydrated wheatgrass, a common ingredient in green food supplements, is more nutritionally rich than the juicing variety. Wheatgrass contains beta-carotene, calcium, chlorophyll, fiber, iron, vitamins B_6, B_{12}, C, and K, folic acid, and trace minerals. Those allergic to wheat or gluten can enjoy wheatgrass without any concern, as wheatgrass contains no allergenic gluten or gliadin.

Barley grass. Barley grass, also found in most green food formulas, contains many of the same nutrients as wheatgrass and helps support the growth of friendly intestinal bacteria in the digestive tract. Both dehydrated wheatgrass and barley grass contain as much vitamin C as oranges (about 60 mg per 100 grams). Vitamin C is important in the formation of collagen, the structural support of connective tissue.

five

Detoxifying Specific Organs

As our environment and food become increasingly saturated with pollutants and chemicals, the body's mechanisms for elimination of toxins can't keep up with the chemical deluge. All organs involved in detoxification, which include the intestines, liver, lymphatic system, kidneys, skin, connective tissue, and respiratory system, can become overloaded. The constant circulation of toxins in the body taxes the immune system, which must continually strive to destroy or eliminate them. It is advisable to take measures to support these detoxification organs and to remove toxins stored in the body. Detoxification therapies designed for specific organs work in conjunction with fasting and the dietary recommendations for general detoxification described in the previous chapter.

The Detoxification Defense System

The detoxification system has two lines of defense: specific organs prevent toxins from entering the body, and other organs neutralize and excrete the poisonous compounds that get through this initial line of defense.

When functioning properly, the body's defenses protect healthy tissues and joints from damage by harmful free radicals or circulating toxins. The following organs and systems are the key components of the detoxification system.

- The gastrointestinal barrier, including the small and large intestines
- The liver
- The lymphatic system, which transports waste products from the cells to the major organs of detoxification
- The kidneys, bladder, and other components of the urinary system
- The skin, including the sweat and sebaceous glands
- The lungs

The gastrointestinal system is typically the first line of defense against toxins. When compromised, the intestinal membrane no longer acts as an effective barrier, and toxins as well as pathogenic microbes can gain access to the bloodstream. This is one facet of how arthritis begins: Undigested food particles, bacteria, and other substances usually confined to the intestines escape into the bloodstream, activating the immune system and initiating inflammation. When the intestines are compromised, the liver, lymphatic system, kidneys, skin, and other organs involved in detoxification become overwhelmed.

The liver bears most of the burden for eliminating toxins. All antigens (foreign substances) are sent to the liver to be neutralized and expelled. By means of enzymes and antioxidants, the liver chemically transforms toxins into harmless substances that can be excreted via the urine or stool. Other toxins are eliminated through the lymphatic system, kidneys, skin, and respiratory system. When the organs of detoxification are not operating efficiently, the result can be poor digestion, constipation, bloating, gas, immune dysfunction, and degenerative illnesses, including arthritis. Detoxification can reduce or eliminate the body's toxic load, restore proper functioning of the immune system, and help alleviate arthritis pain and inflammation.

Toxicity and the Intestines

Most of the body's digestion and absorption of nutrients occurs along the 25-foot-long passageway that comprises the small and large

> Detoxification can reduce or eliminate the body's toxic load, restore proper functioning of the immune system, and help alleviate arthritis pain and inflammation.

intestines. Keeping this passageway clean, free of toxic buildup, and alive with healthy digestive microbes is vital for efficient nutrient absorption.

Digestion begins in the mouth with proper chewing and digestive enzymes secreted by the salivary glands. From the mouth, food travels to the stomach, where hydrochloric acid activates pepsin to break down proteins into absorbable molecular components. The partially digested food then moves to the upper part of the small intestine, where digestion continues with enzymes (produced by the pancreas) and bile. In the next section of the intestine (the jejunum), sugar-digesting enzymes are secreted. The majority of nutrients from food are absorbed into the blood from the small intestine. The large intestine's primary function is to absorb water (about 1 quart a day) and some minerals. Undigested material is then stored until it can be eliminated.

In the early 1900s, most people in the United States had a brief intestinal transit time; it normally took 15 to 20 hours from the time food entered the mouth until it was excreted as feces. Today, many people have a seriously delayed transit time. It may take as long as 50 to 70 hours for food to make the journey from the mouth to excretion. Constipation and sluggish transit time allow the stool to putrefy, harmful microorganisms to flourish, and toxins to be reabsorbed by tissues and lymph vessels, triggering inflammation throughout the body. In addition, undigested proteins that aren't broken down into their constituent amino acids (due to inadequate levels of hydrochloric acid) produce toxins that can escape into the blood or lymph fluids. Inadequate digestion of dietary protein often results in insufficient quantities of free amino acids, which affects levels of hormones, digestive enzymes, and other substances important for proper immune function and overall health.

Mucoid Plaque

Intestinal mucus can become too thick due to poor eating habits, especially the consumption of fried or processed foods; this makes the stools gummy, causing them to stick to the intestinal walls. Mucus also leaves a residue as it passes, which builds up and eventually hardens into plaque. This plaque can be up to an inch thick in a toxic colon. This false lining in the intestines reduces the diameter of the intestinal passageway, leaving only a narrow opening through which waste can travel. As this lining builds up, it also blocks absorption of essential nutrients into the bloodstream and offers a hiding place for toxins, bacteria, yeast, and parasites harmful to human health. These toxins and abnormal lifeforms can kill off the friendly bacteria, such as *Lactobacillus acidophilus*, that inhabit the intestines, leading to an imbalance in intestinal microflora (see "Friendly and Unfriendly Bacteria," page 92).

The large and small intestines constitute the largest immunological system of the body and act as the active front of the immune system, trapping and eliminating pathogens and harmful debris. If the intestines are overburdened, their capacity to protect the body from destructive substances is compromised.

Toxins that build up in the colon pass through the intestinal wall and

The digestive system. Digestion begins in the mouth, then food travels to the stomach (1), where it's further broken down by gastric juices. Next, the partially digested food goes to the small intestine (2), where enzymes from the pancreas (3) and bile produced by the liver (4) act upon the food to extract nutrients for absorption into blood and lymph cells. The unusable food materials are sent to the large intestine (5) for evacuation from the body.

accumulate in the lymphatic system, the network of vessels and nodes that clean and drain the body of unwanted substances. Once the lymphatic system becomes overwhelmed, it, in turn, releases the overflow into the liver, blood, skin, and other organs of detoxification. Once this happens, symptoms will result, such as lack of energy, skin rashes, bloating, gas, digestive problems, and joint pain.

Factors That Harm the Intestines

The following factors can contribute to the formation of mucoid plaque, disturb the balance of intestinal microflora, and cause a toxic bowel.

- Acid diet: Acid-forming foods, such as sugars, processed grains, eggs, and meat, contribute to the formation of intestinal plaque.

Friendly and Unfriendly Bacteria

An estimated 100 trillion bacteria live in the intestines of each human being. Certain bacteria, such as *Lactobacillus acidophilus* and *Bifidobacterium bifidum*, are friendly bacteria that support numerous vital physiological processes. They protect against overgrowth of yeasts and parasites and ensure that bowel movements are regular and frequent. Other bacteria, such as *Citrobacter* spp., *Klebsiella* spp., and *Clostridium* spp., are considered unfriendly because they produce a variety of toxic substances. A healthy proportion of microorganisms in the colon is 85% friendly to no more than 15% unfriendly. Unfortunately, the proportions are reversed in most people, especially if they are eating a standard American diet. A number of factors can throw off the balance of intestinal flora, including stress, use of antibiotics and other drugs, and processed foods.

- Processed foods: Foods made from bleached white flour, such as white bread, pastries, and cakes, contribute to the buildup of intestinal plaque. These foods are almost totally devoid of fiber. In addition, because most of their nutrients have been removed by processing, these foods tend to deprive the body of enzymes and other wholesome nutrients. Enzymes are specialized living proteins that break down food and change it into a form the body can absorb. Without adequate enzymes, food tends to putrefy in the intestines rather than being digested and absorbed.

- Stress: Stress can cause excess acid in the intestine, contributing to the formation of intestinal plaque. Tension causes the walls of the bowel and sphincter muscles to constrict, hindering the passage of fecal material.

- Allergies: The intestines may produce mucus in response to a food allergy, which can cause symptoms including constipation, cramps, bloating, and diarrhea.

- Parasites and yeast: Parasites commonly enter the body through contaminated food or water. Intestinal parasites can induce a wide variety of reactions, including swelling of joints, asthma, skin rashes, and changes in weight.[1]

- Antibiotics: Although commonly prescribed by physicians to kill harmful bacteria, antibiotics don't distinguish between unfriendly and friendly microbes and, unfortunately, kill both indiscriminately. Antibiotics are also fed to poultry

 For more information on **food allergies and arthritis**, see chapter 9, Allergies and Arthritis, pages 166–180. For more about the **role of bacteria and yeast** in intestinal dysbiosis, see chapter 6, Eradicating Bacteria and Yeast, pages 155–133. For more on **parasites and intestinal dysbiosis**, see chapter 7, Eliminating Parasites, pages 134–148.

and beef cattle in alarming amounts, and this practice causes substantial antibiotic residues to remain in meat and other animal products consumed by most Americans,[2] contributing to the demise of friendly intestinal microbes.

- Steroids and birth control pills: These can also cause an imbalance of healthy bacteria.

Alternative Medicine Therapies for a Toxic Colon

Cleansing the intestines to remove accumulated toxins is vital for arthritis sufferers in order to modulate the immune system and stop the chronic inflammatory response that accompanies an overburdened detoxification system. Repopulating the intestines with friendly bacteria is also important for maintaining healthy digestive functioning.

Colon Hydrotherapy

Colon hydrotherapy (colonics or colonic irrigation) can help to reduce levels of rheumatoid factor and antinuclear antibodies, which are often elevated in autoimmune illnesses. Colon hydrotherapy involves the gentle infusion of warm, filtered water into the colon. Although it can be slightly uncomfortable for some people, colon hydrotherapy is unsurpassed in its ability to detoxify the colon, correct disordered intestinal bacteria (dysbiosis), and treat intestinal permeability (leaky gut syndrome). It also tones the muscles of the colon and stimulates peristalsis (the wavelike contractions of the intestines), which propels food through the digestive tract and prevents the buildup of destructive wastes.

Normal colon function yields two to three bowel movements per day, following meals. The average American eliminates less than once per day, which means that most people are actually constipated. With constipation, the stool is hard and dry. Hardened fecal stones (fecoliths) get caught in the folds of the colon, contributing to toxic buildup. In traditional cultures, where 5 to 10 times more unprocessed fiber is eaten than in the standard American diet, the stool is typically larger and softer, and elimination occurs more frequently. There is a corresponding lower incidence of colon cancer and other gastrointestinal diseases in these cultures.

For more information on the **comprehensive digestive stool analysis**, see chapter 3, Diagnosing Arthritis, pages 39–65. For more about **leaky gut syndrome**, see chapter 8, Alleviating Leaky Gut Syndrome, pages 149–165. For more on **rheumatoid factor** and **antinuclear antibodies**, see chapter 3, Diagnosing Arthritis, pages 39–65.

How's Your Digestive Function?

A comprehensive digestive stool analysis consists of nearly two dozen tests performed on a stool sample. The tests reveal how efficiently food is being digested and how well nutrients and fats are absorbed. It also assesses adequacy of fiber in the diet, the status of digestive enzymes, the balance of friendly to unfriendly bacteria, and the presence of yeasts, such as candida. An imbalance in any of these areas can contribute to inflammation and arthritis.

The Colonic Procedure. Colonic hydrotherapy begins with the insertion of a small rectal tube (speculum) into the patient by the therapist, nurse, or physician. The colon hydrotherapy machine is a closed system. Water, oxygenated water, food-grade hydrogen peroxide, ozone, botanical antimicrobials, nutritional supplements, or a solution of friendly intestinal flora (probiotics) is gently infused into and out of the intestines. The temperature, water pressure, and flow are continuously monitored throughout the treatment. The colonic machine is self-sanitizing, featuring a built-in check valve that prevents wastewater from returning and contaminating the water source. All instruments used in the treatment are sterile and disposable, eliminating any possible contamination of the patient.

The water pressure used during the colonic treatment is a safe and gentle 5 pounds per square inch. The treatment usually lasts about an hour, which includes time for evacuating the bowels after the treatment.

A series of 8 to 12 colonic treatments is often prescribed, depending on the person's diagnosis. The medications or therapeutic substances infused during the colonic are changed often so as to expose the disease-causing microorganisms in the colon to the widest spectrum of disease fighters, guaranteeing maximum eradication. We recommend using healthy bacteria during colon hydrotherapy (at the end of the treatment), because it's much more effective than taking oral supplements.

CAUTION Pregnant women and people with severe heart disease, appendicitis, aneurysm, gastrointestinal hemorrhage, severe hemorrhoids, colon cancer, intestinal wall herniation, severe colitis, and intestinal blockages should not undergo colon hydrotherapy.

Enemas

Enemas can easily be done at home. Adding medicinal herbs or the friendly bacteria *Lactobacillus acidophilus* makes an enema even more effective. Enemas help purge both the colon and liver of accumulated toxins, dead cells, and waste products.

Colon-Cleansing Programs

Begin a colon-cleansing program by combining ½ teaspoon psyllium seed powder, 1 teaspoon vitamin C powder, and 8 ounces of water, drinking it immediately after mixing the ingredients and following it with another 8 ounces of water or herb tea. Do this once daily. After two days, begin taking a combination of herbs such as barberry, wormwood, and cascara sagrada, which help to destroy unfriendly bacteria and stimulate elimination through the colon. Also, begin a regimen of supplementation to help rebuild a healthy intestinal lining, including L-glutamine, plantain, slippery elm, ginkgo, and skullcap. Continue taking the herbs and supplements daily for a month, then reduce to one or two times per week.

Increased interest in colon health has led to a surge in the development of over-the-counter colon-cleansing products. Most of these products utilize supplements containing a combination of herbs, nutrients, enzymes, and toxin absorbers designed to help remove the mucoid plaque lining in the colon and enhance digestion and absorption of nutrients. Many of these supplements include ingredients that also cleanse the liver, gallbladder, and lymphatic system. If they're quality products, they'll also recommend a diet of organic whole foods high in natural fiber and dark green leafy vegetables.

The Origins of Colon Hydrotherapy

Accounts of bowel cleansing date back to ancient Egypt. *The Ebers Papyrus*, an ancient Egyptian manuscript on health and spirituality, contains hieroglyphs that depict the use of gourds and rushes as a rudimentary enema bag to infuse liquids into the colon through the anus. *The Essene Gospel of Peace* contains a translation from the ancient Hebrew Dead Sea Scrolls that describes the use of goatskins and reeds to perform an enema as both a medical and spiritual cleanser.[3] About eight decades ago, natural healthcare pioneer John Harvey Kellogg, M.D., of Battle Creek, Michigan, used colon therapy to avoid surgery in a majority of patients afflicted with gastrointestinal diseases.[4] The popularity of colon therapy reached its zenith in the 1920s and 1930s. At that time, colonic irrigation machines were a common sight in hospitals and physicians' offices. Although interest declined with the advent of pharmaceutical and surgical treatments, colon therapy is once again gaining in popularity and is now commonly used by alternative medicine practitioners.[5]

 For instructions on preparing a **coffee enema**, see "How to Administer a Coffee Enema" in this chapter on page 100.

Probiotics

Intestinal cleansing removes both unfriendly and friendly bacteria. It is therefore important to repopulate the intestines with friendly bacteria

Conditions Helped by Colonic Therapy

- Autoimmune diseases, including ankylosing spondylitis and rheumatoid diseases
- Psoriatic arthritis and gout
- Fibromyalgia
- Parasitic infections
- Candida overgrowth
- Irritable bowel syndrome
- PMS and hormonal problems
- Acne, psoriasis, and eczema
- Headaches, especially migraines
- Chronic colds, allergies, and other immune disorders
- Gallbladder afflictions
- Liver disease

afterward, particularly *Lactobacillus acidophilus* and *Bifidobacterium bifidum*. Cabbage is one of the best food sources of friendly bacteria; it can be eaten raw, juiced, or used as the fermented Oriental product called kimchi. Other foods that can help revitalize the colon and encourage the growth of friendly bacteria include rice protein, chicory, onions, garlic, asparagus, bananas, yogurt, and kefir (fermented milk). Be sure to use only organic, plain yogurt or kefir with no sugar or artificial sweeteners. Probiotic supplements can also be useful. It's best to choose a nondairy formula; look for these in the refrigerated section in most health food stores.

The Overburdened Liver

The liver, located beneath the right lower part of the rib cage, is the largest organ in the body and one of the most complicated, rivaled only by the brain. The liver collects and removes foreign particles and chemicals from the blood and detoxifies these poisons through three systems: the Kupffer cells; phase I and phase II biotransformation systems, involving over 75 enzymes; and production of bile. Each system feeds into the others, and all three must be operating at full efficiency for proper detoxification.

Approximately 3 pints of blood pass through the liver each minute for filtering. The Kupffer cells are stationary white blood cells that engulf foreign matter in the blood before it passes through the rest of the liver. When the liver is damaged, toxic, congested, or sluggish, the Kupffer cells become overburdened and the filtration system breaks down, allowing increased levels of antigens, foreign proteins, bowel microorganisms, and dietary waste products to pass through the liver and enter the general circulatory system. Inflammatory agents called cytokines are also released, contributing to the development of inflammation and arthritis.

The most complex of the liver's detoxification mechanisms are

Success Stories: Eliminating Mucoid Plaque Helps Ease Joint Pain

After years of poor diet, constipation, and stagnation, the colon wall accumulates a layer of debris, mucus, impacted feces, minerals, and microorganisms. It resembles a greenish black snake and has the texture of rubber cement. Although many conventional gastroenterologists dismiss the existence of mucoid plaque, we've observed it on several occasions. Richard, 48, had chronic psoriasis and psoriatic arthritis and a history of only two bowel movements per week. We recommended colonic hydrotherapy along with a detoxification diet to start his program. During his fourth colonic treatment, mucoid plaque was dislodged from Richard's colon and expelled. Through colon therapy, nutritional supplements, and adherence to the arthritis diet, Richard experienced a reduction in joint pain and psoriasis and eventually a complete remission of all symptoms.

Orlando, 60, developed joint pain and stiffness, which was particularly unbearable in his spine, when he was 35 years old. The pain soon inhibited his daily activities and interfered with his job. Conventional doctors put him on prednisone, NSAIDs, and gold injections, which brought temporary relief from his joint pain but soon resulted in gastrointestinal disturbances. Orlando decided to seek the advice of an alternative medical practitioner. We reviewed his case and immediately placed him on a restrictive diet that eliminated his favorite snack, hot dogs, and his evening glass of wine. Removing these two items from his diet resulted in a slight improvement in his symptoms and convinced him that exploring alternative medicine might be worthwhile. We then started preparing Orlando for a supervised fast. First, he began to drink fresh vegetables every day and slowly cut back on his intake of solid foods. After he was comfortable on that regime, he began his supervised weeklong water fast. The entire fasting period lasted 40 days and included a daily colonic. During one colonic treatment, a large section of mucoid plaque was passed. Shortly after this session, Orlando reported a surge of energy and reduction of joint pain. He was immediately able to resume a more active life, including athletic pursuits such as biking, swimming, and running. Today he's an active athlete and competes in triathlons.

referred to as the phase I and phase II biotransformation systems. When a toxic chemical, such as alcohol, enters the liver, reactions begin that attempt to break down these chemicals into harmless substances. Phase I is the oxidation phase, in which the original offending substance is broken down by enzymes into intermediate substances. Then the phase II enzymes act to combine these decomposed substances with other molecules (such as sulfur, glutathione, and glycine) to make them more water-soluble and easier for the body to excrete.

Bile, a yellowish brown, orange, or green fluid, is excreted by the liver, stored in the gallbladder, and pumped into the small intestine as needed.

Bile emulsifies or breaks down fat and prevents putrefaction of intestinal contents. The overall goal of the liver's detoxification systems is to convert toxins into a water-soluble form for easy elimination from the body via the stool.

Detecting Defective Detoxification

Defects in the body's ability to activate detoxification pathways create an accumulation of toxins or a slowed excretion rate. Overactivation of phase I results in excessive production of free radicals and toxic by-products. In addition, if phase II is sluggish, the intermediate products created by phase I remain in the system instead of being quickly eliminated. The intermediate substances produced by the phase I reaction can be even more toxic to the system than the original substances and can cause damage to the liver cells. In the case of alcohol, the breakdown products are the highly toxic acetaldehyde and highly reactive chemicals containing oxygen.[6]

Natural health-care practitioners often test patients to evaluate the status of phase I and phase II pathways by using the functional liver detoxification profile. This test involves ingestion of caffeine, aspirin, and acetominophen, followed by collection of saliva and urine samples. Known breakdown products are measured in the samples, helping to determine the liver's ability to efficiently process these substances. If the phase I and phase II systems aren't working well, patients are considered to be "pathologic detoxifiers." An overwhelming percentage of the arthritis patients we've tested show imbalances in their liver detoxification pathways. Causes for this problem include regular use of aspirin, acetaminophen, and other NSAIDs, as well as deficiencies in folic acid, vitamins B_{12}, B complex, and C, and the amino acids glutathione, cysteine, and methionine.

Liver Detoxification Therapies

Balancing the phase I and phase II processes of the liver is extremely important for those with arthritis. Techniques that can help cleanse, tone, and repair damaged liver cells include a liver flush, coffee enemas, castor oil packs, and specific herbs, plants, and foods for liver support.

Liver Flush

A liver flush stimulates the elimination of wastes from the body, increases bile flow, and improves overall liver function. Here are some instructions for preparing and administering a liver flush.

1. Make 1 cup of freshly squeezed juice from organic lemons and/or limes. The number of lemons or limes needed will vary depending on the size of the fruit. Dilute with 1 cup of filtered water.

2. Add the juice of 1 clove of garlic and a small amount of ginger juice. Use a 1- to 2-inch piece of raw ginger root and either put it through a juicer or grate it, then press the shreds with a garlic press to get juice.

3. Add 1 tablespoon of high-quality, organic extra virgin olive oil and blend or shake thoroughly.

4. Drink this juice in the morning and don't eat any food for 1 hour afterward.

5. After an hour has elapsed, drink two cups of a detoxifying herbal tea. You can purchase detoxifying teas in health food stores or make your own by combining equal parts of dandelion, burdock root, fennel, and peppermint. Steep 1 teaspoon of this blend in 1 cup boiling water for 5 minutes, then drink.

6. Do the flush for 10 days, discontinue for 3 days, then resume for 10 days (this is one cycle). Repeat for another cycle.

Coffee Enema

Coffee contains specific chemicals that have been shown to be liver protective.[7] Research by Max Gerson, M.D., of the Gerson Institute, who was recently inducted into the Orthomolecular Medicine Hall of Fame, led to the use of coffee enemas to stimulate liver detoxification. A coffee enema, easily done at home, can help purge the liver of accumulated toxins, dead cells, and waste products. The enema is prepared by brewing organic caffeinated coffee through a natural brown filter, letting it cool to body temperature, and delivering it via an enema bag (see "How to Administer a Coffee Enema," page 100).

Castor Oil Packs

Castor oil comes from the bean of the castor plant, *Oleum ricini*. The plant itself is quite poisonous, but the oil pressed out of the bean is safe to use, since the toxic constituents remain in the seeds. The Egyptians used castor oil as a laxative for cleansing the bowels and as a scalp rub to make hair grow and shine. When rubbed into sore muscles and joints just before infrared heat treatment, it is said to reduce the pain and swelling of rheumatism and arthritis. Castor oil packs have been used traditionally for many conditions, including liver problems, constipation,

How to Administer a Coffee Enema

It's best to do coffee enemas in the morning, since they can cause insomnia when used near bedtime, especially in individuals sensitive to caffeine. Eat a piece of fruit before the coffee enema to activate your upper digestive tract. Keep all equipment clean and sanitized. Coffee enemas can be useful in minimizing the headaches, fever, nausea, intestinal spasms, and drowsiness that often accompany detoxification programs.

1. Brew 4 cups of organic coffee and allow it to cool to body temperature.
2. Lubricate the rectal enema tube with K-Y Jelly, aloe vera gel, or another lubricant. Hang the enema bag above you, but no more than 2 feet from your body; the best level is approximately 6 inches above your intestines. Lying on your right side, draw both legs close to your abdomen.
3. Insert the tube several inches into your rectum. Open the stopcock and allow the coffee to run in very slowly to avoid cramping. Breathe deeply and try to relax.
4. Retain the solution for 12 to 15 minutes. If you have trouble retaining or taking the full amount, lower the bag; if you feel spasms, lower the bag to the floor to relieve the pressure. After about 20 seconds, slowly start raising the bag toward its original level. You can also pinch the tube to control the flow. Move to the toilet to release any excess liquid.

and other ailments involving elimination, as well as nonmalignant ovarian fibroid cysts and headaches. The oil helps to draw out toxins, release tension, and improve blood circulation, especially in the lower abdomen (see "Castor Oil Pack Instructions," page 101).

Dietary Recommendations to Support the Liver

Foods that help the liver include cabbage and all cruciferous vegetables (such as brussels sprouts, cauliflower, and broccoli), which aid the liver in both phase I and phase II detoxification. Brussels sprouts are the best of the cruciferous vegetables for the liver, according to John Bastyr, N.D., the founding father of Bastyr University of Naturopathic Medicine, in Seattle, Washington. Other helpful foods include onions, garlic, leeks, and chives. All of these foods for the liver contain sulfur.

Beets contain high levels of betaine, a powerful lipotropic agent, meaning it increases the flow of bile. Black radish and artichokes contain cynarin, which has liver-protective properties similar to milk thistle. Olive oil promotes the production of bile in the liver and also protects it from harmful microorganisms. Many aromatic cooking herbs and spices also aid the liver in its detoxification process. Outstanding among them is rosemary, which assists in the production and movement of bile through the liver and gallbladder. Dill, caraway, and fennel aid in phase II detoxification.

Therapeutic Herbs for the Liver

Milk thistle (*Silybum marianum*): For centuries, European herbalists have used the bioflavonoid silymarin, found in milk thistle, for restoring liver function. Bioflavonoids are plant pigments with beneficial properties; they protect against damage from destructive free radicals in the body and enhance the activity of vitamin C. Silymarin accelerates the process of regenerating damaged liver tissue, thereby freeing the organ to carry out its key functions. It has been proven effective against acetaminophen and petrochemical solvent poisoning.[9] It's best to use milk thistle standardized to 70% to 80% silymarin content.

Katuka (*Picrorhiza kurroa*): This tiny plant grows in the Himalayas at altitudes between 9,000 to 15,000 feet. Its active ingredient has been found comparable or superior to silymarin. Clinical trials on patients with OA, rheumatic pains, ankylosing spondylitis, and psoriasis have shown a favorable response.[10]

Dandelion (*Taraxacum officinale*): As a liver and digestive tonic, as well as blood cleanser and diuretic, dandelion aids in detoxification of the body. As testimony to dandelion's powerful influence on the liver, severe hepatitis has been reversed in as short a period as a week by dandelion tea along with dietary restrictions.[11] Given that chemical or heavy metal toxicity is frequently involved in arthritis, dandelion can help cleanse the body and support the liver in its elimination functions. As a digestive tonic, dandelion may also help with the gastrointestinal complaints associated with arthritis.

Green tea: Green tea is rich in catechins, a bioflavonoid used by European naturopaths and medical doctors to treat chemical hepatitis,

Castor Oil Pack Instructions

1. Fold a flannel sheet to fit over your whole abdomen.

2. Cut a piece of plastic 1 to 2 inches larger than flannel sheet.

3. Soak the flannel sheet in gently heated castor oil. Fold it over and squeeze until some of the liquid oozes out, then unfold.

4. Prepare the surface where you will be lying, covering it with a large plastic sheet and an old towel to prevent staining.

5. Lie down on the towel and place the oil-soaked flannel sheet over your abdomen. Place the fitted plastic piece over the flannel sheet, then apply a hot water bottle over the area.

6. Wrap a towel under and around your torso.

7. Rest for 1 to 2 hours.

8. Rinse off the oil with a solution of 3 tablespoons baking soda to 1 quart water.

9. Repeat one to three times per week, or as instructed by your health-care practitioner.

How Traditional Chinese Medicine Views the Liver

The idea of a congested or sluggish liver is an ancient concept in traditional Chinese medicine (TCM; SEE QUICK DEFINITION). The signs of a sluggish or congested liver can manifest as PMS, fatigue, lethargy, an inability to properly digest foods (particularly fats), multiple allergies, environmental and chemical sensitivities, constipation, and arthritis.

TCM maintains that various emotions are connected to different organs. The liver is considered the reservoir of anger toward other people or toward the self. Anger affects the liver's ability to govern the flow of qi (vital life force energy), blood, and vital nutrients to ligaments, tendons, sinews, joints, bones, and muscles. One of the main Chinese herbs used in liver ailments as well as arthritis is gardenia. It is known as the "happiness herb" because it has an ability to loosen emotions like anger, which have been stuck due to chronic liver congestion.[8] In TCM, the liver is associated with the wood element and is represented by the color greenish yellow. Leafy greens and other substances of that color are considered beneficial for toning and boosting liver function.

A Chinese doctor once told us that he recommended eating asparagus to all his patients because asparagus will bring joy and happiness and release anger in the liver. This is fascinating, as most patients with arthritis have a deficiency in a detoxifying enzymatic reaction called sulfoxidation, which is necessary for digesting sulfur-containing foods, like asparagus. A self-test to see if the sulfoxidation pathway is operating normally is to eat asparagus and then note the odor of your urine after consumption. If your body is having difficulty processing sulfur, it will cause a distinctive odor.

 Traditional Chinese medicine (TCM) originated in China over 5,000 years ago and is a comprehensive system of medical practice that heals the body according to the principles of nature and balance. A TCM physician considers the flow of vital life force energy (qi) in a patient through close examination of the patient's pulse, tongue, body odor, voice tone and strength, and general demeanor, among other elements. Underlying imbalances and disharmony in the body are described in terminology analogous to the natural world (heat, cold, dryness, or dampness).

cirrhosis, and other environmental and viral forms of liver disease. Catechins can be taken as a nutritional supplement.[12]

Other herbs: Most herbs and plant foods contain important phytonutrients (*phyto* means "plant"), substances that have health-protecting qualities. Burdock, goldenseal, baptisia, smilax, Oregon grape root, and echinacea all contain phytonutrients that act as Kupffer cell stimulants. We've documented improved liver function after using these herbs in our medical clinic.[13]

Success Story: Detoxification
Heals Juvenile Rheumatoid Arthritis

Cam, age seven, woke up the day after her birthday party vomiting and running a high fever. Her mother wasn't surprised by her illness; the day before, Cam had overdosed on excitement, birthday cake, and ice cream. Cam's symptoms were alleviated by taking acetaminophen to reduce the fever, but her mother noticed that Cam continued to feel fatigued and appeared abnormally pale. A few weeks later, Cam's fever returned, coupled with joint and muscle pain and a dry, hacking cough. She was taken to the family pediatrician, who, upon running a complete blood count test, found a high level of white blood cells, suggesting a possible infection. He prescribed antibiotics, and Cam and her mother returned home to wait anxiously for her recovery. But the recovery never came; Cam's fever and migrating joint pain persisted after several months.

Additional blood tests showed that Cam's platelet count was dangerously high. (Platelets are disk-shaped cells produced in bone marrow and released into the blood, where they are essential for clotting). Her platelet count was 922 (normal is 130 to 400), suggesting either severe anemia, chronic infection, or inflammatory conditions. Her red blood cell count was 9.8 grams per deciliter (normal being 10.3–14.9 g/dl), confirming a moderate case of anemia. An infectious disease specialist initially diagnosed Cam's problems as long-term pneumonia and prescribed a five-day cycle of antibiotics. But Cam's joint pain continued to become more debilitating.

Because Cam's physical complaints and anemia matched the symptoms of RA (70% of RA patients have anemia), a rheumatologist joined her medical team. But each test for RA came back negative, and her doctors, unable to conclusively confirm RA, decided that a bacterial or viral infection must be responsible. Cam was placed on prednisone (an anti-inflammatory steroid), methotrexate (a cancer chemotherapy drug used on RA patients to decrease inflammation), and antibiotics.

By this time, Cam was no longer an active and vibrant seven-year-old. She could no longer walk by herself and even had problems standing. She had lost 12 pounds and had developed a rash on her thighs and abdomen. Profuse night sweats made it difficult for her to sleep, and she was always exhausted. The steroid therapy helped ease the pain in her joints for a while, but it caused many side effects.

When we first met her, Cam's face was bloated (moon-shaped) from the disease and the prednisone. Her symptoms—joint and muscle pain, night sweats, and fevers—still suggested RA, although her conventional doctors had diagnosed her with infectious arthritis, since her rheumatoid factor (SEE QUICK DEFINITION), at 32, was normal (normal range is 0 to 39). However, natural medical practitioners pay close attention to the low end and the high end of what is conventionally considered normal. To us, Cam's value of 32 was approaching the high end. We decided to test for possible parasitic infections, heavy metal toxicity, and delayed food allergies, all contributing factors in RA that are commonly overlooked by conventional doctors.

Darkfield microscopy showed that Cam's immune system was compromised. She had low numbers of red blood cells, and they were abnormally clumped together like rolls of coins. Red blood cells are unable to deliver oxygen to the tissues or export toxic waste products out of the body when they're bunched together in rows; a condition referred to rouleau. Another indicator that Cam's body was unable to fight pathogens was the abnormally large and sluggish appearance of her white blood cells, a common side effect of the prescription drugs methotrexate and prednisone. We also found metabolic by-products (due to poor diet or faulty breakdown of waste products) that appeared in the darkfield screen as red and yellow crystals with sharp edges. These crystals can accumulate in joints, muscles, and tissues, causing irritation and pain.

Blood and hair analysis confirmed that Cam had heavy metal toxicity. We found high levels of copper, cadmium, nickel, and aluminum—heavy metals that contribute to liver problems and autoimmune diseases, including RA. Cam also had parasites and the yeast *Candida albicans*, probably due to the antibiotics and her nutritionally poor diet. Taxing her already crippled immune system were food allergies to major components of Cam's diet: wheat, milk, fish, chicken, lamb, cauliflower, celery, squash, and bell pepper. Cam ate the basic unhealthy standard American fare, including hot dogs, fast foods, sodas, and lots of processed food.

Our nutritionist put Cam on an allergen-free diet, restricting wheat products and emphasizing organic vegetables, soy products, small amounts of organic meat, and low carbohydrates. To counteract her anemia, her new diet was rich in organic iron from sources such as organic beets and leafy greens, and she supplemented with spirulina or blue-green algae. To ensure that she received enough essential fatty acids, we suggested that her mother give her a salad dressing made from olive oil, flaxseed oil, lemon juice, oregano, and garlic.

Cam was advised not to eat fast foods, sodas, or other processed foods. If she craved a soda, we recommended that she add a little seltzer water to her herbal tea instead. All food preservatives, chemicals, additives, and dyes were to be avoided. We also recommended using a filter for drinking and bathing water, because toxic chemicals can be absorbed through the skin as well as ingested. Cam's system was so sensitive that she couldn't tolerate the normal levels of toxins most people encounter and accommodate every day.

We also started Cam on a protocol of intravenous vitamin and mineral therapies to support her liver function, reduce inflammation, prevent cellular damage, and stimulate the growth of connective tissue and cartilage. The solution contained sterile water, potassium chloride, vitamin C, magnesium sulfate, heparin, selenium, manganese, zinc, chromium, B complex, B_6, and taurine. Cam received intramuscular injections (one per week) of vitamin B_{12}, folic acid, and a liver extract that supports the liver and helps with anemia.

In addition, Cam took the following supplements.

- A keratin polymer to help chelate (bind and remove) heavy metals and metabolic wastes

- MSM (methylsulfonylmethane) and shark cartilage to repair damaged cartilage, stimulate the immune system, and relieve pain

- Malic acid to reduce pain in connective tissues

- Micellized vitamin E for antioxidant support (micellized nutrients are more rapidly absorbed through cell membranes)

- Vitamin B_{12} as methylcobalamin for cellular energy

- Folic acid for nutritional support and to replenish folic acid levels depleted by methotrexate

- Digestive enzymes to be taken with meals to help digestion, and to be taken again on an empty stomach to help alleviate joint pain

- Vitamin C, vitamin B$_6$, and pantothenic acid to support the adrenal glands, under stress from constant steroidal drug intake
- Yunnan Paiyao, a blend of Chinese herbs, to support the easy flow of blood to the muscles and joints and alleviate gut permeability

For Cam's anemia, her conventional physician had prescribed ferrous sulfate, a form of iron that contributes to free radical production and is harmful to joints. We replaced it with ferrous fumarate, a nontoxic form of iron, and also gave her yellow dock, an herb with high iron content.

Several therapies were used to help with her detoxification process. We prescribed a combination of weekly visits to a physiotherapist and nightly baths using Epsom salts and baking soda to relax her aching muscles and joints, and pull toxins out through the skin. In addition, every night before bedtime Cam's mother massaged her with a mixture of warmed sesame oil for increasing essential fatty acids and rebuilding cartilage, mustard oil for stimulating joints by increasing circulation, and cayenne pepper, a mild analgesic for pain relief.

After four months on the regimen, Cam started to have pain-free days and less inflammation. She was then able to gradually decrease her intake of conventional medications. Cam continued on these therapies for over a year, during which time her symptoms slowly receded. She stopped having night sweats and fevers, and her joint pain lessened, although she still experienced occasional stiffness. A follow-up urine analysis showed that her body was adequately absorbing essential nutrients. It took two and a half years on the diet and nutritional therapies to raise her red blood cell count into the normal range. Her parents were tremendously relieved to see their daughter active and running around the playground again. Now a young adult, Cam reports that if she does too much and stays up late several nights in a row, she experiences the return of some of her symptoms, including fatigue and joint pain. Therefore, she has to maintain a fairly strict regimen of healthy eating and getting enough rest to feel top-notch.

The Stagnated Lymphatic System

Lymph is a clear to milky fluid containing nutrients that must be delivered to cells. It also carries waste products and cellular debris that accumulate in the tissue spaces between cells to the bloodstream for elimination. The lymphatic system is the body's master drain, collecting and filtering the lymph fluid. Interspersed throughout the lymph channels are the lymph nodes, clusters of immune tissue that work as filters to remove foreign and potentially harmful substances from the lymph fluid. Each lymph node contains scavenger cells (macrophages and reticulo-endothelial cells) that destroy toxins and microbes. Lymph nodes are clustered in strategic junctures of the body, such as the head and neck, the armpits, and the groin. The gastrointestinal tract, including the appendix, contains a tremendous quantity of lymph nodes called the gut-associated lymphoid tissue (GALT), a primary filter for the bloodstream.

Unlike the circulatory system, which uses the heart to pump the blood, the lymphatic system doesn't have its own pump. Instead, it depends on movement of skeletal muscles during normal day-to-day activities, exercise, and breathing, as well as massage and other lymphatic drainage techniques. As the muscles contract and relax, they push the lymph fluid along; backflow is prevented by valves throughout the lymphatic system. The lymph is full of

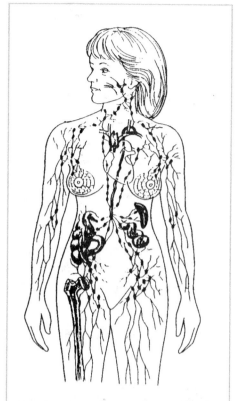

Lymph nodes are clusters of immune tissue that work as filters by removing foreign and potentially harmful substances from the lymph fluid. Lymph nodes are part of the lymphatic system, which is the body's master drain.

nutrients on their way to the cells and waste products that must be removed. Any interference with this flow can create serious problems for the body.

Stagnant lymphatic fluid changes in consistency, going from clear and thin to thick and cloudy in the early stages of toxicity. If the lymph remains stationary, it will progress to a glutinous consistency similar to thick cream, and eventually cottage cheese. Viscous lymphatic fluid becomes an oxygen-deprived sludge that impedes the flow of nutrients to the cells and barricades toxic substances from exiting the extracellular spaces. Lack of nutrients to tissues combined with the stagnation of waste products leads to degenerative diseases, including cancer and arthritis. Lymphatic stagnation can be caused by allergenic and mucus-forming foods, chronic constipation, musculoskeletal imbalances, lack of exercise, improper breathing, prescription drugs, and impairment of local or systemic circulation due to complications of diabetes or arteriosclerosis.

Therapies for Improving Lymphatic Drainage

It is of paramount importance to prevent stagnation of the lymphatic system. This ensures that the lymph fluid continues to circulate freely throughout the body and that the body is properly detoxified. Techniques that encourage lymphatic drainage include manual lymph massage, light beam therapy, dry skin brushing, exercise, and herbs.

Manual Lymph Drainage

Manual lymph drainage is a specially designed massage technique that uses gentle, stationary circular motions on the lymph nodes, palpating with the tips or the entire length of the fingers. These motions act like an external pump that pulls lymphatic fluid through the lymph channels and enhances the release of toxins. Lymph drain massage should not be confused with conventional massage techniques, as it relies on gentle and directed manipulations designed to induce lymph flow. The lymph should only be massaged lightly, as too much pressure can cause thickening. Lymph drain massage is a commonly prescribed technique in Europe, especially in Germany, Austria, France, and the Scandinavian countries. It is also growing in popularity in the United States.

Do-at-Home Lymph Massage

While not intended as a substitute for lymph drain massage, a self-massage technique may be helpful in stimulating the flow of lymph. Doing one leg at a time, elevate the leg and gently massage up from your ankle, around your knee, and up toward your hip, massaging the front and back of your leg. This technique moves lymph fluid in the direction it should naturally flow. The ideal time to perform this type of massage is at the end of the day's activities.

Light Beam Therapy

High-tech lymphatic drainage uses various types of light beam generators to break up lymph blockage. The light beam generator looks like a flashlight with a long, extensible hose. Practitioners use this handheld device to focus energy on blocked lymph areas. The energy from the generator breaks the electrical bonds that hold clusters of lymph protein molecules together, thus unclogging stagnated lymph fluid. This therapy is often used to enhance the benefits of lymph massage. It is also very effective as a therapy for lymphedema, a condition wherein over-accumulation of lymphatic fluid causes swelling.

Dry Skin Brushing

Dry skin brushing improves flow in the lymphatic system by stimulating the lymph nodes under the skin. This technique is based on the theory that underlies acupuncture, which states that there are an estimated 3 million nerve points spread over the surface of the skin, 700 of which are nodal, meaning they can serve as treatment nodes in acupuncture. By applying friction to the skin with a soft, natural-fiber brush (called a dry skin brush, available at most health food stores), a loofah, or a tightly rolled towel, one can stimulate all of these nerve points, which correspond to specific organs, glands, and muscles.

The physical motion of dry skin brushing moves lymph fluid through the lymphatic channels to encourage drainage and prevent stagnation. Blood and lymphatic circulation and metabolism are stimulated in all organs and tissues as well. Brushed skin is better able to eliminate toxins from the body, as oils (sebum) and dead skin are removed and pores are unclogged. Toxins are transferred into the main lymphatic drainage ducts, which go directly to the liver for elimination. Qi, or vital life force energy, can move freely through the meridians, thus relieving the pain caused by obstruction. Additionally, white blood cells (lymphocytes) migrate into the skin after brushing, enhancing the function of the immune system.

To perform dry skin brushing, begin gently brushing from the ends of the arms with long strokes that sweep toward the trunk of the body. Do all sides of the arms. Then brush the head and neck with downward strokes toward the clavicle (collar bone). Brush the feet and legs upward toward the groin area; be sure to brush all areas of the legs. As you brush the trunk, use upward-sweeping motions toward the heart. The ideal time to perform dry skin brushing is prior to showering. When you're finished, jump into the shower to remove the dead skin cells. Be sure to clean the brush thoroughly with soap and water and then hydrogen peroxide after each use.

Exercise

Any exercise helps to pump the lymph, because of the contracting and relaxing motions of the muscles. The rate of lymph flow increases dramatically during physical activity. Light bouncing on a mini trampoline is especially effective in helping to restore lymph flow. The mini trampoline has a flexible jumping surface measuring 28 to 40 inches in

Lymph movement can also be aided by contrast hydrotherapy (alternating hot and cold water), yoga, qigong, and massage. For more information about **physical therapies**, see chapter 14, Exercises and Physical Therapies, pages pages 295–320.

diameter and set 6 to 9 inches off the ground. Bouncing on the mini trampoline allows rapid changes in gravity to act as a powerful lymphatic pump, causing expansion of lymph ducts and channels for increased circulation. As you land on the mini trampoline, your body is pulled down with twice the force of gravity, which makes this practice more effective than running for stimulating the flow of lymph.[14] This exercise can be tailored to an individual's fitness level, and can yield results in just 5 to 10 minutes per day.

Herbs That Stimulate Lymphatic Drainage

Poke root (Phytolacca americana): Poke root is used to stimulate white blood cells (B and T lymphocytes) to assist the immune system in fighting off viruses, such as Epstein-Barr, and is a powerful remedy in laryngitis, swollen tonsils, and sore throat. Poke root is also used when lymph nodes throughout the body are swollen; it's one of the most potent herbs for lymphatic drainage. Caution: Poke root can be highly toxic. Use only under medical supervision.

Cleavers (Galium aparine): Also known as goose grass or bedstraw, cleavers is a safer alternative to poke root. Cleavers reduces swelling and edema and is also a kidney tonic. It removes "damp congestion," the traditional Chinese medicine designation for the pain associated with arthritis, and helps cleanse the lymphatic system. Fresh, preserved cleavers juice can be added to vegetable juice or carrot-apple-ginger juice, or you can make a spring tonic by combining cleavers with dandelion greens and chickweed.

Use poke root only as directed by an experienced health-care practitioner. It can be toxic or fatal in relatively small doses. Toxic symptoms include a burning sensation in the mouth and stomach, drowsiness, weakness, sweating, prostration, dyspnea (labored breathing), and respiratory paralysis.

Supporting the Portals: Kidneys, Skin, and Lungs

An effective detoxification protocol must include therapies that enhance the body's ability to expel waste products through all the detoxification pathways. The exit routes, or portals—the kidneys, skin, and lungs—must be supported to ensure that toxins are efficiently removed. If there is an imbalance in these organs, toxins can be reabsorbed, compromising detoxification and impeding the healing process.

Kidneys

The kidneys assist the body in removing nitrogenous wastes originating from protein metabolism, xenobiotics (environmental estrogens), drug residues, and a host of other water-soluble toxins. They also regulate sodium and potassium levels, as well as blood pressure. During detoxification, it's important to keep the urine diluted by drinking at least 2 quarts of filtered water per day. Concentrated urine contains high levels of toxins, especially during detoxification, and these can cause kidney damage. Periodic laboratory measurements of kidney and liver function during a detoxification program are a necessity.

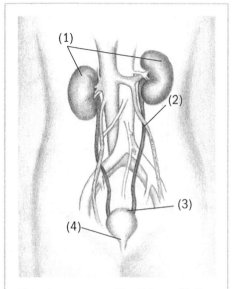

The urinary system: The kidneys (1) filter water-soluble toxins and other wastes from the blood. These substances are excreted as urine, which is sent through the ureter (2) to the bladder (3) for temporary storage until it can be expelled from the body through the urethra (4).

Botanical diuretics assist the kidneys in excreting waste; some increase blood flow to the kidneys, while others work by inhibiting the reabsorption of water, which increases urinary output. Botanical diuretics are also helpful in reducing uric acid levels; this is especially important for those suffering from gout.

Dandelion *(Taraxacum officinale):* Dandelion leaves are an excellent diuretic and also support the liver.

Parsley *(Petroselinum sativa):* Much more than just a plate garnish, parsley is used to support kidney function because of its diuretic action. Include fresh parsley juice in vegetable juices and eat it regularly as a vegetable.

Horsetail *(Equisetum arvense):* Also called scouring rush because it was used by native peoples to scour dishes, horsetail is an excellent diuretic and also contains the mineral silica, a critical nutrient for bone, muscle, and cartilage formation. Silica has a long history of use in rheumatism.[15]

Skin

The skin is the largest organ of the body. Often referred to as "the third kidney," it's the first line of defense against external pathogens. The pores and glands of the skin are important organs of elimination through which toxic chemicals can be excreted via either sweat or sebum (oil secreted by the skin).[16] Chemical toxins, such as formaldehyde, phenol, various insecticides, chlorine, and petroleum products, may be implicated in the development of immune system deregulation, which leads to rheumatoid diseases. In addition to entering the body through inhalation, these chemicals can be absorbed through the skin, by drinking tap water, or during bathing.[17]

Dry Skin Brushing. To enhance the skin's ability to detoxify, use a dry skin brush or loofah sponge. Brush the skin with long strokes toward the heart, then bathe or shower. This helps remove the top layer of dead skin cells and stimulates lymphatic drainage (see page 109 for more information on dry skin brushing).

Sauna (Heat Stress Detoxification). Using a sauna can effectively clear the body of fat-soluble toxins. The heat of the sauna helps arthritis by making the muscles, joints, and sinews more pliable and by increasing blood flow to the joints. Studies of fat biopsies before and after a heat stress detoxification protocol revealed an average of 21.3% reduction in body levels of 16 toxic chemicals, including PCBs and PBBs, with a 64% to 75% reduction in harmful toxins.[18] The study found that toxins in patients continued to decrease for up to four months after discontinuing heat and detoxification therapy. Detoxification programs that included fasting, juicing, sauna therapy, exercise, and lymphatic drainage produced a reduction of various pesticide residues ranging up to 66%.[19]

Sauna Brew

This herb tea is recommended for people using sauna therapy. The tea expedites sweating, especially if consumed as a hot tea before and during the sauna treatment, thereby enhancing the removal of toxins from the body. Patients have commented that this blend also tastes exceptionally good. Combine equal parts of the following herbs.

- Cinnamon (*Cinnamomum zeylanicum*)
- Ginger (*Zingiber officinale*)
- Boneset (*Eupatorium perfoliatum*)
- Yarrow (*Achillea millefolium*)
- Peppermint (*Mentha piperita*)
- Elder (*Sambucus nigra*)

Use 1 tablespoon of the herb mixture per cup of tea. Pour 1 cup of steaming hot water over the herbs, cover, and allow to steep for 20 minutes.

Lungs

During the energy crisis in the 1970s, U.S. building construction practices changed; homes, offices, schools, and most buildings were sealed tightly and better insulated. This saves a great deal of energy but tends to trap indoor air pollution, including pollens and other allergens, oils, and dry-cleaning fluid (a known liver toxin). Toxic chemicals such as benzene (a carcinogen) are released from paint, new carpets, drapes, and upholstery. Formaldehyde vapors rise up from plywood, new cabinets, furniture, carpets, drapes, wallpaper, and paneling. All enter the body through the lungs.

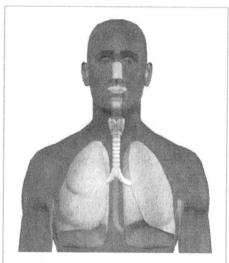

The lungs and respiratory system are important avenues of detoxification.

Herbs for Lung Detoxification. Herbs are frequently used to target specific aspects of lung contamination and detoxification.

- Fenugreek and horehound help decrease production and thickness of mucus secretions.
- Wild cherry bark is an expectorant that helps remove mucus and reduce congestion.
- Mullein, elecampane, and grindelia strengthen lung tissue.
- Eucalyptus and thyme oil are antiseptics that kill microbial organisms; a combination of these herbs can be taken as a tincture.

Inhalation Therapy. Steam inhalation can be very helpful for detoxifying the lungs. Add two to three drops of eucalyptus and thyme oils to a pot of boiling water, remove the pot from the stove, and place your head above the steam. Create a tent by covering your head with a towel, and inhale the steam vapors. Be sure to keep your head far enough above the steam so as not to get burned.

Exercise. Exercise helps the lungs by increasing the perfusion of blood,

 For more information about **yoga breathing techniques**, see chapter 14, Exercises and Physical Therapies, pages 295–320.

which enhances intake of oxygen and qi (vital life force energy) and increases elimination of waste products through exhalation. Aerobic exercise, such as running, cycling, and walking, can help clear the lungs. However, aerobic activity needs to be done in fresh, clean air; running in a polluted environment only increases the overall body burden of toxins and should be avoided. Yoga breathing techniques are excellent for cleansing the lungs and increasing oxygen levels in the body. They are especially useful for arthritis patients, who may be in too much pain to do aerobic exercise.

six

Eradicating Bacteria and Yeast

There are close to 400 species of bacteria in the gastrointestinal tract. Under normal conditions, friendly bacteria (such as *Lactobacillus acidophilus* and *Bifidobacterium bifidum*) predominate and contribute to digestion and the overall health of the body. However, dysbiosis, an intestinal imbalance, has become increasingly common. When a person is afflicted with dysbiosis, pathogenic bacteria dominate their intestine, impairing digestion, absorption of nutrients, and the normal elimination cycle. These bacteria also provoke allergic reactions to food and contribute to erosion of the intestinal membrane and infiltration of inappropriate substances into the bloodstream, a condition referred to as leaky gut syndrome.

Dysbiosis is a major cofactor in the development of many health problems, including rheumatoid arthritis, acne, chronic fatigue, depression, digestive disorders, bloating, food allergies, PMS, and cancer. Of the pathogenic

> **IN THIS CHAPTER**
>
> - The Detoxification Defense System
> - What Causes Intestinal Imbalance?
> - The Role of Intestinal Toxins in Arthritis
> - Bacteria and Arthritis
> - Success Story: Treating Candida Relieves Juvenile Arthritis
> - Illuminating the Candida Connection

> Dysbiosis is a major cofactor in the development of many health problems, including rheumatoid arthritis, acne, chronic fatigue, depression, digestive disorders, food allergies, PMS, and cancer. Until this condition is addressed, it's unlikely that people with arthritis will completely reverse their problem.

bacteria most significantly implicated in arthritis, three are of special interest—klebsiella, proteus, and the yeastlike fungus candida. Until they are eliminated and intestinal balance is restored, it's unlikely that people with arthritis will completely reverse their problem.

What Causes Intestinal Imbalance?

The standard American diet (SAD) is largely responsible for dysbiosis. It is a sad diet indeed, for it has not only led to a nation with a staggering number of obese individuals but it has also caused chronic aberrations in the digestive flora. This diet is typically high in commercial meat products, which contain large amounts of chemical residues from the pesticides and herbicides used in livestock feed, along with hormones and antibiotics used to make the animals grow larger and more rapidly. Ingestion of antibiotics, either through food products or prescribed medication, severely alters the intestinal flora by killing off bacteria, including beneficial microorganisms.[1] As the bacterial communities repopulate after prolonged use of antibiotics, the colonic environment favors the growth of disease-causing organisms in lieu of the healthier bacteria. Consuming large quantities of sugar and refined carbohydrates and relatively few whole foods and vegetables also adds to the negative effects on the intestinal environment.

Incomplete digestion is also a problem. The body depends on the stomach's digestive juices and enzymes (SEE QUICK DEFINITION) secreted by the

Alternative Medicine Therapies for Bacteria and Yeast

- Arthritis diet
- Dietary recommendations
- Ayurvedic antifungal therapies
- Herbal remedies
- Nutritional supplements
- Probiotics

pancreas to properly break down food. However, many people have a deficiency of both hydrochloric acid (the stomach's main digestive acid) and pancreatic enzymes, which leads to incomplete digestion. When foods are not digested properly, especially amino acids (from proteins), they putrefy in the intestines and release toxins into the system. For example, the amino acid ornithine is ingested as part of a normal diet. If it is not broken down completely, however, it undergoes unfavorable chemical changes, converting into a toxic substance called putrescine,

Enzymes are specialized living proteins fundamental to all processes in the body. They are necessary for every chemical reaction in the body and for the normal activity of our organs, tissues, fluids, and cells. Enzymes are essential for the production of the energy required for all cellular functions, and they enable the body to digest and assimilate food. Different enzymes do different jobs: proteases digest proteins, amylases digest carbohydrates, lipases digest fats, cellulases digest fiber, and disaccharidases digest sugars. Enzymes also assist in clearing the body of toxins and cellular debris.

which then degrades into polyamines, such as spermadine, spermine, and cadaverine. These endotoxins tend to be elevated in individuals with arthritis.

Leaky Gut

In the unhealthy state of dysbiosis, the cellular "glue" that keeps the mucosal membrane of the intestines intact is slowly attacked and eventually develops gaping holes, initiating leaky gut syndrome. The substances that were once sealed off from the body can then easily pass through the intestinal wall and trigger inflammatory cascades, allergic reactions, and more

For an in-depth discussion of **leaky gut syndrome**, see chapter 8, Alleviating Leaky Gut Syndrome, pages 149–165.

serious illnesses, such as arthritis. As intestinal "garbage" escapes into the bloodstream, the immune system attacks what it perceives as antigens (foreign bodies) and inflammation results. Inflammation leads to gastrointestinal disorders (bloating, flatulence, heartburn, diarrhea, and constipation),[2] as well as arthritis,[3] diabetes,[4] heart disease,[5] and other illnesses.

The overall body burden of circulating immune complexes increases as a result of leaky gut syndrome. Some of the toxic by-products produced by pathogenic microorganisms are carcinogens. They damage brain and nervous system tissues, and interfere with neurological functions. Intestinal endotoxins also block the body's energy production pathways, par-

QUICK DEFINITION

The **Krebs cycle** (also known as the citric acid cycle) is a metabolic process that occurs in the mitochondria, small organelles in each cell of the body. It is an essential step in cellular respiration (the exchange of oxygen and carbon dioxide between the cell and the environment). Foods consumed are transformed by digestion into smaller molecules, such as glucose, fatty acids, and amino acids; these are further converted into carbon compounds called pyruvates and acetates. In the Krebs cycle, acetates and pyruvates are converted into carbon dioxide and four pairs of electrons. The energy found in these electrons is eventually stored in adenosine triphosphate (ATP). ATP is the molecular fuel that provides energy to every cell.

ticularly the Krebs cycle (SEE QUICK DEFINITION), which occurs in the mitochondria (energy-producing centers) of all the body's cells.

The Role of Intestinal Toxins in Arthritis

Toxins produced in the intestines contribute to the arthritis process by stimulating inflammatory cascades in the body. Inflammation is triggered by endotoxins, candida, bacteria such as streptococcus, and various food allergens. Although inflammation is a natural protective mechanism, it can lead to tissue and joint damage if it becomes chronic.

Intestinal toxins trigger inflammation by stimulating a noncellular part of the immune system known as the complement pathway. This refers to a series of 30 proteins that are activated in a chain reaction when the immune system senses a foreign protein (antigen). The complement system's legitimate job is to amplify inflammation, summoning additional white blood cells to the tissues to aid in the removal of foreign matter. When the inflammatory response gets out of control, however, the condition shifts into a disease process and healthy cell structures are broken down by the excessive white blood cell activity. As the white blood cells release powerful peroxides (like hydrogen peroxide) to oxidize invaders, healthy tissues are oxidized as well.

The liver is also involved in the inflammatory response. Under normal conditions, the liver traps about 99% of the bacteria that escape from the intestines. These intestinal endotoxins activate the liver's Kupffer cells, which causes a release of interleukin-2. Interleukin-2 activates other white blood cells to act aggressively to remove waste products from the tissues. If, however, the liver is overburdened, weakened, or compromised by poor diet, excessive toxins, or other factors, it becomes less efficient at processing circulating immune complexes. These complexes then escape the liver's filtering system and enter the body's connective tissues, producing inflammation and eventually tissue damage. Another side effect of increased toxins and subsequent white blood cell infiltration is an elevation in the number of free radicals. The free radicals generated by the white blood cells can quickly deplete the body's supplies of antioxidants and initiate inflammation and damage throughout the body.

Bacteria and Arthritis

In the 1970s, the British immunologist Alan Ebringer, M.D., a member of the department of rheumatology at both Middlesex Hospital and Kings College in London, suggested a correlation between ankylosing spondylitis (a type of arthritis that affects the back and spine), a specific bacteria, and a specific human gene. Dr. Ebringer discovered that 96% of ankylosing spondylitis patients carry the genetic marker HLA-B27.[6] When the HLA-B27 gene is expressed or activated, it forms a particular pattern on the surface of the cell. These patterns act as a signaling device to the immune system and help immune cells differentiate between healthy cells and those which should be destroyed. Klebsiella bacteria have cell surface markers very similar to the pattern on human cells with the gene HLA-B27, a phenomenon called molecular mimicry. The similarity acts as an effective camouflage technique for the bacteria, allowing them to hide from the host's immune system. However, once the immune system recognizes the bacteria and begins to attack them, it then also attacks body tissues with similar cell surface markers.[7] The body's reaction to its own tissues as something foreign constitutes an autoimmune disease, a potentially serious health problem.

Dr. Ebringer found that many ankylosing spondylitis patients have intestinal overgrowth of klebsiella and high blood levels of klebsiella antibodies, and that klebsiella antigens (proteins recognized by the immune system as foreign substances) cross-react with HLA-B27, initiating

Causes of Enzyme Depletion

Enzyme depletion is an important factor in intestinal imbalance and may be caused by a number of factors:

- Pesticides and chemicals in foods
- Hybridization and genetic engineering of plants
- Bovine growth hormone (BGH) used in raising livestock
- Pasteurization
- Irradiation of food
- Excess intake of unsaturated and hydrogenated fats
- Cooking at high temperatures
- Microwaving
- Radiation and electromagnetic fields
- Geopathic stress zones (harmful subterranean and man-made energies)
- Fluoridation of water
- Heavy metals
- Mercury amalgam dental fillings
- Root canals and hidden dental infections

inflammation and leading to bacterial reactive arthritis. This condition arises when the immune system begins to attack the klebsiella bacteria and simultaneously begins attacking the body's own tissues. In essence, Dr. Ebringer proposed that klebsiella microbes present in the bowel act as triggers for the development of ankylosing spondylitis. Dr. Ebringer also found that men generally have more klebsiella in their bowels than women, and this, he thought, may explain why ankylosing spondylitis is almost three times more prevalent in men than it is in women. His research further indicated that klebsiella can inhabit areas of the body other than the digestive system, triggering a process of tissue self-destruction. Other bacteria, such as salmonella, yersinia, and shigella, can also trigger inflammatory reactive arthritis.

Ankylosing spondylitis patients suffer increased stiffness and pain in the back, spine, and buttocks, particularly in the low back in the morning. Chronic inflammation in this region of the body leads to the development of bone bridges, or osteophytes; eventually these can take an otherwise mobile joint and ankylose or fuse it. Dr. Ebringer contended that ankylosing spondylitis is actually the end-stage disease of repeated episodes of inflammation caused by klebsiella bacteria.

Evidence also exists that RA may be linked with the enterobacteria *Proteus vulgaris* and *Proteus mirabilis*. These bacteria have similar markers to surfaces of cells that carry the HLA-DR4 gene. High levels of antibodies to *Proteus* spp. have been found in RA patients.[8] It's possible, Dr. Ebringer speculated, that the reason two-thirds of sufferers of RA are women is because *Proteus* spp. also causes urinary tract infections, which women are far more susceptible to than men (due to of the anatomical proximity of the anus to the vaginal opening).

Our clinical research shows that many other microorganisms are associated with the development of RA. For instance, many children afflicted with juvenile arthritis tend to have a predominance of streptococcus in their colon. These patients often have high levels of antibodies to streptococcus bacteria, which, incidentally, may also be derived from infected root canals and underlying gum disease. When we interview patients shortly after they've had dental work, we commonly find that they have a strong exacerbation of symptoms, such as an increase in stiffness and joint swelling, along with an elevation of inflammatory markers.

Other microorganisms that have been linked to the development of RA include mycoplasma,[9] mycobacterium, ureaplasma, and chlamydia.

Microorganisms Implicated in the Development of Arthritis

Severe Pathogens

Streptococcus spp.
Yersinia enterocolitica
Shigella spp.

Campylobacter spp.
Yersinia pseudotuberculosis
Salmonella spp.

Dysbiotic Organisms (organisms of low intrinsic virulence that can induce disease, especially in a host with compromised immune function)

Hemolytic Escherichia coli
Citrobacter freundii
Bacteroides fragilis
Enterobacter spp.
Klebsiella spp.
Aeromonas spp.
Mycobacteria spp.
Chlamydia spp.

Mucoid Escherichia coli
Bacillus spp.
Morganella spp.
Pseudomonas spp.
Proteus spp.
Mycoplasma spp.
Ureaplasma spp.

Fungi/Yeast

Candida spp.
Geotrichum spp.
Fungal conidia

Rhodotorula spp.
Trichospora spp.

Diagnosing Overgrowth of Pathogenic Bacteria

Often, streptococcus, mycoplasma, mycobacterium, ureaplasma, and chlamydia can be detected by PCR (polymerase chain reaction). This laboratory method utilizes the enzyme DNA polymerase to identify precise areas of the DNA of bacteria, viruses, and other infectious disease agents. However, in many instances the disease mechanism is a hyperactive immunologic reaction to a past infection, which triggers an autoimmune disease rather than a direct infection of the joint by the organism. In some instances, the infectious agent is present in the body but continually changes form to evade the immune system. This makes detection difficult. Even when the organism can't be detected by medical testing, the immune system still recognizes that the organism is present and attempts to eradicate it, leading to a hyperimmune response.

Another method of diagnosing pathogenic bacteria is a comprehensive digestive stool analysis. This group of nearly two dozen tests per-

For more detailed information on the **comprehensive digestive stool analysis**, see chapter 3, Diagnosing Arthritis, pages 39–65. For detailed **dietary recommendations for arthritis**, see chapter 12, The Arthritis Diet, pages 225–256. For **colon-cleansing programs**, see chapter 5, Detoxifying Specific Organs, pages 88–114.

formed on a stool sample reveals how effectively the body is digesting food and absorbing nutrients. It also determines the proportion of friendly versus unfriendly bacteria in the intestines, the presence of bacteria and yeasts (such as candida), and whether the diet contains adequate fiber. All of these factors must be considered when treating arthritis.

The Anti-klebsiella Starch-Free Diet. Dr. Ebringer discovered that klebsiella (like candida) thrives on a diet rich in refined carbohydrates and starch. A reduction or elimination of starchy carbohydrates, such as rice, potatoes, and flour products, as well as refined sugars and fruit juices, reduces the number of klebsiella in the intestines. Subsequently, fewer antibodies to this bacteria are produced, which otherwise would cause inflammation when the body attacks itself (the inflammatory cascade). Dr. Ebringer contended that this low-starch diet leads to a reduction in the total amount of IgA (a specific antibody associated with the gastrointestinal tract) in the blood, thereby decreasing inflammation and symptoms of ankylosing spondylitis.

The diet allows unrestricted consumption of protein, eggs, fruits, and vegetables, particularly the nonstarchy vegetables (dark leafy greens, such as kale, Swiss chard, and broccoli). Our modifications of this diet include adding digestive enzymes (to properly break down the starches, proteins, and other substances) and antimicrobial therapy (such as herbs that fight microbes and colon-cleansing programs) to kill the klebsiella bacteria. Following these dietary recommendations, along with the arthritis diet, will help the body fight off any kind of invading microorganism.

Success Story: Treating Candida Relieves Juvenile Arthritis

Essie, 16, was diagnosed with juvenile rheumatoid arthritis (RA). Her family history included a cousin who had also suffered from juvenile arthritis and an aunt with lupus (an autoimmune condition characterized by skin lesions). Her initial symptoms occurred suddenly and included fatigue, musculoskeletal pain, nausea, and loss of appetite. Essie's pediatrician had put her on a course of antibiotics, which provided her with no relief whatsoever. She was then treated with a series of drugs, including NSAIDs, prednisone, and gold injections, among others. The medications caused a number of severe side effects—nausea, chronic headaches, liver inflammation, anemia, and fatigue—and didn't alleviate her original symptoms.

When we first examined Essie, she had large synovial pouches (areas of swelling containing joint fluid) at her wrists, elbows, knees, and ankles. Blood tests revealed an elevated erythrocyte sedimentation rate and elevated rheumatoid factor, both diagnostic indicators for RA.

In addition to diagnostic tests already done by Essie's conventional physicians, we ran a food allergy test (IgG ELISA), which showed that she was sensitive to barley, wheat, buckwheat, broccoli, grapefruit, oranges, beef, and lamb. She consumed wheat, broccoli, and orange juice in large quantities. A hair analysis to test for heavy metals revealed high levels of copper, mercury, and aluminum. The test also indicated that Essie was deficient in two trace minerals, molybdenum and germanium.

Another blood test signaled high levels of the immunoglobulin IgM, indicating an infection of the yeastlike fungus *Candida albicans*. Her IgM antibody level was 51.5; a normal level is less than 12.5. A urinalysis showed an ele-

 Homeopathy was founded in the late 1700s by German physician Samuel Hahnemann. Today, an estimated 500 million people worldwide receive homeopathic treatment; in Britain, homeopathy enjoys royal patronage. Homeopathy is now practiced according to two differing concepts. In classical homeopathy, only one single-component remedy is prescribed at a time, in a potency specifically adjusted to the patient; the physician waits to see the results before prescribing anything further. In complex homeopathy, a prescription involves multiple substances given at the same time, usually in low potencies.

vated level of leukocytes (white blood cells); protein in her urine, as well as blood; high specific gravity (indicating excess sediments in the urine and kidney stress); and trace amounts of ketones (indicating excess protein in the urine). These test results made us suspect bladder inflammation or a urinary tract infection.

Using a darkfield microscope, we examined Essie's blood. Her red blood cells were slightly low in number, confirming the diagnosis of anemia, and were abnormally clumped together. We also saw long tubules in her blood, which usually indicate the presence of parasites or other infectious microorganisms. Red and yellow crystals in her blood corresponded to her joint pain. Finally, her blood contained high levels of yeast forms, confirming the presence of candida.

The last test we ran was a stool analysis, which showed that Essie was producing insufficient amounts of digestive enzymes and hydrochloric acid (the primary stomach acid). We also found occult (hidden) blood, an indication of bleeding in the intestinal tract, perhaps caused by her drug therapy. She had none of the friendly bacteria *Lactobacillus acidophilus*, indicating an imbalance in her intestinal flora, and tested positive for parasite infection.

Clearly, we needed to address not just Essie's arthritis symptoms but her underlying health problems as well. Our goal was to reduce the number of drugs she was taking, which were adversely affecting her. We needed to treat the candida and parasite infections, rebuild her digestive system, decrease the pain and swelling in her joints, and decrease her fatigue and other symptoms.

To begin, we gave Essie an intravenous infusion of vitamins, minerals, antioxidants, and amino acids to build up her depleted nutrient reserves and to support her liver function. We started her on several homeopathic remedies for her food allergies and joint pain.

To treat candida, we gave Essie a probiotic supplement containing the friendly bacteria *Lactobacillus acidophilus* and *Bifidobacterium bifidum*. Friendly bacteria are beneficial microbes inhabiting the human gastrointestinal tract, where they are essential for proper nutrient assimilation. Friendly bacteria are also natural antagonists for candida, and supplementing with them helps normalize intestinal flora.

We recommended vitamin C, pantothenic acid, and raw adrenal concentrate for adrenal support. For immune support and to address Essie's fatigue, we recommended a multivitamin-multimineral, echinacea, shiitake mushroom, burdock root, licorice, and digestive enzymes. For joint support, Essie took calcium, magnesium, boron, and vitamin D.

We recommended a number of dietary changes for Essie. Clearly, she needed to avoid the foods that she had tested positive to on the allergy test. We also advised her to avoid nightshade vegetables (tomatoes, bell peppers, white potatoes, and eggplant) as these seem to aggravate arthritis symptoms. She was to follow a vegetarian diet high in dark green leafy vegetables, with lots of steamed vegetables of different colors. Also, she could have free-range organic turkey, chicken, and fish, each once a week. We encouraged her to eat several small meals throughout the day and to chew each bite thoroughly to ease the stress on her digestive system. It's also important for arthritis patients to get the right oils and essential fatty acids to decrease inflammation. To this end, we recommended that Essie use a dressing made with organic flaxseed and olive oils (both excellent sources of healthy oils), lemon juice, and herbs on her salads and vegetables.

Essie also began physical therapy and visited a chiropractor and massage therapist weekly. We taught her mother to do reflexology (SEE QUICK DEFINI-TION) and massage treatments at home. We also used Reiki and similar techniques to help balance her energy.

After several months on this treatment protocol, Essie's attitude and energy levels were greatly improved. She had adjusted to her healthy diet and her bowel movements were much more regular, indicating that her gastrointestinal tract was improving. We started her on antiparasitic herbs at this stage. After another month, Essie was able to stop the medications she had been taking for her arthritis. After a year and a

Reflexology is based on the idea that there are reflex areas in the hands and feet that correspond to every part of the body, including the organs and glands. By applying gentle but precise pressure to these reflex points, reflexologists can release blockages that inhibit energy flow and cause pain and disease. Practitioners often focus on breaking up crystals of lactic acid and calcium accumulated around any of the 7,200 nerve endings in each foot. Eunice Ingham, a physiotherapist, pioneered the discipline in the United States in the late 1930s. She mapped out reflex points on the feet and developed techniques for inducing healing effects in those areas by working on the feet.

half on the program, Essie was pain-free except for occasional bouts of inflammation due to stress or lapses in her diet. Her candida infection was also under control, and she felt considerably better in general.

Illuminating the Candida Connection

While many species of microorganisms can overgrow in the body and cause an increase in intestinal permeability, of prime concern is *Candida albicans*. This is a yeastlike fungus found widely in nature—in the soil, on vegetables and fruits, and in the human body. It is frequently present in small quantities in the intestines and vagina. Candida overgrowth, a condition called candidiasis, can become pathogenic and cause allergic reactions throughout the body. These reactions can lead to a wide range of symptoms, including depression, fatigue, weight gain, anxiety, rashes, headaches, and muscle cramping.

Predisposing factors for candidiasis include the use of steroid hormone medications such as cortisone or corticosteroids, which are often prescribed for skin problems; prolonged or repeated use of antibiotics;

Candida—A Stealth Pathogen

That *Candida albicans* (or other *Candida* species) can pass through the intestines and into general blood circulation was first established many years ago, yet in conventional medical circles, the importance of candida involvement in health is still largely undervalued. In 1969, W. Krause, Ph.D., demonstrated that intact *Candida albicans* organisms are capable of escaping the intestinal tract and reaching the blood and urine in humans.

After he was carefully screened for any prior illness or exposure to candida, Dr. Krause ingested a large dose of *Candida albicans* orally. In a surprisingly short time, just a few hours later, he developed numerous symptoms, including headaches and fever. The scientists working with Dr. Krause were able to culture candida organisms from his blood and urine, and the colonies were found to be identical to the strain administered.[10] Dr. Krause's bold experiment proved that it is possible for candida to cross the gastrointestinal tract in a viable form and cause systemic illness in healthy patients.

The researchers also concluded that use of antibiotics may be a common precursor in cases of systemic candidiasis and increased intestinal permeability. Despite Dr. Krause's experiment, the conventional medical arena is not convinced that candida can systemically translocate to distant sites in the body as a kind of "stealth pathogen" and cause illness.

oral contraceptive use; estrogen therapy; and a diet high in sugar, both natural and refined. Certain illnesses, such as AIDS, cancer, and diabetes, which are accompanied by extreme immune suppression, can also increase susceptibility to candida overgrowth.[11]

Candida changes form as it develops and sends hyphae (microscopic rootlike filaments) through the intestinal wall, similar to the way English ivy grows up a wall and adheres to the bricks. This analogy is helpful in understanding how candida produces illness. The ivy's rootlets infiltrate the mortar between the bricks and severely damage it; if unchecked, it can eventually disintegrate the mortar. Similarly, candida's rootlike filaments become attached to the intestinal wall and loosen the intracellular "cement" (the connective tissue between cells), create holes through the cell membranes, and release toxic waste products that circulate throughout the system. This results in joint and connective tissue damage through overstimulation of the immune response (specifically, the complement system).

Yeasts, such as candida, contain decarboxylases, enzymes that convert (and putrefy) amino acids (protein building blocks) into vasoactive amines (such as putrescine from arginine and ornithine, and indican from tryptophan), which cause alterations in the permeability of blood vessels and other tissues and affect how easily materials penetrate cell membranes. Vasoactive amines can dissolve the intestinal membrane that

> Elevated levels of candida in the body is highly relevant for people with arthritis. Muscle aches, pain and swelling in the joints, loss of energy, and chronic muscular tightness—in other words, the key symptoms of arthritis—are all symptoms of *Candida albicans* overgrowth.

holds the cells of the gastrointestinal system together and cause leaky gut syndrome.

Candida albicans can also produce over 400 mycotoxins, any of which can cause systemic illness. Mycotoxins are fungal poisons, and in the specific case of candida overgrowth, they are fragments from dead yeast cells or toxic chemicals released into the blood as a by-product of the yeast's metabolism. Some of these mycotoxins, like acetaldehyde and alcohol, can produce feelings akin to being hungover, which many patients affected with candida tend to experience. One mycotoxin in particular, gliotoxin, has been shown to suppress the immune system, particularly the ability of the white blood cells to engulf foreign material. It suppresses the thymus gland, lymph nodes, spleen, and bone marrow's production of white blood cells.[12] Gliotoxin also interferes with normal glutathione metabolism within the cell.[13] The depletion of glutathione not only robs the person of this important antioxidant needed for liver detoxification, it also contributes to other systemic illnesses associated with low levels of glutathione, such as allergies and symptoms of chemical hypersensitivity.

Candida and Arthritis

Although activation of the complement system rids the body of invading foreign organisms, overactivation by a candida infection can cause significant damage to healthy body tissues. Candida stimulates the immune system to summon aggressive white blood cells. Once stimulated, these white blood cells destroy all cells in the area, candida and other pathogens as well as the body's own cell membranes and tissues. In patients with arthritis, significant damage occurs in the joints because the lining of the joints and cartilage are broken down.

Though the predominant fungal species that causes these health problems is *Candida albicans*, other organisms that contribute to arthritis include *Candida tropicalis*, *Candida krusei*, *Trichosporon* spp., *Geotrichum* spp., *Rhodotorula* spp., and fungal conidia. In addition to candida and fungal forms present in the intestines, many other infective agents can initiate joint inflammation, even though they originate in other areas of the body. Some examples include chronic bacterial inflammation of the sinus cavities, infections of the gums and teeth (including abscesses, cavities, and root canals), and inflammation of the adenoids or tonsils. All provide constant sources of bacteria that can initiate or worsen any arthritis already present.

Diagnosing a Yeast Overgrowth

The following tests can be used to diagnose overgrowth of *Candida albicans*.

Symptom questionnaire: William Crook, M.D., author of *The Yeast Connection*, popularized the idea that candida can create numerous health problems. During the course of his research, Dr. Crook developed a reliable questionnaire for assessing potential candida involvement in a patient's health. Among the questions are the following (positive answers may indicate a yeast infection):

- Have you taken repeated courses of antibiotics or steroids (for example, cortisone)?
- Have you used birth control pills?
- Have you had repeated fungal infections (jock itch, athlete's foot, ringworm, vaginal yeast infections)?
- Do you regularly have any of these symptoms: bloating, headaches, depression, fatigue, memory problems, impotence or lack of interest in sex, muscle aches with no apparent cause, brain fogginess?
- Do you experience symptoms of PMS (premenstrual syndrome)?
- Do you have cravings for sweets, products containing white flour, or alcoholic beverages?
- Do you repeatedly experience any of these health difficulties: inappropriate drowsiness, mood swings, rashes, bad breath, dry mouth, postnasal drip or nasal congestion, heartburn, urinary frequency or urgency?

Candida antibody titer. Rather than measure the level of candida directly, this blood test analyzes the body's reaction to the presence of candida as indicated by levels of the antibodies IgA, IgM, and IgG. The test is useful but not totally reliable. If positive, it can indicate past or present candida infection somewhere in the body, but it may not indicate intestinal overgrowth. A negative result could mean that although candida is present, the body's immune mechanisms didn't react appropriately to create the antibodies against candida. This occurs in individuals with a compromised immune system.

Comprehensive digestive stool analysis. This is a complete survey of the contents of the patient's stool sample. It can indicate digestive strengths or weaknesses and pinpoint causes of dysbiosis, including yeast overgrowth and parasitic infestation.

Darkfield microscopic blood analysis. This method evaluates living whole blood cells under a specially adapted microscope that projects a dynamic image, magnified 1,400 times, onto a video screen. The presence of fungal forms can be verified by the use of yellow phosphorescent cellulose-binding dye, which helps to identify yeast.

Ridding the Arthritic Body of Candida

Successful treatment of candidiasis requires the reduction of factors that contribute to candida overgrowth, along with strengthening of immune function. Diet, nutritional supplements, herbal and Ayurvedic remedies, acupuncture, and enzyme therapy can be used to help accomplish these ends.

Controlling chronic candidiasis seldom takes less than three months, and it may take much longer. However, many patients experience relief from some symptoms after only one week. For example, Adriane, 45, had joint swelling, fatigue, bloating after eating, and an inability to think clearly. She came to see us for help in discontinuing some of the NSAIDs and other drugs she was taking for arthritis. After a full examination, we found that she had a high level of *Candida albicans* (4 out of a possible score of 5). Adriane agreed to start an anticandida diet individually tailored to her specific food allergies. Three days after starting this diet, Adriane noticed that although she still had some joint pain, her stomach was much less bloated after eating and she was able to think more clearly. It took Adriane two years to completely resolve her arthritis, but she got the candida under control in one month.

Dietary Recommendations
Reduce dietary sugars: Yeast thrives on any kind of sugar, so to overcome candidiasis, sugar must be avoided in all its various forms. These include sucrose, dextrose, fructose, fruit juices, honey, maple

Why Friendly Bacteria are Essential to Your Health

L. acidophilus and other friendly forms of bacteria have been studied for their beneficial effects on health. Newborns given *L. acidophilus* shortly after birth encouraged growth of normal intestinal flora and reduced the incidence of inflammatory diseases and opportunistic infections. *L. acidophilus* prevents the attachment of harmful bacteria to human intestinal cells, thus providing a barrier against these bacteria in the digestive system. The pathogenic bacteria affected include *Escherichia coli*, *Salmonella typhimurium*, *Yersinia pseudotuberculosis*, and *Campylobacter pylori*, a common bacteria that causes acid peptic disease. *L. acidophilus* helps to maintain the levels of healthy bacteria while discouraging the growth of pathogenic bacteria. One of the common side effects of treatment with antibiotics is that both friendly and pathogenic bacteria are killed off, opening the door to yeast infestation and gastrointestinal distress, particularly diarrhea. According to several studies, supplementing with lactobacillus and other probiotics can restore the normal intestinal microflora damaged by antibiotics.[16]

syrup, molasses, milk products (which contain lactose), most fruits (except berries), and potatoes (their starch converts into sugar). Those with candidiasis should also avoid all alcohol since it's composed of fermented and refined sugars.

Consume foods rich in friendly bacteria: Unsweetened organic yogurt, high in natural probiotics, can be useful to help reestablish friendly bacteria. However, arthritis patients sensitive to dairy products are advised to avoid yogurt. Freeze-dried acidophilus supplements derived from nondairy sources, available in capsule or powder form, are also effective, and naturally fermented foods, such as sauerkraut and kimchi, are high in beneficial bacteria.

Minimize intake of nonorganic animal foods: Consumption of meat, dairy products, and poultry can foster candida growth due to the large amount of antibiotics used in animal feed. For example, the antibiotic tetracycline is regularly used as a growth enhancer in poultry; traces of this antibiotic remain in the poultry tissue and are passed on to those who consume it. Antibiotics kill off all microflora, both friendly and unfriendly, living in the colon and give opportunistic organisms such as candida a chance to repopulate areas once dominated by beneficial bacteria. If you choose to eat animal products, use organic, hormone- and antibiotic-free meat, dairy products, or poultry whenever possible.

Reduce intake of foods with yeast: Although *Candida albicans* is not the same as the yeast used in foods such as bread, a cross-reactivity between yeasts and fungi frequently occurs. All foods containing yeast should be avoided, such as baked goods, alcohol, vinegar, and all vinegar-containing condiments. Rice cakes and rye crackers are good bread substitutes. Make your own vinegar-free salad dressing with lemon juice instead of vinegar; lime or vitamin C crystals can also be used to replace vinegar, as each can impart a suitably tangy taste.

Avoid molds: Exposure to molds increases candida symptoms. These include food molds (found in cheeses, grapes, mushrooms, and fermented foods) and environmental molds (found outdoors and in wet climates, damp basements, and plants).

Ayurvedic Antifungal Therapies: Ayurvedic medicine (SEE QUICK DEFINITION) considers candidiasis to be a condition attributed to the accumulation of *ama*, or internal congestion, which is caused by the improper digestion of foods. Ayurvedic suggestions for controlling candida combine the ingestion of grapefruit seed oil and tannic acid, which act as antifungals and antibiotics, and acidophilus, which helps restore the balance of friendly bacteria in the intestines. Long pepper, ginger, cayenne,

Tea Tree Oil—An Effective Germ-Fighter

The essential oil extracted from the leaves of the tea tree (*Melaleuca alternifolia*) is effective against numerous conditions, including candidiasis, acne, insect bites, sunburn, athlete's foot, cuts, muscle aches, and shingles. Tea tree oil has been studied specifically for its effects against candida.[20] In a 1995 study published in the *Journal of Applied Bacteriology*, scientists at the University of Western Australia tested eight components of tea tree oil against infectious microorganisms, including *Candida albicans, Escherichia coli, Pseudomonas aeruginosa,* and *Staphylococcus aureus.* The researchers concluded that no single element in tea tree oil confers its remarkable germ-fighting ability; rather, the interaction of at least eight distinct chemicals in the oil seemed to produce the effects.[21] Tea tree oil can be used at full strength or diluted in water or another oil.

Ayurveda is the traditional medicine of India, based on many centuries of empirical use. Its name means "end of the Vedas" (India's sacred scripts), implying that a holistic medicine may be founded on spiritual principles. Ayurveda describes three metabolic, constitutional, and body types (*doshas*), in association with the basic elements of nature in combination. These are *vata* (air and ether, rooted in the intestines), *pitta* (fire and water, rooted in the stomach), and *kapha* (water and earth, rooted in the lungs). Ayurvedic physicians use these categories (which also have psychological aspects) as the basis for prescribing individualized formulas of herbs, diet, massage, breathing techniques, meditation, exercise, yoga postures, and detoxification programs.

and the Ayurvedic herbs trikatu and neem should be taken 30 minutes before meals to increase immunoglobulin and digestive functions. A Panchakarma program, which involves herb supplements, individualized diet, massage, breathing techniques, meditation, exercise, yoga postures, and detoxification programs, can also be useful.

Herbal Remedies for Candidiasis. Herbs are often used to kill harmful yeasts and to shore up immune function. Herbs containing berberine (an alkaloid) have proven to be particularly useful for candida.[14] These include goldenseal, Oregon grape root, and barberry. Berberine acts as a natural antibiotic against candida overgrowth, normalizes intestinal flora, helps digestive problems, and stimulates the immune system. Other herbs helpful for candidiasis include artemisia, quassia bark, red clover, pau d'arco, citrus seed extract, thyme oil, oregano oil, tea tree oil, and garlic.

 Tea tree oil is meant for topical, not oral, use.

Nutritional Supplements for Candidiasis

Probiotics: High doses of probiotics, or friendly bacteria, such as *Bifidobacterium bifidum* and *Lactobacillus acidophilus*, *Lactobacillus bulgaricus*, *Lactobacillus plantarum*, and *Lactobacillus salivarius*, are available as nutritional supplements. Recolonizing the intestines with friendly bacteria can help prevent illness by depriving pathogenic bacteria of the opportunity to flourish and overgrow.

Caprylic acid: This medium-chain fatty acid found in coconut oil is an effective antifungal agent.[15] Caprylic acid is readily absorbed into the body and should be taken in coated tablets or in a sustained-release form that ensures release in the small intestine rather than the stomach. Consuming virgin coconut oil can also be helpful.

Garlic: Louis Pasteur, the nineteenth-century formulator of the modern germ theory, recognized the antibiotic properties of garlic. Although now eclipsed by penicillin and other antibiotics, garlic often is more effective and more versatile in treating fungal, bacterial, and viral infections.[17] Allicin, the active antifungal component in garlic, attacks the surface of the candida cells, alters its fat content, and oxidizes a group of its essential enzymes.[18] Allicin is potent—only a small concentration is needed to kill candida—and garlic has the added benefit of stimulating the immune system.

Oil of oregano: Oil of oregano has been shown to have specific anticandida effects.[19] Distilled from *Origanum vulgare*, a species of oregano that grows prolifically on Mediterranean hillsides, it's used to treat topical and internal candidiasis. Its powerful antimicrobial properties come from a combination of carvacrol, a naturally occurring antiseptic, and thymol, which is also found in thyme. Carvacrol is a phenol that rivals in strength the synthetic phenol carbolic acid, once used to sterilize medical instruments. For internal candida infections, a relatively small amount of oil of oregano is needed to kill the overgrown fungi. But while this amber-colored liquid may look mild, it has a strong and almost spicy flavor. We recommend mixing it with vegetable juice.

 CAUTION Through darkfield microscopy, we've seen an increase in the fragility of red blood cells in patients who stay on isolated caprylic acid for more than two months; perhaps the same factors that attack candida also begin to attack blood cell membranes. We use caprylic acid only for short-term intervention and rely on dietary and lifestyle changes for a long-term cure. This problem does not occur with the use of virgin coconut oil.

Eliminating Parasites

Parasites can often be a major factor underlying unexplained health problems, including allergies, fatigue, chronic intestinal dysbiosis, and joint pain, and the possibility of parasitic infestation should be considered in all cases of arthritis. In this chapter, we explain how a parasite infestation may be a causative factor in arthritis, leading to inflammation and deterioration of the joints. We also outline how alternative medicine can help eliminate parasites through colon cleansing, herbs, and diet and thus alleviate arthritic problems.

What Is a Parasite?

A parasite is an organism that feeds off other organisms, usually to the host's detriment. When parasites are present in the body, they usually reside in the intestines, but several species migrate during certain life stages to the blood, lymph, heart, liver, gallbladder, pancreas, spleen, eyes, and brain, as well as inside the lining of the joints.

More than 300 kinds of parasites can live in the human body. They generate numerous symptoms, including headaches, back pain, energy loss, spaciness, vomiting, weight loss, colitis, gas, uncontrolled appetite, acne, and joint and muscle pain. Conventional medical practitioners usually mistakenly associate these symptoms with other illnesses and rarely consider testing for parasites as a possible cause for these symptoms.

In the United States, the most common parasites, apart from head lice, are microscopic protozoans. These include *Giardia lamblia*, which is found in contaminated water and is a common cause of traveler's diarrhea;[1] *Entamoeba histolytica*, which can cause dysentery and injure the liver and lungs; *Blastocystis hominis*, which is increasingly linked to acute and chronic illnesses; *Dientamoeba fragilis*, which is associated with diarrhea, abdominal pain, anal itching, and loose stools; and *Cryptosporidium* spp., which are particularly dangerous to those with compromised immune function. Arthropod parasites—mites, fleas, and ticks—can carry smaller parasites that are also infectious to humans. Of particular interest to arthritis patients is *Borrelia burgdorferi*, a parasite that causes Lyme disease, a condition with many arthritis-like symptoms. Larger parasites include pinworms, tapeworms, roundworms, hookworms, filaria (threadlike worms that inhabit the blood and tissues), and flukes (which invade the liver). Parasites are difficult to diagnose and often evade detection, especially when they're outside the gastrointestinal tract.

Parasites Associated with Arthritis

- Blastocystis hominis
- Brachiola algerae
- Chilomastix mesnili
- Cryptosporidium spp.
- Cyclospora cayetanensis
- Dientamoeba fragilis
- Endolimax nana
- Entamoeba histolytica
- Giardia lamblia
- Strongyloides stercoralis
- Toxocara canis

The Link Between Parasites and Arthritis

Parasites cause joint pain in two ways: by directly invading a joint, and through the production of toxic waste products that increase the body burden of circulating immune complexes, initiating an exaggerated immune response. The possibility of parasitic infestation should be considered in all cases of arthritis.

Medical researchers around the world have reported on the correlation between parasites and arthritis. Some species of parasites once thought to exist only in nonhuman hosts have now been found to cause

> Parasites can often be a major factor underlying unexplained health problems, including allergies, fatigue, chronic intestinal dysbiosis, and joint pain; the possibility of parasitic infestation should be considered in all cases of arthritis.

RA in humans. Researchers in Austria found *Toxocara canis*, which usually infects dogs, foxes, and cats, to be the causative agent of dozens of cases of RA.[2] *Brachiola algerae*, a parasite found in mosquitoes and cultured in mice, has also infected skeletal muscle in humans.[3] A report from Germany cites a case where a child who exhibited arthritis-like symptoms was cured after he was treated for the common intestinal parasite cryptosporidium.[4]

Scottish researchers reported that rheumatic syndromes occur in a variety of parasitic diseases. They suggest that effective diagnosis of a parasitic origin is hampered by the confusion caused when, due to travel and immigration, afflicted patients may live far from the usual geographic area of a particular parasite.[5] Doctors in India describe a case of arthritis where larvae of *Strongyloides stercoralis*, which can live both inside and outside the body, were isolated in the stool and duodenum of an arthritis patient. The patient's symptoms were resolved by anthelmintic (antiparasite) treatments.[6] In the United States, *Cyclospora cayetanensis*, carried by fruit, has been linked to many food poisoning outbreaks and also has been associated with a variety of long-term illnesses such as Guillain-Barre syndrome and arthritis.[7]

Success Story: Reversing Arthritis by Eliminating Parasites

Harold, 35, came into our office so disabled by arthritis that he needed a cane to walk. He complained of intense pain in his lower back, neck, and hips. His arms and legs were weak and often tingled or felt numb, and the pain in his knees, which had been relieved years earlier by orthopedic surgery, had returned. Gastrointestinal problems also afflicted Harold; he had abdominal pain and recurrent diarrhea that contributed to his incessant fatigue. He wrestled with bouts of depression, sinus infections, facial dermatitis, and toothaches brought on by bacterial infections hiding in the deep pockets of his gums. Harold was also anemic, an uncommon condition in men, although often present in arthritis patients.

As a child, Harold had asthma, hay fever, and eczema. Suspecting that food allergies contributed to his current respiratory problems, he started avoiding dairy products, coffee, cheese, and pasta and also took nutritional supplements. To relieve his pain, he tried yoga, gentle stretching, and breathing exercises three times a week, but he still felt that his health was worsening as his arthritis spread from his lower back to his hips and neck.

Initial laboratory tests showed that Harold had an elevated erythrocyte sedimentation rate (ESR). This is an indicator of chronic infection and inflammatory conditions. Harold had a history of arthritic symptoms and a genetic predisposition (the gene HLA-B27) for ankylosing spondylitis. Some bacteria, through molecular mimicry, are able to reproduce a specific pattern determined by the HLA-B27 gene, and avoid activating an immune response through this mechanism. Specifically, the bacteria klebsiella has been implicated in triggering ankylosing spondylitis.

Ankylosing spondylitis patients (of which there are three times more men than women) typically suffer from stiffness and pain in the lower back and spine as a result of joint inflammation. Stiffness can then spread to the ribs, shoulders, hips, and knees and is often accompanied by mild fatigue, loss of appetite, and anemia. Once the inflammation becomes chronic, the bone and cartilage begin to deteriorate and bone bridges (osteophytes) form; these can eventually fuse joints and parts of the spine, rendering the person immobile.

Through a stool analysis, we found that Harold had elevated levels of *Klebsiella* spp. and *Citrobacter freundii*, intestinal bacteria believed to induce autoimmune responses through molecular mimicry. *Citrobacter* spp. also creates antigens that are similar to those of *Salmonella* spp. and *Escherichia coli*, causing intestinal inflammation and, in some cases, leaky gut syndrome. Harold's stool analysis revealed dysbiosis—an unbalanced ecology of microorganisms in his gastrointestinal tract. Ratios of short-chain fatty acids (normally produced by friendly bacteria) were unbalanced. Under normal conditions, healthy microflora breaks down soluble fibers into short-chain fatty acids, which are then used as food by the cells of the colon. But in a dysbiotic state, pathogenic bacteria don't produce these fatty acids, instead producing toxic by-products that impair digestion. Harold also had low levels of chymotrypsin, a key enzyme (secreted by the pancreas) that prompts the breakdown of proteins into smaller compounds. Decreased levels of chymotrypsin in fecal samples suggest incomplete digestion and malabsorption of proteins.

Harold's stool analysis revealed high levels of *Blastocystis hominis*. This parasite has been linked to chronic fatigue, arthritis, and rheumatoid complaints, as well as diarrhea, abdominal cramps, nausea, and flatulence. It usually resides in the intestines but can migrate (via leaky gut syndrome) to other vital organs and the synovial fluid of the joints. A sample of synovial fluid was extracted from Harold's knee and was examined under a darkfield microscope. *Blastocystis hominis* and yeasts normally found in the gastrointestinal tract were detected in the fluid. When parasites migrate outside the intestines, they stimulate the immune system, which then initiates an overzealous autoimmune response that turns against itself, attacking healthy cells.

When a person suffers from leaky gut syndrome, the structural integrity of the intestines breaks down, allowing the intestines to leak these molecules across the intestinal membranes. Harold's stool analysis revealed the presence of *Citrobacter* spp. and *Klebsiella* spp., both of which are linked to the development of leaky gut syndrome.

We started Harold on the following antiparasitic protocol.

- Grape seed extract
- An herbal combination of barberry root, citrus seed, Chinese goldenseal rhizome (*Coptis*), garlic bulb, black walnut green outer hull, Rangoon creeper fruit (*Quisqualis indica*), quassia wood, cascara sagrada bark, Chinese wormwood flowering tops (*Artemisia annua*), and volatile oils of thyme, oregano leaf, tea tree, and clove
- Daily enemas with a few drops of the essential oils of red thyme, marjoram, and oregano

After four months on this treatment, Harold no longer experienced joint pain. We referred him to a naturopathic physician closer to his hometown for maintenance consultations. This case shows that careful microscopic analysis of the synovial fluid is mandatory in all cases of arthritis, especially ankylosing spondylitis and RA. Parasites and bacteria must always be considered possible contributors to the onset of arthritis.

Diagnosing Parasite Infestations

If you suspect you may have parasites (symptoms include headaches, back pain, energy loss, spaciness, vomiting, weight loss, colitis, gas, uncontrolled appetite, acne, and joint or muscle pain), make sure your testing facility follows the investigational guidelines set by the U.S. Centers for Disease Control in the *Manual of Clinical Microbiology*.[8] In general, parasites can be very difficult to positively diagnose. Conventional physicians will often order a simple stool analysis, and if the results are negative, parasites are ruled out. However, in many cases the parasites are present but have avoided detection.

Several methods of testing are used to diagnose parasites.[9]

- Macroscopic and microscopic analysis of tissue samples: This procedure, which has a long history of use, allows for the immediate identification of all the parasites present in mixed infections, as well as evaluation of the parasite load. It is a cost-effective method that relies ultimately on the skill of the observer to detect and identify parasite stages.

- Parasite antigen detection: This method is useful for directly diagnosing occult, or hidden, infections.

- Parasite DNA/RNA: This is a sensitive procedure for detecting specific parasites and can also identify sibling species.

- Host antibody detection: This method is an indirect tool for detecting the presence of parasites by evaluating the host's response to infection.

Additional screening tools used in alternative medicine to diagnose the presence of parasites include applied kinesiology, electrodermal screening (EDS), and darkfield microscopic blood analysis. Regarding the latter, we have observed the presence of long tubules in the blood of many arthritis patients and contend that these have a high positive correlation with a diagnosis of parasites.

Applied kinesiology is the study of the relationship between muscle dysfunction (weak muscles) and related organ or gland dysfunction. Applied kinesiology employs a simple strength resistance test on a specific indicator muscle related to the organ or part of the body being tested. If the muscle tests strong (maintaining its resistance), it indicates health. If it tests weak, it can mean infection or dysfunction. When testing for parasites, the practitioner challenges a strong muscle while the patient holds a vial containing parasite specimens; the muscle will weaken if one of these parasites is causing their health problem.

In EDS, a blunt, noninvasive electric probe is placed at specific points on the patient's hands, face, or feet corresponding to acupuncture points at the beginning or end of energy meridians. Minute electrical discharges from these points serve as information signals about the condition of the body's organs and systems. The key idea with EDS is that it is a data acquisition process in which the trained practitioner conducts an "interview" with the patient's organs and tissues, gathering information about the basic functional status of those systems and their energy pathways. As such, EDS is an investigational, not diagnostic, device because it requires the practitioner's knowledge of acupuncture, physiology, and therapeutic substances to interpret the energy imbalances, establish their precise focus, and select the most appropriate therapeutic response. EDS testing may utilize vials containing specimens of various parasites to test the meridians of the patient; if parasites are a factor, there will be a corresponding weakened EDS reading.

 For more information about **testing for parasites**, see chapter 3, Diagnosing Arthritis, pages 39–65.

Natural Parasite Elimination Techniques

We recommend a period of general body detoxification according to the protocols explained in chapter 4, General Detoxification, prior to starting a parasite removal program. We start a specific parasite elimination protocol only after the patient has been on a detoxification and rebuilding program for at least one to two months. This enables patients to experience a higher level of wellness before undergoing the health challenges that can occur during a parasite elimination program. In addition, if the immune system is strengthened due to detoxification, a nutritious diet, and healthy lifestyle changes, the body may eliminate parasites on its own, without further intervention.

During a parasite elimination program, it's common to have an unpleasant die-off reaction (Jarisch-Herxheimer reaction). Typically the die-off symptoms may include malaise, fever, coated tongue, and gastrointestinal disturbances. The Jarisch-Herxheimer reaction can also cause a flare-up of preexisting conditions, including joint pain, headaches, bloating, itching, and mood swings. Bear in mind that these are, in fact, good signs, indicating that the parasites are dying off.

Parasites can be difficult to eradicate. As the adult forms are killed, they often form spores or eggs that are deposited in body tissues, hatching after two to three weeks. Therefore, the parasite cleansing program needs to be in effect for at least one to two months to effectively break this cycle.

After finishing a parasite cleanse, diagnostic tests should be repeated every two months until the results are clearly negative three consecutive times. In addition, pay attention to any increase in previous symptoms. Although self-treatment is possible, we advise that all patients have a knowledgeable health-care practitioner follow their progress; be sure this practitioner is familiar with parasite life cycles, testing, and cleansing procedures.

Colon-Cleansing Programs

There are a number of colon-cleansing programs available to help remove pathogenic microorganisms and other toxic materials from the intestines. Colonic irrigations and enemas, in which water or some other fluid is used to flush out the lower portion of the colon, can help restore intestinal health.

Colonic irrigation, performed in a clinic with special equipment, involves the gentle infusion of the large intestine with water or a solution of medicinal herbs. This procedure is used by many natural health-care practitioners to help rid the body of parasites. A 20- to 30-minute cleansing of the colon with pure filtered water, ozonated water, or water infused with hydrogen peroxide is followed by infusion with powerful botanical medicines. The herbs are retained in the large intestine for several minutes to allow for maximum antimicrobial effect.

Natural Parasite Elimination Techniques

- Colon cleansing
- Herbs for parasites
- Dietary changes
- Kitchen and culinary hygiene

Parasite cleansers taken orally are also helpful in the eradication of parasites. They include psyllium husks, agar-agar, citrus pectin, papaya extract, pumpkin seeds, flaxseeds, comfrey root, beet root, and bentonite clay (take bentonite only in combination with another substance, such as psyllium). To help flush the intestines, you might also take extra vitamin C to increase bowel tolerance. The amount needed will vary from one individual to another. To achieve bowel tolerance, take increasing amounts of vitamin C until your stools become very loose. Then cut back the amount until the stool firms slightly and continue with that dose for two weeks. Note, however, that vitamin C taken at the same time as wormwood (an antiparasitic herb) makes wormwood ineffective, so use them at different times of the day.

Food-grade hydrogen peroxide can be added to an enema as an

antiparasitic agent. Add ¼ cup of peroxide per 2 quarts of fluid. We've been successful using hydrogen peroxide (diluted before use) either as an enema or in the last 5 to 10 minutes of a professionally administered colonic treatment. We use food-grade hydrogen peroxide because drugstore brands typically contain impurities not appropriate for internal use. Ozonated water (SEE QUICK DEFINITION) is another safe and effective enema for treating parasites. The ozonated water destroys the parasites as well as the hard covering that surrounds their cysts or eggs, which are highly resistant to many forms of treatment.

 Ozone (O_3) is a less stable, more reactive form of oxygen, containing three oxygen atoms (O_2, containing only two atoms, is the more usual form). The third oxygen atom causes ozone to more readily react with, or oxidize, other chemicals. In oxidation, the extra oxygen atom breaks off, leaving ordinary oxygen, thereby favorably increasing the oxygen content of body tissues or blood. Medical-grade ozone is used as part of oxygen therapy to increase local oxygen supply to lesions, speed wound healing, reduce infections, and stimulate metabolic processes. Ozone may be administered intravenously or by injection or applied topically in a solution with water or olive oil; it may also be taken orally or rectally as ozonated water.

A third approach is to perform an enema with essential oils. Combine 2 drops each of the essential oils of thyme, oregano, and marjoram in a 2-quart container of water. This will make two complete enemas, each utilizing a full 1-quart bag of water. To ensure complete eradication, we usually recommend two to three enemas per week for a period of four weeks, followed by a test for ova and parasites, then a repetition of the enemas and oral antiparasitics if the test result is positive or inconclusive.

Herbs for Parasites

Herbs have been used for their antiparasite activity for thousands of years in cultures around the world. In many instances, they are safer and more effective than prescription drugs.

Pumpkin seeds (Cucurbita pepo): Purgative herbs, such as pumpkin seeds, act as mild intestinal cleansers. Pumpkin seeds contain cucurmoschin, which helps destroy tapeworm and other intestinal parasites and has been studied for its antifungal activities.[10]

Garlic (Allium sativum): Raw garlic and garlic extract have been shown to destroy common intestinal parasites, including roundworms, hookworms, yeasts, and other types of fungi. Garlic destroys pathogenic cells but doesn't harm the cells of the body. The small molecules of the active

How to Do an Antiparasite Enema

1. Measure 2 quarts of purified filtered water; do not use tap water. Bring the water to a boil, then remove from the heat.

2. Add the following to the water: 4 teaspoons powdered goldenseal root, 4 teaspoons powdered thyme, the juice from 2 cloves of garlic, and 2 teaspoons of tea tree oil. Let the solution steep and cool to body temperature, about 20 minutes, in a covered container.

3. Empty your bowels and bladder prior to the enema. Lubricate the enema speculum (the small tube inserted into the anus) with K-Y jelly, aloe vera gel, or another lubricant, enabling it to easily enter the anus without abrasion. Keep a towel under your buttocks to collect run-off stool.

4. Hang the enema bag above your body so that gravity assists the fluid flow. Assume the fetal position and lubricate your rectum. Place the enema speculum into your rectum. Turn and roll to lie on your back with your knees up. Use one hand to keep the speculum in and the other to control the flow valve.

5. Allow the liquid to slowly flow into your colon; stop the flow every few seconds to allow yourself to adjust to the pressure. Allow the fluid to enter until you feel a slight cramping or discomfort.

6. When you feel full, remove the speculum, hold your sphincter muscles tight, get up, and sit on the toilet. Release your bowels and remain on the toilet seat until all the water has been evacuated.

7. Repeat the enema process until you've used all the water. Clean yourself up, soak the enema speculum in bleach water, and clean the area.

8. Do this procedure two to three times a week for four weeks.

constituents in garlic are able to cross cell membranes and combine with sulfur-containing molecular groups in parasites, interfering with their metabolic processes. Healthy cells in the body contain glutathione, a powerful antioxidant that offsets the destructive effects of the allicin and other active antimicrobial constituents of garlic. In addition, garlic activates the normal activity of the immune system,[11] and it's been shown to be specifically effective against candida, as well as antibiotic-resistant bacteria.[12] In our practice, we use freshly juiced garlic for treating parasites, *Candida albicans*, and other infectious microbes. (The juice should be refrigerated after pressing.) We add 2 to 3 teaspoons of the juice to a 2-quart enema bag and infuse this mixture into the patient's colon at the end of a colonic. Since garlic is fairly caustic and can injure tissues if used in a highly concentrated form, be sure to sufficiently dilute it.

Goldenseal *(Hydrastis canadensis):* The alkaloid compound berberine, found in particularly high concentrations in the root of the goldenseal plant, inhibits the growth of several common parasites that invade the intestines, vagina, and oral cavity, including *Entamoeba histolytica, Giardia lamblia,*

CAUTION Before beginning any parasite elimination program, consult a qualified health-care professional. Do not undertake any parasite detoxification program if you are pregnant.

Erwinia carotovora, Leishmania donovani, and *Streptococcus mutans.*[13] In one study, children with giardiasis were given either berberine sulfate (a standardized goldenseal extract) or the drug Flagyl. After 10 days, both substances produced similar results: 90% of the berberine-treated group no longer had giardia in their stools compared to 95% of the Flagyl-treated group. Unlike the Flagyl-treated group, however, those receiving berberine suffered no negative side effects.[14]

Thyme *(Thymus vulgaris):* The principle chemical components found in thyme are the volatile oils phenol, thymol, and carvacrol.[15] Thymol is one of the most potent antimicrobial substances known and even surpasses many of the strongest antibiotics. Thymol's antimicrobial activity is 18 times more powerful than phenol, the major antiseptic used in commercial germicidal cleansers like Lysol, and it can destroy parasites, worms, fungi, bacteria, and many viruses.[16]

Grapefruit *(Citrus paradisi):* Grapefruit seed extract (GSE), made from grapefruit seeds and pulp, has demonstrated extensive antibacterial and antifungal activity. Studies conducted by the U.S. Food and Drug Administration, the Pasteur Institute in Paris, and various universities have investigated the use of grapefruit seed extract against a wide variety of bacterial, fungal, and viral infections, including giardia, amebic dysentery, *Escherichia coli,* candida, herpes, and salmonella.[17] Made from grapefruit seeds and pulp, the medical virtues of GSE were identified in 1964 by Florida physician Jacob Harich, M.D., and later marketed as Citricidal. GSE contains bioflavonoids (vitamin C enhancers) and hesperidin, a natural immune booster, and is effective against candidiasis and parasites.

Epazote *(Chenopodium ambrosioides):* Also called wormseed or Mexican tea, epazote has traditionally been used in the Caribbean and Central America for worms, and it has been scientifically studied for its effectiveness as an antiparasite treatment.[18] We've observed that among the Indians in Mexico, epazote is regularly used as a preventive measure against parasites. It's prepared as a mild tea for children and a stronger one for adults. If parasites are already a problem, a very thick brew of epazote is prepared and taken by the spoonful.

Wormwood *(Artemisia absinthium):* Wormwood has a long history of use as a vermifuge, or worm expeller, hence its common name, wormwood. It was prized by Hippocrates for its ability to expel worms. It's especially effective against giardia and other protozoa, but some caution is advised. It may initially worsen symptoms and cause minor intestinal irritation. It may be toxic if used alone in large quantities, so it's usually mixed in formulas with citrus seed extract and other antiparasitic herbs, such as black walnut hulls and ground cloves, which offset its possible toxic effects. Such herbal combinations should only be used with professional guidance from a licensed health-care practitioner. Chinese wormwood (*Artemisia annua*), used in the treatment of malaria, is often utilized to kill intracellular parasites.

Effective Formulas for Parasites

Herbs: Grapefruit seed extract, artemisia, anise, cinnamon, marjoram, thyme, oregano, black walnut, cloves, gentian root, and ginger are among the most effective antiparasitic herbs. Berberine, an alkaloid compound particularly antiparasitic, is present in the roots of many herbs, including goldenseal root, Oregon grape root, and barberry bark.

Laxative tea: Drink senna, Turkey rhubarb root, or cascara sagrada tea to help eliminate breakdown products from the parasites.

Epsom salts: Epsom salts (magnesium sulfate) are a strong laxative. Use according to package directions.

Ayurvedic Herbs for Parasites

The traditional Indian medical science of Ayurveda has several natural remedies that address specific parasite infections. Bitter melon (*Momordica charantia*) is a cucumber-shaped fruit that's best used cut up and eaten in small pieces with other vegetables because of its bitter taste. Consuming one or two bitter melons a day for 7 to 10 days, then repeating this after one month, can be effective in the treatment of pinworms. If pinworms are present, small white worms will be seen in the stool a day after eating bitter melon. The active constituent momordicin may be responsible for bitter melon's antiworm effects.[19]

The Ayurvedic herbs vidang (*Embelia ribes*), and kamila (*Mallotus philippensis*) are most effective for roundworms and tapeworms. Mix the them together and take 1 teaspoon twice per day in fruit juice. Continue for 10 days, watching the stool for evidence for worms and eggs. Stop for one week, then repeat the protocol.

Small protozoan parasites, such as giardia, amoebas, and cryptosporidium, require a longer course of treatment lasting several months. The Ayurvedic herbs most effective for these microscopic intruders are bilva (*Aegle marmelos*), neem (*Azadirachta indica*), and herbs, such as goldenseal (*Hydrastis canadensis*) and coptis (*Coptis trifolia*), which contain beberine and can be taken in combination. Ayurvedic herbs are usually administered as combination formulas. Seek guidance from an Ayurvedic practitioner for dosage and instructions for use.

Ayurvedic physicians believe that the health of the immune system must also be addressed to support the body's defense against parasites. Herbs useful for this task include ginseng, ligustrum berries, and schizandra berries. Nutritional support for enhancement of the intestinal microflora is also important for the overall program; psyllium husks, turmeric, and *Lactobacillus acidophilus*, among others, are useful in this regard.

Dietary Changes

If an intestinal parasite infection is diagnosed or suspected, we advise you to eliminate all uncooked food from your diet and to cook all meats until well-done. Parasites are often passed along through consumption of raw foods, especially animal products such as raw fish in sushi and sashimi. Soak all vegetables, including those organically grown, in salted water (1 tablespoon salt to 5 cups of water) for at least 30 minutes before cooking to kill parasites and their eggs. Avoid junk food and all processed food, as these lower immunity and make it more difficult for the body to fight off parasites.

Digestive Enzyme Supplements: Pepsin, hydrochloric acid, and digestive pancreatic enzymes, as well as bromelain and papain, can help break down the cell walls of parasites and should be taken as supplements both with and between meals. When taken with meals, they aid with digestion; when taken between meals, they help destroy parasites and other cellular debris.

Probiotics: Supplement your diet with friendly bacteria, such as *Bifidobacterium bifidum*, *Lactobacillus acidophilus*, *Lactobacillus bulgaricus*, *Lactobacillus plantarum*, and *Lactobacillus salvarius*. *L. plantarum* is the most effective of these in treating parasites. Treatment may last from 8 to 12 weeks. Recolonizing the intestines with friendly bacteria can help prevent illness by depriving the parasites of the opportunity to flourish and overgrow.

Antiparasitic foods: Certain foods inhibit parasite growth, including garlic, onions, papaya, pineapple, pumpkin seeds, figs, pomegranate seeds, and the seeds of the Rangoon creeper fruit (*Quisqualis indica*). Since most commercial fruit is irradiated, the amount of enzymes found in fresh pineapple and papaya, unless organic, is minimal. Their enzymes are

How to Avoid Parasites

Taking precautions will help you avoid parasites.

Food

- Don't eat raw beef or pork; both can be loaded with tapeworms and other parasites.
- Don't eat raw fish (such as in sushi); you're more likely to get worms if you do.
- When handling raw meat or fish (including shrimp), wash your hands afterward, and in particular, don't put your hands near your mouth before washing them.
- Use separate cutting boards for meat and vegetables. Spores from meat can seep into the board and contaminate vegetables or anything else you put on the board.
- Wash utensils thoroughly after cutting meat.
- Wash fruit, vegetables, eggs, and meats thoroughly with a diluted bleach solution, particularly salad items, as they often harbor parasites (see "Kitchen and Culinary Hygiene" for details on how to prepare the solution).
- Don't drink untreated water from streams, rivers, lakes, and other natural water sources.

Pets

- Don't sleep near pets; they harbor many worms and other parasites.
- Deworm your pets regularly and keep their sleeping areas clean.
- Don't let pets lick your face.
- Don't let pets eat off your dishes.
- Don't walk barefoot around animals.

When Traveling

- Don't drink the local tap water. Use filtered or bottled water instead.
- Start taking herbs or other preventive medications two weeks before traveling and continue them while you travel.

General

- Always wash your hands after using the toilet.
- Wash your hands after working in the garden; the soil can be contaminated with spores and parasites.

important, as they can help break down parasites inside the body. Pomegranate juice can aid in the expulsion of worms , and wheat germ can be used to inhibit various amoebas from binding to target cells in the intestines.

Kitchen and Culinary Hygiene

You can take simple steps to purify raw fruits and vegetables, eggs, and meats of contaminants, including possible parasites. The following technique will rid these foods of harmful toxins, chemicals, sprays, and other poisons. It will also reduce your chances of picking up parasites and noticeably improve the flavor and shelf life of foods.

- Combine ½ teaspoon of bleach with 1 gallon of water. Be sure to use old-fashioned, pure bleach, not chlorine. Soak all fruits, vegetables, meats, and eggs in this solution for the times listed below.

- Divide your foods into the following categories and soak each no longer than the time listed: thin-skinned berries (10–15 minutes), heavy-skinned fruits (15–30 minutes), leafy vegetables (10–15 minutes), root vegetables (15–30 minutes), eggs (20–30 minutes), meats (5–10 minutes per pound).

- Prepare a fresh bleach solution for each category of food and dispose of the solution after use.

- Soak all foods in a fresh water bath for 10 minutes after they've soaked in the bleach solution. Soaking food in a bleach solution isn't your only food-cleansing option. Commercial fruit and vegetable washes are widely available at health food stores. These contain natural emulsifiers that liquefy dirts, oils, and parasites, which cling to the surface of fruits and vegetables, so they can be easily rinsed away.

eight

Alleviating Leaky Gut Syndrome

A healthy intestinal tract is a dual-functioning system: It allows for the maximum absorption of nutrients while also inhibiting the absorption of toxins into body tissues. If, however, the structural integrity of the intestinal lining breaks down, a condition known as intestinal permeability, or leaky gut syndrome, develops. This breakdown allows undigested food proteins and other toxins to enter the bloodstream. When this happens, several things can occur.

The immune system recognizes these particles as foreign substances and sends white blood cells to attack them. This attack produces an increase in free radicals and chemicals released by the white blood cells, which further activates the immune system, causing irritation and inflammation in the area of the attack.

If a high volume of particles continues to flood across the intestinal membranes, the immune system becomes overzealous and begins to attack not only the particles that escape through the leaky gut but also the healthy tissues of surrounding organs and joints. The immune system then becomes deregulated and starts to

---

IN THIS CHAPTER

- Success Story: Treating Leaky Gut Reverses Arthritis
- Healthy and Unhealthy Intestines
- Causes of Leaky Gut Syndrome
- Alternative Medicine Therapies for Leaky Gut Syndrome

consider the body's own tissues as an invader. This continuous attack on the body furthers inflammation and contributes to the escalation of arthritis.

As toxic substances continue to leak from the intestines and enter the bloodstream, they can build up in the body, overwhelming the liver. When the liver is overwhelmed, it can't efficiently break down these substances and an important phase of detoxification shuts down. (For more information on the detoxification phases, see chapter 5, Detoxifying Specific Organs, page 88.)

Leaky gut can also trigger food allergies. Intestinal permeability allows larger-than-normal food proteins to be absorbed before they're completely broken down. Once they leave the intestines, where they're harmless, the immune system sees them as foreign invaders and begins to make antibodies against them. Eventually, autoantibodies are created and a food allergy is born, triggering an inflammatory response whenever the offending food is consumed.

Intestinal dysfunction, allergies, and painful inflammation seem to operate in a loop, each triggering the next. Until the loop is permanently disrupted, the cycle repeats itself with increasingly serious and painful consequences for people with arthritis. In this chapter, we'll investigate the causes of leaky gut syndrome and recommend dietary and lifestyle changes that help relieve this condition without depending on drugs.

Success Story: Treating Leaky Gut Reverses Arthritis

Susan, 49, was diagnosed with aggressive rheumatoid arthritis and experienced pain and swelling in the joints of her neck, shoulders, wrists, feet, and elbows. She also complained of fatigue, memory and balance problems, anxiety, nausea, poor digestion, irritable bowel, bleeding gums, premenstrual syndrome (PMS), chronic sinus infections (postnasal drip, earache, and a persistent cough), difficulty breathing, and frequent urination at night.

Originally, Susan came to us because she wanted to start a supervised fast and detoxification program. She had previously tried this approach at a health spa and found that it greatly relieved her chronic pain. Fasting is commonly used in our clinic with the goal of correcting digestive imbalances and reducing joint pain. Before one of our patients begins a fast and detoxification program, we do a complete workup to develop an individualized protocol that will be best for that person. We tested

Susan for food allergies and found that she had a sensitivity to almost every food group. Such severe food allergies usually indicate leaky gut syndrome, which we confirmed in Susan through an intestinal permeability assay.

We then checked on the health of her liver. According to a functional liver detoxification profile, her liver was so overloaded with toxins that an important phase of detoxification (SEE QUICK DEFINITION) had effectively shut down. Susan's test results showed that her liver could adequately complete phase I of detoxification but broke down in phase II. Her supplies of glutathione sulfate were depleted (the reading was a 4; normal results fall somewhere between 15 and 70), and as a result, high levels of intermediate toxins were slipping back into her bloodstream without undergoing complete detoxification. The Kupffer cells in her liver, which help with cleansing the blood, were also inactive. Toxins were accumulating in her bloodstream and disturbing her connective tissue and immune and endocrine systems, causing inflammation and illness.

A nutritional profile and hair analysis revealed that Susan was dangerously low in antioxidants. She ranked only in the tenth percentile for antioxidant levels, while the seventy-fifth percentile and greater is considered normal. She was particularly deficient in selenium (an important constituent of glutathione peroxidase, which helps the liver detoxify toxins), copper (necessary for healthy structural tissues, joints, and muscles), zinc (an immune system booster), vitamins B_2 and B_{12}, chromium, and calcium.

Due to the high amount of foreign particles that escaped her intestines due to leaky gut syndrome, Susan's liver was overwhelmed and used up its supply of the antioxidants needed to effectively accomplish phase I and phase II detoxification. As a result, vital processes dependent upon antioxidant activities began to slow down.

Susan's low energy level was attributed to anemia resulting from

Alternative Medicine Therapies for Leaky Gut Syndrome

- Fasting
- Dietary guidelines
- Herbs and botanicals
- Digestive enzymes
- Nutritional supplements

 QUICK DEFINITION In liver detoxification, **phase I** and **phase II** refer to the natural two-step process the liver conducts to rid the body of toxins. During phase I, the liver converts toxic compounds into intermediate components. In phase II, the liver combines these components with glutathione sulfate, forming substances that can be eliminated from the body. They are then delivered to the colon or bladder for excretion.

deficiencies in vitamin B$_{12}$ and hypoglycemia due to low blood sugar and a deficiency of chromium, which stabilizes blood sugar production. It was also linked to antioxidant deficiency. Cellular energy production depends upon a rich supply of antioxidants, which help carry out important phases of the Krebs cycle, the process by which the body's cells produce energy.

Susan's secondary symptoms of anxiety and PMS suggested imbalances of the adrenal glands caused by stress. Stress causes the adrenal glands to release cortisol, which stimulates the fight-or-flight response. Chronic stress causes the release of excess amounts of cortisol, which leads to muscle fatigue and immune dysfunction and adversely affects metabolism and the transport of nutrients in the body. A deficiency in calcium (an essential cofactor in nerve function and energy production) further weakened Susan's adrenal system.

We started Susan on a complete and individualized program of tissue detoxification with specific therapies focusing on her intestines, liver, connective tissues, and adrenals. To treat Susan's intestinal permeability, we prescribed the following supplements.

- Glutamine: This essential amino acid aids in rebuilding gastrointestinal cells.
- Fiber: To cleanse and strengthen Susan's intestines, we recommended a combination of psyllium, oat bran, pectin, guar gum, goldenseal powder, geranium, and okra powder.
- Colon-cleansing treatments: To help reestablish healthy intestinal flora, we suggested colonics that infused the friendly bacteria *Lactobacillus acidophilus* during the last 5 minutes of therapy.
- Castor oil packs: This therapy was recommended to relieve Susan's joint pain and for relief of her PMS symptoms (see "Castor Oil Pack Instructions," in chapter 5, Detoxifying Specific Organs, page 101).

Next, we worked on cleansing Susan's liver and restoring its ability to detoxify her body. We gave her lipotropic factors (SEE QUICK DEFINITION) containing the liver-detoxifying agents inositol, phosphatidylcholine, and methionine. Herbal lipotropics included milk thistle, celandine, fringetree, black radish, and beet extract. To restore vitality to her liver, we needed to increase her levels of sulfur-containing amino acids, which are integral to detoxification. We instructed her to drink vegetable juice daily, including vegetables in the cabbage family (which are high in sulfur), parsley, and dandelion roots and greens. Parsley and dandelion are also high in sulfur and act as diuretics, helping to clear toxins from the kidneys.

To replenish Susan's supplies of antioxidants we prescribed the following supplements.

- Vitamin E: Offers anti-inflammatory action that suppresses the breakdown of cartilage while stimulating cartilage growth.

- Carotenoid complex: For antioxidant and anti-inflammatory support.

- Buffered vitamin C: Vital for tissue repair, and when taken in combination with vitamin E, contributes to the stability of cartilage.

- Quercetin: Heals leaky gut and stabilizes gut immune regulation and histamine release.

- Pycnogenol: Extracted from pine bark or grape seeds; contains flavonoids to strengthen tissue integrity.

- Essential fatty acids: A combination of fish oil and flaxseed oil to be used as an anti-inflammatory and to sooth to the gastrointestinal tract.

To improve Susan's stress level, we scheduled sessions in a flotation REST tank to reduce anxiety. To lower her levels of stress hormones and heal her adrenal glands, she took an herbal combination containing Siberian ginseng (*Eleutherococcus senticosus*), ashwaghandha, rehmannia, and Panax ginseng. She took licorice root (*Glycyrrhiza glabra*) to support her adrenal glands and liver; licorice is also a powerful anti-inflammatory. She also supplemented with glucosamine to help rebuild her joints and cartilage.

Susan undertook a fast to further detoxify her system. She then resumed a normal diet, being careful to avoid foods she was allergic to or that might exacerbate her arthritis symptoms. After six

 Lipotropic factors are substances that help detoxify the liver by removing and preventing fatty deposits; some of the most important lipotrophic factors are inositol, phosphatidylcholine, and methionine. Inositol (a fiber component) is considered a B vitamin and works closely with choline, especially in cases of liver disorders, diabetes, and depression; it helps remove fats from the liver, preventing stagnation of liver fats and bile. Phosphatidylcholine, also known as lecithin, is a combination of choline, phosphate, and two fatty acids; it's needed to maintain cell membranes and to help reduce multiple liver symptoms from hepatitis, cirrhosis, and fatty liver from alcohol or diabetes. Methionine (an amino acid) helps the liver detoxify; it's also integral to cartilage and can help improve the strength of joint tissues.

months, another round of testing revealed that her leaky gut was resolved, as well as the irritable bowel, PMS, and asthma. Yearly checkups have

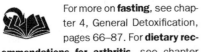

For more on **fasting**, see chapter 4, General Detoxification, pages 66–87. For **dietary recommendations for arthritis**, see chapter 12, The Arthritis Diet, pages 225–256.

shown continued improvement, but Susan has to maintain her arthritis-friendly diet and supplementation or her inflammation returns. She walks comfortably now and no longer suffers debilitating pain in her joints.

Healthy and Unhealthy Intestines

Most patients with RA have some degree of digestive difficulty. It's common for leaky gut and irritable bowel symptoms to precede the onset of arthritis and other inflammatory conditions, such as fibromyalgia.[1] In a healthy intestine, large molecules can't escape between the cells of the intestines because of the tight seal created by the intracellular barrier. However, when this intracellular barrier is compromised, large molecules can escape into the bloodstream, triggering a series of harmful biochemical events. For example, the inflammatory marker TNF-alpha, which contributes to inflammation, has been linked to increased intestinal permeability.[2]

In the intestines, the total surface area capable of absorbing nutrients is about the size of a tennis court. The small intestine absorbs about 95% of the fats and 90% of amino acids we consume as food. Food is first churned in the stomach, where it's broken down by digestive enzymes and hydrochloric acid. (If digestive enzymes and hydrochloric acid are deficient, as they often are in arthritis patients, digestion is incomplete.) The food mass is then moved into and through the small intestine by peristalsis, wavelike contractions of intestinal walls. Fingerlike projections called villi and smaller subprojections, or microvilli, line the small intestine wall and provide a twentyfold increase in the absorptive surface area.

In healthy intestines, semidigested food stays inside the intestines, which is lined with a protective mucous layer (glycocalyx). The only substances absorbed are completely digested nutrients. In the leaky gut, however, larger molecules of incompletely digested foods are able to escape through the damaged intestinal cell membranes. These particles are recognized by the immune system as invaders and stimulate the formation of circulating immune complexes, which initiate inflammation throughout the body.

It takes approximately one to six hours for food to transit through the small intestine. The semifluid bolus of digested food then passes

Most patients with rheumatoid arthritis have some degree of digestive difficulty. It's common for leaky gut and irritable bowel symptoms to precede the onset of arthritis and other inflammatory conditions, such as fibromyalgia.

through the ileocecal valve from the small intestine into the large intestine. Once in the large intestine, or colon, water is reabsorbed from the digested food and the remaining contents form the feces, which consist of indigestible cellulose fibers, friendly and unfriendly microbes, and potentially harmful bile that contains the liver's processed toxins. Average transit time through a healthy large intestine is 12 hours. In patients with chronic constipation, however, transit time may increase to 72 hours or longer. This delayed transit time increases reabsorption of toxic waste products into the body.

Causes of Leaky Gut Syndrome

A majority of arthritis patients have some degree of abnormal digestive function, such as indigestion and constipation, and leaky gut syndrome is also common.[3] Common causes of leaky gut syndrome include a diet high in fried foods, processed foods, inorganic meat products, and simple carbohydrates, as well as excessive alcohol intake. Ironically, medications such as NSAIDs, often used to relieve symptoms of discomfort associated with arthritis, also cause severe leaky gut. Toxins, viruses, candida, and parasite infestation are sometimes implicated as well.

NSAIDs

NSAIDs (nonsteroidal anti-inflammatory drugs) are conventional drugs given to reduce inflammation, pain, and joint stiffness associated with OA and RA, lupus, and other similar conditions. Side effects commonly associated with NSAIDs include rashes, edema, vertigo, nausea, vomiting, and potentially fatal gastrointestinal hemorrhages. NSAIDs may cause gastrointestinal malfunction and irritation, which are leading contributors to leaky gut syndrome. They have been known to create holes in the gastrointestinal wall, particularly that of the stomach, even at normal therapeutic doses in some individuals. When the intestines are irritated and duodenal lesions occur, brought on by NSAID toxicity, the stage is set for leaky gut syndrome.

> Although NSAIDs may initially help with pain due to their anti-inflammatory action, they actually *advance* the overall pathology that causes chronic arthritis, making the disease process worse over time.

Research has uncovered several specific mechanisms that lead to the breakdown of the intestinal wall by NSAIDs. These include damage to the mucosal lining, damage to the mitochondria (energy production centers of the cells), breakdown of intercellular integrity, recirculation of the liver's waste products, and activation of neutrophils caused by the escape of bacteria and large molecules of undigested food through the compromised intestinal barrier.[4] It is important to note that although NSAIDs may initially help with pain due to their anti-inflammatory action, they actually *advance* the overall pathology that causes chronic arthritis, making the disease process worse over time.

Lectins

Lectins are protein fragments of incompletely digested foods that bind with specific sugars on the surface of all cells of the body. They tend to stick like Velcro to the lining of the gastrointestinal tract, where they irritate the tissues and can destroy cell membranes. Further, lectins flatten out the intestinal villi, decreasing absorption of nutrients.

One treatment that can help patients deal with lectins is the use of "decoy sugars," which act by attracting and neutralizing dietary lectins before they can attach themselves to the intestinal lining. (Dr. Zampieron coined the term "decoy sugars" to reflect their ability to "trick" the lectins into moving away from the gut lining.) The correct decoy sugar to use depends on the person's blood type. For instance, the supplement NAG (N-acetyl-D-glucosamine) is useful for blood type A, while the sugar fucose (from the herb bladderwrack) works well for blood type O. Both are readily obtainable in health food stores.

Habitual Alcohol Use

Elevated intestinal permeability has been found to be present in a high percentage of alcoholics and is a major factor involved in the development of alcoholic liver disease. Ethanol and its metabolic derivatives, acetaldehyde in particular, disrupt the tight junctions in the cells lining the intestines and increase membrane permeability to large molecules.[5] To reduce the risk of leaky gut syndrome, it is advisable for patients with arthritis to abstain from alcohol consumption.

Toxins

When gastrointestinal mucous cells are exposed to various toxins, the tight junctures between them widen and allow for the absorption of larger molecules. These molecules translocate from the gut and migrate to other areas of the body, causing inflammation.[6]

Viruses

Viruses use many methods to cause increased intestinal permeability. For example, rotaviruses have proteins on their outer surface that are capable of opening the cellular space usually sealed by the tight junctures between the gastrointestinal mucous cells.[7] In our clinic, patients often report the start of arthritis symptoms after a prolonged flulike illness that adversely affected their digestive system.

Yeast infections

Candida and other forms of yeast can grow on the mucosal lining of the intestines and send out mycelia, rootlike structures that can puncture the intestinal lining, causing leaky gut syndrome to develop. An overgrowth of candida and translocation of the yeast into distant parts of the body (generally due to leaky gut syndrome) causes many arthritis-like symptoms, such as joint pain and stiffness, inflammation, and loss of energy, as well as allergies, headaches, immune suppression, and liver dysfunction.

 For more on **candida's role in arthritis**, see chapter 6, Eradicating Bacteria and Yeast, pages 115–133.

Causes of Leaky Gut Syndrome

- Aspirin and other NSAIDs
- Lectins (harmful protein fragments) from incompletely digested food
- Habitual alcohol use
- Toxins
- Viruses
- Standard American Diet (SAD)
- Candida and parasite

Alternative Medicine Therapies for Leaky Gut Syndrome

Treating leaky gut requires a multiple-therapy approach. Fasting, detoxification, and dietary changes can help ease the stress on the digestive system and begin the healing process (see chapter 4 [page 66] and chapter 5 [page 88] for more details). Herbs, enzymes, and nutrients can then tonify and soothe inflamed tissues and normalize digestion. And stress reduction is also important to decrease the release of stress hormones, which can cause inflammation.

Fasting

Scientific studies have shown fasting to be beneficial in treating leaky gut syndrome and rheumatoid arthritis.[8] It is an inexpensive, rapid, and effective therapy for eliminating toxins from the body, and it allows damaged intestines to regenerate by decreasing their exposure to food allergens and dietary lectins. White blood cell activity increases during fasting, more efficiently removing circulating immune complexes (CICs) from the gastrointestinal lining, joints, and body tissues, which in turn reduces leaky gut issues and inflammation.[9]

 For a complete guide to **detoxification and fasting**, see chapter 4, General Detoxification, pages 66–87.

Dietary Tips to Reduce Leaky Gut Syndrome

Consume organically grown foods whenever possible. Conventionally grown food can have high levels of antibiotic residues, pesticides, and herbicides. Avoid alcohol and any foods you have any sensitivity to—this will be determined by noting your reaction to various foods or by IgG food allergy testing (see "IgG ELISA Test," page 59). Eliminate sugar, all processed and refined foods, and artificial sweeteners, colorings, flavorings, and preservatives. Eat with awareness. Instead of gulping down food on the run, sit down and take your time while eating. Chew slowly and thoroughly until the food is liquefied. Begin the digestive process in a calm, thoughtful state, with an appreciation of the sensory qualities of the food. Consider using chopsticks instead of a knife and fork to induce a more contemplative approach to eating. If you eat with your right hand, switch to your left. Put down your fork between bites and take smaller bites. When you're eating, do nothing else—don't watch television; don't read. Drink only a small volume of liquid with meals, because large amounts will dilute your digestive juices, rendering digestion less effective.

Bitter Herbs and Disgestive Enzymes for Tonifying the Digestive System

Bitter herbs and digestive enzymes can help strengthen the digestive and enzymatic functions of the intestines and tonify the digestive system.

Bitters, including bitter herbs, have been used for thousands of years as a digestive tonic in many traditional cultures. Bitter-tasting herbs trigger nerves in the tongue that stimulates the release of digestive enzymes in the mouth. Bitter flavors also enhance the release of hydrochloric acid in the stomach, increase the liver's production of bile, and stimulate the appetite. They promote production of saliva and gastric juices and accelerate emptying of the stomach, thus triggering the pancreas to begin releasing digestive enzymes. Bitter herbs are useful for sluggish digestion, heartburn, dyspepsia, bowel tension, flatulence, and bloating.[10]

An excellent bitters herbal combination includes extracts of ginger root, cardamom seed, centaury, astragalus root, fennel seed, rosemary leaf, and gentian root. Bitters should be used as a tea or liquid extract, because they need to be tasted in order to be effective. You can also prepare a bitters salad with dandelion leaves, escarole, endive, and other bitter salad greens. These can be combined with romaine, green leaf, and red leaf lettuce, and dressed with olive oil, flaxseed oil, spices, and lemon juice. This type of salad triggers the entire digestive system to function more effectively. Commercial bitters formulations are available as well; you can find Swedish bitters in health foods stores, and most liquor stores sell several varieties of bitters, including Fernet Branca and Angostura, which are alcoholic beverages.

People with arthritis are often deficient in digestive enzymes. Digestive enzymes have a dual role: If taken along with food, they improve digestion and help heal a leaky gut. If taken on an empty stomach, they can be used for their anti-inflammatory action. Digestive enzymes break down large food molecules, decrease the amount of food allergies, inactivate dietary lectins, stimulate digestion, and halt

Testing for Intestinal Permeability

A specific laboratory test, the intestinal permeability assay, can measure the degree to which leaky gut is present. In this test, the patient drinks a liquid that contains a combination of two large sugar molecules, mannitol and lactulose. For the most part, these sugars are not absorbed through the intestine; they pass through the colon and are excreted in the stool. However, if the person has leaky gut syndrome, some of these large sugar molecules leak through the intestines and into the blood. They are then filtered out by the kidneys and exit the body through the urine. The amount of lactulose and mannitol that is collected in the urine provides a reliable assessment of the condition of the intestinal wall. Elevated levels of both of the test sugars in the urine indicates increased permeability.

For more **dietary recommendations for arthritis**, see chapter 12, The Arthritis Diet, pages 225–256.

or alter the growth of dysbiotic microorganisms in the gut. In essence, they help arrest the processes responsible for arthritis. Digestive enzymes can be taken as a dietary supplement. Papain from papaya and bromelain from pineapples are effective vegetarian digestive enzymes.

Pancreatic enzyme supplements aid in the body's natural production of its own enzymes. The pancreas can recycle and recirculate pancreatic enzyme extracts, so not only do they support digestion while it's occurring in the small intestine, they also support future digestion and tonify the pancreas and small intestine.

Demulcent Herbs and Foods

A demulcent is an herb or food that has a protective effect on the mucous membranes. Demulcents contain large amounts of mucilaginous materials—gummy, slimy substances that have a direct action on the lining of the intestines, soothing irritation. Mucilage-containing demulcents minimize irritation down the whole length of the bowel, reducing the sensitivity of the digestive system to gastric acids, relaxing painful spasms, and decreasing leaky gut and digestive inflammation and ulceration.[11]

Marshmallow *(Althea officinalis)*: Marshmallow root contains 25% to 35% mucilage and can be used for any inflammation of the gastrointestinal system. It is usually taken as a tea or liquid extract.

Slippery elm bark *(Ulmus fulva)*: Bark from the branches of the slippery elm tree is a demulcent helpful for the respiratory and gastrointestinal systems. It has traditionally been used for ulcers, colitis, irritable bowel, infections, and diarrhea.[12]

Cabbage juice: Juice from raw organic green cabbage contains high amounts of glutamine, an essential amino acid that aids in the metabolism of gastrointestinal cells. Cabbage juice can be made in combination with other plant foods that are effective in reconstructing a healthy gut mucosa, such as chickweed and plantain. Mix them together to make an excellent healing tonic.

Okra *(Hibiscus esculentus)*: This mucilaginous vegetable contains constituents that soothe and restore the irritated gastrointestinal tract. When okra is cooked, it releases its mucilaginous agents, giving it a slimy texture; this characteristic is good for thickening soups and stews.

Fenugreek *(Trigonella foenum-graecum)*: Use of this medicinal plant dates back to the Egyptians and the Greek physician Hippocrates. Fenugreek seeds contain 28% mucilin and are an excellent demulcent. They have a maple-syrup odor and can be steeped as a tea or used in capsules.

Anti-Inflammatory and Astringent Herbs

Anti-inflammatory herbs help reduce localized tissue swelling and inflammation in the gut. Astringent herbs tighten and tonify tissues, thus sealing the permeable intestines.

Ginkgo biloba: The ginkgo tree is one of the oldest tree species on our planet, having existed for over 200 million years. Its survival over those many aeons is attributable, in part, to its resistance to infection and parasites, which also lend it some of its remarkable health-supporting qualities. Its leaves contain biochemical compounds responsible for ginkgo's healing properties. Clinical and laboratory tests have shown that *Ginkgo biloba* extract (standardized to 24% ginkgo flavoglycosides) protects the integrity of the mucosal lining of the intestines by reducing the oxidative damage due to free radical activity.[13] Ginkgo is also helpful for many health problems associated with inadequate blood supply, since it increases circulation to the small capillaries throughout the body.

Khella *(Ammi visnaga):* The use of khella has been part of Bedouin folk medicine for centuries. Khellin, the chief active component of khella, inhibits the release of histamine, which induces an inflammatory response. Khella also has antispasmodic properties and supports the detoxification activities of the kidneys.[14] The allopathic antihistamine drug cromolyn sodium is based on this ancient remedy.

Chinese skullcap *(Scutellaria baicalensis):* This herb has significant antiallergenic and antioxidant properties. Its active constituents, baicalin and the flavonoid wogonin, are responsible for its anti-inflammatory action. Chinese skullcap has been shown to block highly inflammatory end products of the arachidonic acid cascade (SEE QUICK DEFINITION) and has specific healing action on gastric mucosa.[15]

Licorice root *(Glycyrrhiza glabra):* A systemic anti-inflammatory, licorice also has beneficial effects on the endocrine system, adrenal glands, and liver. Its anti-irritant effect on the gastrointestinal system is thought to be due to

 The **arachidonic acid cascade** is a chemical reaction occurring when excessive arachidonic acid stored in cell membranes is converted into molecules such as prostaglandins and leukotrienes, which may cause many negative physiological reactions. These include bronchial constriction (in asthmatics), intestinal permeability, water retention and swelling, allergies, inflammation, and, ultimately, tissue destruction. Arachidonic acid is a fatty acid found primarily in animal foods such as meat, poultry, and dairy products. When the diet is high in arachidonic acids, they're stored in cell membranes and then transformed into the prostaglandins and leukotrienes that instigate inflammation.

flavonoid compounds called steroidal saponin glycosides, which exert a protective effect.[16] Licorice root has also been shown to reduce the gastric bleeding caused by NSAIDs, often prescribed for arthritis.

Meadowsweet *(Filipendula ulmaria):* Meadowsweet contains anti-inflammatory glycosides, tannins, mucilage, and flavonoids, all of which aid in the treatment of ulcers and other inflammatory conditions of the gastrointestinal system. The astringent properties of meadowsweet act to strengthen the bonds in the connective tissue between cells, thus solidifying the protective intestinal barrier and helping to decrease leaky gut syndrome. It also has powerful free radical scavenging properties.[18]

Chamomile *(Matricaria chamomilla):* Chamomile's Latin name, *Matricaria chamomilla*, means "mother of the gut." This herb has traditionally been used to relieve anxiety, sleep disorders, muscle tension, and digestive distress. In Germany, chamomile is licensed as an over-the-counter drug for internal use against gastrointestinal spasms and inflammatory diseases of the intestinal tract. Two chemicals extracted from chamomile, azulene and bisaboline, have been studied for their anti-inflammatory effects.[19]

Goldenseal *(Hydrastis canadensis):* One of the most widely used American herbs, goldenseal is a tonic remedy that stimulates the immune response and destroys germs, due to the presence of berberine.[20] Goldenseal has astringent effects that aid digestive problems, such as peptic ulcers and colitis, and it promotes the production and secretion of digestive juices. It is useful for helping to reestablish healthy gut mucosa. Because overharvesting of goldenseal is a major problem, we often recommend the use of berberine-rich substitutes, such as barberry and Oregon grape root.

Other Nutrients for Leaky Gut

Quercetin: A naturally occurring bioflavonoid found in many species of plants, including oaks, onions, and blue-green algae, quercetin has powerful antioxidant and anti-inflammatory properties and is used to treat arthritis, autoimmune diseases, asthma, cataracts, and leaky gut syndrome.[21] By decreasing the rapid opening of mast cells and basophils (white blood cells that release histamines), quercetin stabilizes the gut and decreases permeability.

Glutamine: This amino acid is an important nutrient for the intestinal mucosa. L-glutamine supports the integrity of the gastrointestinal system's protective layer of mucus[22] and reduces movement of pathogenic bacterial forms through a leaky gut and into general circulation,[23] whereby they are deposited in joint tissue, instigating or aggravating arthritis. Glutamine is used in the synthesis of N-acetyl-D-glucosamine (NAG), an important nutrient that's fundamental to the production of the protective mucous lining in the digestive and respiratory tracts, and as such is the first line of defense against leaky gut syndrome. Glutamine supplementation also increases levels of glutathione, an important antioxidant that's instrumental in the liver's detoxification processes.

Glutathione: Glutathione is a tripeptide (a small protein made up of three amino acids) that regulates the activity of antioxidants, such as vitamins A, C, and E. Glutathione stores become depleted when an overabundance of free radicals are present in the body. This condition, known as oxidative stress, negatively affects the musculoskeletal, nervous, immune, and endocrine systems and underlies many of the symptoms associated with arthritis.[24] In the liver, glutathione combines with toxins and ensures their elimination from the body. In addition, glutathione strengthens red blood cell membranes and supports the immune regulation performed by white blood cells. Although taking glutathione directly as a supplement may be beneficial, some studies have shown that absorption of oral glutathione supplements is limited.[25] The best way to elevate glutathione levels is to increase the precursors that the body needs to manufacture glutathione, including foods in the cabbage family, onions, and garlic, as well as glutamine.

N-acetyl-D-glucosamine (NAG): This sugar compound is important in the formation of glycocalyx, a specialized mucus that coats the delicate

Chinese Herbal Combination for Leaky Gut

Traditional Chinese medicine (TCM) offers several patent formulas that have a soothing effect on the digestive system.

Curing Pill Formula: This herbal combination helps cramping, abdominal pain, diarrhea, irritation, and mucousy stools. It is made up of many ingredients, including coix seed, *Atractylodes macrocephala*, chrysanthemum flowers, and citrus peel.

Yunnan Paiyao: Notoginseng is the main ingredient in this valuable first-aid remedy for internal and external bleeding. When taken internally, Yunnan Paiyao is used to treat gastrointestinal inflammation and bleeding ulcers.

intestinal tissues and acts as a first line of defense against bacteria, fungi, and viruses as they attempt to adhere to the cell surface and invade the intestinal walls. NAG also functions as a decoy sugar, attracting and binding dietary lectins, thus preventing them from attaching to the gut.[26] People with a compromised gastrointestinal lining, including a majority of arthritis patients, are more likely to experience gastrointestinal irritation caused by food allergies, dietary lectins, and bacterial, fungal, and viral organisms. NAG promotes the growth of friendly bacteria and is quickly digested by healthy intestinal bacteria.

Essential fatty acids (EFAs): Inflammation is strongly influenced by the kind of fats and oils that are ingested. A significant reduction in lab indicators of inflammation after using omega-3 fatty acids has been verified in clinical studies.[27] These beneficial fatty acids are found in fish oils and certain vegetable oils, such as flaxseed and hemp seed oil. Borage seed oil and evening primrose oil are also useful; they contain an omega-6 fatty acid known as gamma-linolenic acid (GLA), which also has anti-inflammatory effects.[28] Those with arthritis should consume at least 4 to 6 tablespoons of these oils daily and also significantly decrease consumption of the "bad" fats found in commercially raised meat products, hydrogenated oils from commercial baked goods, and margarine.

 For more on **herbs and nutrients helpful in treating arthritis**, see chapter 13, Supplements for Arthritis, pages 257–294.

Vitamins and minerals: Several vitamins, minerals, and nutraceuticals have been shown to decrease oxidative stress,[29] which is one of the main causes of intestinal damage. (Nutraceuticals are foods that confer health benefits beyond their basic nutritional value.) The nutrients zinc, selenium, vitamin C, vitamin E, carotenes, vitamin A, enzymes such as superoxide dismutase (SOD) and catalase, and the amino acid N-acetyl-L-cysteine are all antioxidants, meaning they've been shown to quench free radicals. Antioxidants help prevent intestinal damage due to oxidation and also decrease inflammation systemically, particularly in the joints and connective tissues.

Probiotics: Each human body contains several trillion beneficial bacteria comprising over 400 species, all necessary for health. Many of these friendly bacteria, also called probiotics, reside in the intestines, where they are essential for proper nutrient assimilation. Probiotics also protect the tight junctions in the intestine from leaky gut caused by the use of aspirin and other NSAIDs.[30] Among the more well-known of these are *Lactobacillus acidophilus* and *Bifidobacterium bifidum*. Prior to 1945 and the introduction of mass-market foods and chemical agriculture, most people normally obtained adequate amounts of probiotics from fresh vegetables. Now, due to soil imbalances caused by commercial farming practices, supplementing with probiotics is beneficial, and it's especially important for those with digestive problems.

Fructo-oligosaccharides (FOS): Another option is FOSs, popularly known as "fast food for probiotics." These simple carbohydrates are found in food sources such as Jerusalem artichokes, onions, barley, honey, asparagus, and garlic. They provide a growth medium for beneficial bacteria in the intestines. There is a continuing debate in the medical community over the use of FOSs as a supplement. We have observed in our clinic that FOS supplements may increase candida

Friendly Bacteria Available as Supplements and Their Benefits

In addition to *Lactobacillus acidophilus* and *Bifidobacterium bifidum*, several other varieties of beneficial bacteria are available as supplements. These are some of the most common probiotic supplements, along with their benefits:

- *Lactobacillus acidophilus* supports the immune system.
- *Lactobacillus bulgaricus* has antiviral activity and produces interferon.
- *Lactobacillus casei* helps treat diarrhea.
- *Lactobacillus plantarum* helps allergies and produces lactolin (a natural antibiotic).
- *Lactobacillus rhamnosus* supports the health of gut mucosa.
- *Lactobacillus salivarius* produces enzymes and B vitamins.
- *Bifidobacterium bifidum* is an anti-inflammatory and provides immune support.
- *Bifidobacterium breve* protects against ulcers and provides immune support.
- *Bifidobacterium longum* produces B vitamins and provides immune support.
- *Streptococcus thermophilus* helps with diarrhea and lactose intolerance.

overgrowth, so we don't recommend their use. To increase the amount of FOSs in your system, eat more fresh fruits and vegetables.

nine

Allergies and Arthritis

Allergies often play a significant role in the onset of inflammation and arthritis. Allergic reactions initiate an increase in inflammatory mediators, such as TNF-alpha (tumor necrosis factor alpha) and IL-1beta (an interleukin).[1] Both rheumatoid arthritis and the inflammation in osteoarthritis can be caused by sensitivities to environmental pollutants and food allergies. Allergies can disrupt normal digestive function, leading to intestinal permeability and an increase in inflammation throughout the body. Allergies, intestinal dysfunction, and painful inflammation operate in a vicious cycle—each one triggering the next. Until the cycle is permanently disrupted, it repeats itself with increasingly serious and painful consequences. Fortunately, alternative medicine offers safe and effective natural therapies to get out of the allergy loop and obtain lasting relief.

Allergies, intestinal dysfunction, and painful inflammation operate in a vicious cycle—each one triggering the next. Until the cycle is permanently disrupted, it repeats itself with increasingly serious and painful consequences. Fortunately, alternative medicine offers safe and effective natural therapies to get out of the allergy loop and obtain lasting relief.

Success Story: Eliminating Food Allergies and Arthritis

Morton, 32, complained of minor muscle and joint pain affecting his neck, fingers, and wrists. For most of the first year of treatment, he followed a healthy, semivegetarian rotational diet (foods are eaten in a four-day cycle to reduce allergic reactions), took nutritional supplements, and was free from joint pain. But in March, there was an unforeseen hiccup.

As he does every year on Saint Patrick's Day, Morton attended a family gathering. And as he does every year, he drank a large amount of stout beer. But this year, Morton didn't wake up with just a hangover the following day; instead, he had severe and disabling arthritis pain unlike his usual symptoms of mild muscle aches. "Is there a possible connection between arthritis and drinking beer?" he asked us.

In addition to standard blood tests, we ran a food allergy test, which indicated that Morton had minor allergies to eggs, green beans, kidney beans, yellow wax beans, oysters, and sesame seeds, and major allergies to brewer's yeast (an ingredient in beer) and baker's yeast. Clearly, Morton was allergic to beer, and his increased beer consumption during his family's annual Saint Patrick's Day celebration was making his arthritis worse.

More precisely, Morton was allergic to the yeast in beer, and yeast is also found in many foods, including vinegar, breads, pickles, ketchup, mustard, mayonnaise, salad dressing, sauerkraut, and certain cheeses. Not only did Morton like his beer, his diet included large quantities of bread and he was fond of salad dressings and condi-

Natural Therapies for Allergies

- Dietary recommendations
- Applied kinesiology
- Supplements and herbs

A Primer on Allergies

An allergy is an adverse immune system reaction—sometimes mild, sometimes severe—to a substance that is harmless to nonallergic people. The offending substance, referred to as an allergen, is often a protein that the body judges to be foreign and dangerous. Common manifestations of an allergic response following exposure to an allergen include fatigue, headaches, sneezing, watery eyes, and stuffy sinuses. Allergies fall into two categories, those caused by environmental factors and those caused by food. The most common source of environmental allergies is plant pollen, particularly from trees, weeds, and grasses. The most common culprits in food allergies are yeast, wheat, corn, milk and other dairy products, egg whites, tomatoes, soy, shellfish, peanuts, chocolate, and food dyes and additives.

Common symptoms of an allergic reaction: Difficulty breathing, congestion, sneezing, coughing, itching, nosebleeds, puffy face, flushing of the cheeks, dark circles under the eyes, runny nose, swelling, hives, vomiting, stomachache, intestinal irritation or swelling, and inflamed, bloodshot, scratchy, or watery eyes.

Common health problems caused by allergens: Acne, allergic rhinitis (inflammation of the mucous lining of the nose), bedwetting, diarrhea, asthma, ear infections, eczema, fatigue, arthritis, chronic runny nose, headache, irritability, hay fever, concentration problems, hyperactivity, and attention deficit disorder. (Note that conventional medicine often ignores food allergies as a causative agent of many of these symptoms.[2])

The Cycle of Food Allergies: There is a strange paradox linked to food allergies. People often crave the very foods that produce an allergic response. When a person stops eating an allergy-producing food to which their body has become addicted, such as coffee or chocolate, they often experience unpleasant withdrawal symptoms, such as fatigue, for about three days. As with other addictions, eating more of the addictive substance can actually improve the situation by suppressing the withdrawal symptoms. This, however, becomes an unhealthy cycle of addiction, craving, and fulfillment that eventually leads to more serious health problems. This suppression of symptoms after consumption of an allergenic food is referred to as masking, because it disguises the true allergic symptoms.

The Allergic Response: Allergens enter the body via breathing, absorption through the skin, eating or drinking, or by injection, as with insect bites or vaccinations. Because the body determines the allergen to be dangerous, it reacts to the substance as an allergic antigen, triggering an inflammatory response. The mobilized immune system then releases antibodies, specific forms of protein designed to deactivate the allergenic antigens, setting in motion a complex series of events involving many biochemical compounds. These chemicals then produce inflammation or other symptoms typical of an allergic response. In general, the allergic response, in the form of inflammation, swelling, or tenderness, is the body's attempt to heal itself from the effect of the allergen. However, if it continues unchecked for too long, health will suffer.

The antibody most commonly involved in the allergic response to pollens and other environmental allergens is IgE, one of five immunoglobulins involved in the immune system's defense response to foreign substances. The main types of immunoglobulins, grouped according to their concentration in the blood, are IgG (80%), IgA (10%–15%), IgM (5%–10%), IgD (less than 0.1%), and IgE (less than 0.01%). Mast cells, which produce the allergic response and are found throughout the body's tissues, come into play next. They tend to be concentrated in the gastrointestinal tract, the reproductive organs, and the linings of the skin, nose, and lungs. When the IgE antibody senses an allergen, it triggers the mast cells to release histamine and 30 other chemicals, and the allergic response flares into action. The IgE molecules also attach themselves, like a key fitting a lock, to the allergens.

Immediate versus Delayed Allergic Reactions: The most common allergic reactions occur immediately after exposure to a certain substance (peanuts, pollen, bee stings, or cats). These reactions are typically caused by IgE immunoglobulins, resulting in a runny nose, watery eyes, itching, and skin rashes; more severe reactions include constriction of the bronchial tubes and difficulty breathing. Delayed allergies are another type of allergic reaction, manifesting up to 72 hours after exposure to a triggering substance. This kind of reaction involves IgG immunoglobulins and can cause a wide array of symptoms, including lethargy, attention deficit disorder, fatigue, hyperactivity, acne, itchy skin, mood swings, insomnia, and arthritis inflammation. Up to 80 different medical conditions—from arthritis, asthma, and autism to insomnia, psoriasis, and diabetes—have been clinically associated with IgG food allergy reactions. IgG-mediated reactions can make immediate (IgE) allergic reactions more severe.[3]

These are some of the most common chemicals released during an allergic response.

- Histamine: This substance causes the blood vessels to widen, enabling more fluid to pass into body tissues and resulting in swelling; it also triggers the smooth involuntary muscles in the lungs, blood vessels, heart, stomach, intestines, and bladder to contract. Histamine causes runny nose; red itchy eyes; hot, tender, or swollen body parts; flushing of the skin; and the other symptoms associated with allergic reactions.

- Heparin: Heparin increases blood flow to the site of inflammation or swelling.

- Platelet-activating factor: This substance causes blood platelets to group together so that they release chemicals to change the diameter of blood vessels, thereby affecting blood pressure.

- Serotonin: This neurotransmitter, found in the brain and mucous membrane of the gastrointestinal tract, is involved in the allergic response to foods.

- Lymphokines: Produced by white blood cells (lymphocytes), lymphokines are involved in intracellular communications.

- Leukotrienes: Found in cell membranes, leukotrienes can initiate spasms, such as the bronchial spasm of asthma.

- Prostaglandins: These hormonelike substances help dilate blood vessels, affect smooth muscle contraction, increase pain in affected areas, and heat up inflamed tissues.

- Thromboxanes: These are chemicals that contract blood vessels and bronchial tubes.

- Bradykinin: Formed locally in damaged tissues, bradykinin supports the cascade of inflammatory symptoms set in motion by the mast cells.

- Interleukins: These are antibodies involved in the activity of lymphocytes.

- Interferons: These antiviral compounds are produced by lymphocytes to regulate the speed of immune responses.

ments like pickles. In essence, Morton craved foods that worsened his arthritis and continually toxified his system. Although the Saint Patrick's Day bash was the proverbial straw that broke the camel's back, his overindulgence also provided us with important information about the cause of his arthritis.

To address Morton's allergies, we recommended he limit his consumption of the foods that aggravated his symptoms. We also gave him homeopathic remedies for yeast and mold. By the time Saint Patrick's Day rolled around again, Morton was able to indulge (slightly) in the festivities with less consequences afterward.

The Allergy Connection

Patients are often surprised to learn that the inflammation associated with arthritis can be caused by environmental pollutants, food sensitivities, and bacteria that have translocated out of the intestinal tract. These antigens cross the gastrointestinal membrane, enter the bloodstream, circulate as injurious immune complexes, and are stored in the joints, where they initiate inflammation. High levels of immune complexes have been found both in the blood serum and in the synovial fluid around the joints of arthritis patients.[4]

Arthritis and allergies are strongly linked in many individuals. A 52-year-old woman who had suffered from inflammatory arthritis for 11 years was tested to see if her symptoms were linked with food sensitivities. She was first evaluated while on her regular diet, then while fasting, and then while being "challenged" with foods known to provoke allergies. While on her normal diet, the woman reported morning stiffness. In contrast, after she fasted for three days, she had no morning stiffness and no swollen joints. When she was given 8 ounces of milk four times a day after the fast, she experienced 30 minutes of morning stiffness, numerous tender joints, and four swollen joints. These symptoms began 24 to 48 hours after ingesting the milk, which clinically indicated an IgG-mediated allergy. This strongly suggests that food sensitivities are associated with arthritic symptoms in this patient.

One experiment published in the journal *Rheumatology* tested the levels of two inflammatory mediators, TNF-alpha (tumor necrosis factor alpha) and IL-1beta (interleukin-1beta), in two groups of people: Group one tested positive to particular foods, and group two had no allergic reactions to foods. All patients refrained from eating the most common aller-

> Allergies play a significant role in the onset of inflammation and arthritis. Both rheumatoid arthritis and the inflammation in osteoarthritis can be caused by sensitivities to environmental pollutants and food allergies.

genic foods for 12 days. After following the restricted diet, group one was given the foods they were allergic to (allergies were established previously) for 12 days, while group two was given corn- and rice-rich foods for 12 days. Then these "challenge" foods (the previously established allergenic foods for group one and rice- and corn-rich foods for group two) were eliminated once again. Clinical examinations were performed after eliminating the specific foods at the end of the challenge phase, and at the end of the reelimination phase. The patients were evaluated for stiffness, pain, number of tender and swollen joint, and several inflammatory markers, such as erythrocyte sedimentation rate (ESR), C-reactive protein (CRP), and serum TNF-alpha and IL-1beta levels.

The results indicated that ESR, CRP, TNF-alpha, and IL-1beta levels, and all of the clinical variables, were increased by the food challenges in group one, while in group two no significant change was seen in any of the variables except pain. In addition, important differences were observed for most of the variables between the two groups. About 72% of group one and 18% of group two experienced disease exacerbation after eating the challenge foods. This study concluded that individualized dietary revisions can help regulate TNF-alpha and IL-1beta levels in selected patients with RA.[5] In our clinical experience, we've found that modification of diet is one of the most important treatments for RA.

What Causes Allergies?

The tendency to develop allergies is due to a combination of genetic and environmental factors.[6] Allergies are often caused by an overload of toxins, which continually stimulates the immune system. Over time, the body's normal feedback mechanisms that turn off the immune system malfunction. The system becomes deregulated and attacks molecules that a normal system would recognize as harmless. There are many factors that may initiate this deregulation, including consumption of junk food and allergenic foods, pesticides and herbicides, pollution, immunizations, steroids, birth control pills, antibiotics, and other pharmaceutical drugs. Allergic reactions cause immunoaggression against everything, including healthy tissue, such as joint tissue in the case of RA.

A repetitive diet, limited to 30 foods or less, can contribute greatly to the development of allergies. Food intolerance can develop when the same food, such as bread, is eaten over and over again. The immune system becomes overexposed to the molecules of this particular food, begins to consider it an invader, and initiates an attack against it. The cells and chemicals involved in this attack then begin to destroy the body's own tissues. The immune system in the gastrointestinal tract normally responds only to pathogens and toxins, remaining unresponsive to food antigens. However, this normal functioning goes out of control when bombarded with a repetitive diet, causing inflammation. This overreaction is linked to the development of gut permeability and food allergies.[7]

Foods Linked to Allergies and Arthritis

Although any food can theoretically trigger an allergic reaction in an individual, these are the most common food allergens for arthritis patients.

- Beef
- Chocolate
- Corn
- Dairy products
- Eggs
- Green beans
- Nuts (especially peanuts)
- Oranges
- Soy
- Sugar
- Wheat
- Yeast (both baker's and brewer's)
- Yellow wax beans
- Nightshades (tomatoes, peppers, eggplant, potatoes, paprika, and tobacco)

The Wheat Connection

Wheat is often a major culprit in the development of arthritic conditions. One study focused on a 15-year-old girl who suffered with synovitis (SEE QUICK DEFINITION) in her knees and ankles for three years. The researchers determined that she had an intestinal disease brought about by sensitivity to wheat gluten. When she eliminated wheat gluten (a lectin) entirely from her diet, the synovitis symptoms disappeared, leading researchers to conclude that her arthritis was associated with a bowel disorder produced by wheat allergies.[8] Arthritis patients with elevated levels of antibodies against gliadin, a wheat protein, tend to have more pronounced inflammation.[9] We

 Synovitis results in painful swelling and inflammation of the membrane (the synovium) surrounding joints. It weakens the bone and joint tissues, destroys cushioning cartilage, and is commonly associated with RA. In an advanced stage, it also kills off healthy red blood cells.

have found that patients who completely eliminate all wheat products from their diet often have a remarkable elimination of many symptoms of arthritis, including joint pain and swelling. We suggest that all arthritis patients try a wheat elimination diet, since there are no adverse effects, and it offers the possibility of a dramatic decrease in symptoms. Wheat products include most breads, cakes, cookies, bagels, pizza crusts, and pastas. All labels must be read carefully, because wheat is often a "hidden" ingredient in dressings, sauces, soups, and many other foods.

Food allergies are quite often caused by molecular subfractions (such as proteins) found in the food, not the whole food itself. Therefore, testing for sensitivities to whole foods may miss the true allergenic substances. For example, testing for whole-grain wheat antigens alone, may not detect an allergy to gliadin, which is only a part of the wheat kernel. The test may read negative for an allergy to wheat, while the person is actually intensely reactive to wheat gliadin. The principal allergenic component of wheat (and also of rye and, to a lesser extent, oats and barley) is gluten, the protein-carbohydrate combination that enables flour to bind when baking. The protein gliadin is the prime allergen within the gluten.

The Milk Connection

Several of the constituents found in milk, including the protein (casein) and the sugar (lactose), are directly linked to the development of a wide range of adverse effects, including allergies, dermatitis, digestive difficulties, and arthritis symptoms. The allergy connection to dairy products is often missed because many products that contain hidden lactose, such as breads, cake mixes, soft drinks, lagers, and processed meats, and inadequately labeled.[10] Eliminating all dairy products and, when possible, products containing lactose from the diet for a period of four to six weeks is mandatory for patients who want to track down possible dietary connections to arthritis.

The Nightshade Vegetable Connection

Vegetables in the nightshade family are strongly linked with arthritis. The nightshade family includes such common vegetables as potatoes, eggplant, peppers (both bell peppers and chiles), paprika, tomatoes, and tobacco. One study observed over 5,000 OA and RA patients who agreed to eliminate nightshade vegetables from their diet. The patients were then tested for both subjective and objective measurements of pain and inflammation. The result was a 70% remission of aches and pains, simply due to avoidance of nightshades.[11] A possible explanation is that chemical alkaloids contained in nightshades are deposited in the connective tissue and stimulate inflammation while also inhibiting the formation of normal cartilage. As a result, cartilage begins to break down and isn't replaced by healthy new cartilage cells.

Many people who don't test positive for nightshade allergies still tend to report a decrease in pain after eliminating nightshades from their diet. One theory to explain this phenomenon suggests that lectins in tomatoes and other nightshades may persist in the body and initiate the formation of circulating immune complexes. Immune complexes are deposited in soft tissues if the detoxification pathways are overburdened, causing an inflammatory response, joint swelling, and pain. It is well worth the effort to completely eliminate these foods for six weeks, then follow up with a challenge test, reintroducing one food at a time for three days, to see if symptoms increase once again. If so, that offending food must be avoided.

For more on **dietary factors in arthritis**, see chapter 12, The Arthritis Diet, pages 225–256.

Testing for Allergies

The problem with diagnosing a food allergy is that reactions are often varied or inconsistent and may take several days to develop after eating an allergy-causing food. How much or how often you eat an allergenic food or how it is cooked may all factor into whether or not you have a reaction. In addition, an additive or ingredient may cause an allergy rather than the food itself. A combination of foods is frequently involved in causing the reaction, and symptoms are often masked by regular consumption of the foods.

Do You Suffer from Food Allergies?

The following questionnaire, developed by osteopathic physician and naturopath Leon Chaitow can help determine if you have a food allergy. If your answer to any question is no, give yourself a score of 0 for that particular question; the other scores are provided with each question.

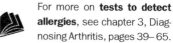

For more on **tests to detect allergies**, see chapter 3, Diagnosing Arthritis, pages 39–65.

- Do you suffer from unnatural fatigue? (Score 1 if occasionally, 2 if three times a week or more.)

- Do you sometimes experience weight fluctuations of four or more pounds in a single day, accompanied by puffiness of the face, ankles, or fingers? (Score 1 if infrequently, 2 if more than once a month.)

- Do you have hot flashes (apart from menopause) or find yourself sweating for no obvious reason? (Score 1 if infrequently, 2 if several times a week or more.)

- Does your pulse race or your heart pound strongly for no obvious reason? (Score 1 if infrequently, 2 if several times a week or more.)

- Do you have a history of food intolerance, causing any symptoms at all? (Score 2 if your answer is yes.)

- Do you crave bread, sugary foods, milk, chocolate, coffee, or tea? (Score 2 if your answer is yes.)

- Do you suffer from migraines or severe headaches, irritable bowel syndrome, eczema, depression, asthma, or muscle aches? (Score 2 if your answer is yes.)

The highest possible score on this test would be 14. If you score 5 or higher, there's a strong likelihood that allergies are part of your symptom picture.

The Elimination Diet

The elimination diet is a test procedure to help identify food allergies. It involves three steps:

1. Eliminate possible allergenic foods for 10 to 14 days.

2. Carefully observe any changes in symptoms.

3. Test the eliminated foods by reintroducing them into the diet, one by one, and noting any return of symptoms.

The foods you choose to eliminate should be those you eat often, especially those you eat daily. Test for wheat and dairy products, foods you crave, and foods that cause any sort of noticeable reaction, such as fatigue or light-headedness. It's important to eliminate all of the suspected foods on your list, as multiple allergies are quite common. If all suspicious foods are not eliminated, it could skew the test results. Also, read the ingredients on any packaged foods very carefully to ensure that you don't inadvertently consume whatever it is you are trying to eliminate (for example, sugar or the flavor enhancer monosodium glutamate). Remember that delayed food allergies can take as long as 72 hours to exhibit symptoms. If you experience symptoms such as irritability, fatigue, headaches, and intense cravings during the elimination period, you may be going through withdrawal, a sure sign that you've been suffering from an allergy.

Blood Test

The IgG ELISA test is a blood test considered by many alternative medicine practitioners to be among the most sensitive and useful in detecting food allergies. (ELISA stands for enzyme-linked immunoserological assay.) For more information on this test, see "IgG ELISA Test," page 59.)

Success Story: Treating Allergies Relieves Painful Joints

Leonard, 47, had suffered with joint and muscle pains for several months, particularly in his hands, wrists, elbows, knees, ankles, back, and neck. His medical history included childhood environmental allergies, and he was still extremely sensitive to pollutants and chemicals. Leonard also suffered from sarcoids (tumorlike growths) in his lungs (most likely from working around asbestos and chemicals for many years), and he was a recovering alcoholic.

We found that Leonard's diet was very poor. He rarely cooked at home, preferring to eat out at fast-food restaurants. His diet consisted predominantly of chicken, shellfish, eggs, whole milk, cheese, French fries, and wheat bread. In addition, Leonard was fond of sodas (drinking 9 to 11 cans per week), sweet desserts, and chocolate. He ate few salads, vegetables, or fresh fruits. Leonard also exercised infrequently.

There was a history of RA in Leonard's family, perhaps indicating a genetic predisposition for the condition. Leonard had numerous physical complaints other than his arthritis symptoms, including itchy eyes and ears, stuffy nose, gastrointestinal problems (gas, bloating, infrequent bowel movements), frequent urination, and periodic bouts of acne.

We did a food allergy test (the IgG ELISA blood test) and found that Leonard had many food sensitivities: almonds, bananas, green beans, kidney beans, yellow wax beans, cheese, eggs, garlic, limes, milk, mustard, oysters, rye, wheat, spinach, yeast (baker's and brewer's), and zucchini. Leonard immediately began working with our nutritionist to change his diet to deal with his sensitivities and improve his nutrient intake.

We also used herbal crystallization analysis (a simple saliva test) to determine which herbs would be most beneficial for Leonard. Based on the results, we gave him an individualized botanical extract containing the following herbs.

- Barberry (*Berberis vulgaris*) root bark: An antibacterial, antifungal digestive tonic and liver stimulant.
- Bayberry (*Myrica cerifera*) root bark: Tonic for the respiratory system and helpful for hay fever, sinus congestion, and colds and flu.
- *Panax ginseng* root: An adaptogenic herb that enhances the overall constitution and strengthens the endocrine glands. (An adaptogen is a natural substance that helps the body adapt to stress.)
- Dandelion (*Taraxacum officinale*) root and leaf: A blood purifier, diuretic, and liver and gallbladder tonic that balances blood sugar.
- Burdock (*Arctium lappa*) root: A blood purifier.
- Yellow dock (*Rumex crispus*) root: A liver tonic and blood purifier that helps skin problems and contains high levels of botanical iron.
- Juniper (*Juniperus communis*): A kidney and adrenal tonic and diuretic that's helpful for gout, diabetes, and hypoglycemia.

We prepared this formula as a nonalcoholic standardized extract, and Leonard took it for four months.

To encourage the detoxification process, we instructed Leonard on the proper way to fast. Regular fasting eases the stress on the gastrointestinal system and allows the body to purge itself of its toxic load. We

Inside Sick Building Syndrome

In the early 1980s, physicians began using the term sick building syndrome (SBS) to refer to a host of symptoms produced by low-grade toxic environmental conditions found in living, work, or office spaces. SBS symptoms are numerous: chest tightness, skin complaints (dryness, itching, abnormal redness), headaches, fatigue, lethargy, coughing, wheezing, asthma, chronic nasal stuffiness, joint pain, infections, emotional irritability, and irritation of the mucous membranes of the eyes, nose, and throat. All of these depress the immune system, rendering the individual susceptible to long-term chronic illness.

Indoor air pollution is widely recognized as a serious environmental risk to human health. Most people in industrialized nations spend more than 90% of their time indoors, where concentrations of pollutants (including toxic chemicals) are often substantially higher than outdoors, leading to chronic exposure to low-grade toxic factors.

Sources of indoor toxic pollution include poorly designed ventilation systems,[12] volatile organic compounds released from particleboard furniture, carpets, glues, paints, toners for copiers and other office machines, and perfumes. Biological agents from mold spores, microbes, mites, or animal dander add to the pollutants and may be partially responsible for symptoms associated with sick building syndrome.[13] People with arthritis should investigate their home and office spaces to determine if the environment is exacerbating their problem. If so, an air filter or plants can help remove toxins from the air. In extreme cases, it may be necessary to live or work in a different space or to make major changes to the indoor environment, such as replacing all carpets with easily cleaned flooring.

also had Leonard undergo regular sauna sessions in order to sweat out additional toxins from his body.

After four months on this program, Leonard was completely pain free, with no stiffness or limitation of movement. His gastrointestinal difficulties were greatly improved, and he vowed to continue with his healthier eating habits. Leonard reported that his environmental allergies were also much better: He was able to withstand greater exposure to pollution or other toxins without going over the edge.

 For information on **fasting**, see chapter 4, General Detoxification, pages 66–87. For more on **saunas and other physical therapies for detoxification**, see chapter 14, Exercises and Physical Therapies, pages 295–320.

Alternative Medicine Therapies for Allergies

Once offending foods are identified, they should be eliminated from your diet. Initially, completely refrain from eating all allergenic foods for 60 to 90 days. After this period, begin to slowly reintroduce them. As allergenic foods are reintroduced, pay close attention to your body over the next 72 hours. If your symptoms reappear, eliminate that food for another two to four weeks, then try again.

Although there is great therapeutic benefit in avoiding foods and chemicals that trigger allergies, rarely is it possible to entirely eliminate them. We use several methods to reduce our patients' allergies and arthritic pain. We often use fasting to reduce allergic reactions and the corresponding arthritic symptoms. During such a fast, the person typically eats only high-nutrient soups, water, and/or vegetable juices. Following this type of diet for four to six weeks decreases the amount of immune complexes (substances formed when antibodies attach to antigens) circulating in the blood. We also use applied kinesiology, supplements, and herbs to alleviate allergies.

Applied Kinesiology

Applied kinesiology, first developed by George Goodheart, D.C., is the study of the relationship between muscle dysfunction (weak muscles) and related organ or gland dysfunction. Applied kinesiology employs a simple strength resistance test on a specific indicator muscle related to the organ or part of the body that is being tested. If the muscle tests strong (maintaining its resistance), it indicates health. If it tests weak, it can mean infection or dysfunction.

A special application that uses kinesiology to detect food allergies is the Nambudripad Allergy Elimination Technique (NAET). Developed by Devi Nambudripad, D.C., L.Ac., this method also helps to eliminate allergies by using acupuncture (or acupressure) and chiropractic. After

Ways to Halt an Allergic Reaction

There are several safe and effective ways to halt an acute allergic reaction before it escalates.

- **Alkaline salts:** Make your own alkaline salts by combining one part potassium bicarbonate (available at any pharmacy) and two parts sodium bicarbonate (baking soda). Take 1 teaspoon of the mixture in a 12-ounce glass of filtered water. Repeat this dose every hour for three hours in the case of an acute allergic reaction, or several times per day if you're on an elimination diet and reintroducing offending foods into your daily meals.

- **Vitamin C:** Use buffered vitamin C, because it doesn't upset the stomach. Take 2 teaspoons in water every 15 to 20 minutes during an acute situation; during a detoxification period, take vitamin C to promote bowel tolerance (the amount that produces loose stools).

- **Antiallergy nutrient cocktail:** For relief of allergic reactions, two to three times a day take powdered and buffered vitamin C (2,000 mg in 8 ounces of water), bioflavonoids (in liquid form, 250 mg), calcium (capsule form, 1,000 mg), magnesium (capsule form, 1,000 mg), and vitamin B_6 (capsule form, 250 mg).

determining the allergy-inducing substances through muscle testing, the patient again holds the offending substance while the NAET practitioner uses acupuncture or acupressure to reprogram the way the body responds to the substance, thereby removing the allergic charge.

Supplements and Herbs

A combination of quercetin and bromelain is one of the most effective supplements available to treat a food allergy. Quercetin is a natural bioflavonoid (SEE QUICK DEFINITION) derived from plants, such as blueberries, cranberries, cherries, or onions. It enhances the body's ability to use vitamin C, increasing its absorption by the liver, kidneys, and adrenal glands. Bromelain, a digestive enzyme derived from pineapple, enhances the absorption of quercetin. Taken together, quercetin and bromelain strengthen the membranes of the body's cells so that they're less likely to be damaged in the presence of an allergen. This, in turn, lessens the severity and reduces the symptoms of allergies.

 A **bioflavonoid** is a pigment within plants and fruits that acts as an antioxidant to protect the body against damage from free radicals and excess oxygen. In the body, bioflavonoids enhance the beneficial activities of vitamin C, and they are often formulated with this vitamin in supplements. Originally called vitamin P, these vitamin C "helper" substances include citrin, hesperidin, catechin, rutin, and quercetin. When taken with vitamin C, bioflavonoids increase the absorption of vitamin C in the liver, kidneys, and adrenal glands. As antioxidants, they also protect vitamin C from destruction by free radicals.

You can reduce your digestive system's reactions to offending foods by using the appropriate enzyme supplements: proteases digest protein, lipases digest fats, amylases digest carbohydrates, lactases digest dairy products, and disaccharidases digest sugars. Supplementing with betaine hydrochloric acid, the primary acid in the stomach, may also help digestive function. As digestion improves, allergic reactions should be minimized or eliminated.

Other nutrients and herbs useful for enhancing tissue repair and regenerating the digestive system include the amino acid L-glutamine, vitamin E, chlorophyll, aloe vera, papaya, slippery elm, and marshmallow root. Probiotics (friendly bacteria) can also help heal the digestive system, thus decreasing allergic reactions to food.

ten

Desensitizing the Autoimmune Reaction

Autoimmune diseases, such as RA, ankylosing spondylitis, juvenile RA, and lupus, involve destruction of healthy cells by the body's own defensive mechanism. In RA, normal cartilage cells become the target of repeated attacks by the immune system, eventually eroding the cartilage and causing joint deformities and disabilities. If the immune system's error in judgment isn't corrected, the attack can progress to the heart, lungs, and other vital organs.

The mechanisms that cause deregulation of the immune response aren't entirely understood. Heavy metal toxicity, leaky gut syndrome, infectious bacteria and parasites, and nutritional imbalances can weaken the body so the immune system becomes overloaded and confused. However, how these and other factors cause the immune system to attack the body's own tissues is not clear. In this chapter, we discuss the components of the immune system and how they interact to fight infections. We explain what is known about the abnormal action of the immune system in autoimmune

IN THIS CHAPTER

- Protecting the Body: The Immune System

- Uncontrolled Inflammation: The Autoimmune Response

- Measuring the Autoimmune Reaction

- Natural Therapies for Calming the Immune System

181

> Autoimmune diseases involve the destruction of healthy cells by the body's own defensive mechanism. In RA, normal cartilage cells become the target of repeated attacks by the immune system.

diseases and address natural therapies that can help regulate the immune system's aggressive behavior without suppressing or altering its necessary defenses.

Protecting the Body: The Immune System

The immune system constantly surveys the body for pathogens (foreign, nonself substances, such as cancerous cells, bacteria, viruses, and parasites). During a normal immune response, leukotrienes and prostaglandins (hormonelike members of the immune system) dilate blood vessels so that white blood cells and other immune components can quickly travel to the area that needs protection. Increased blood flow causes swelling, redness, and heat. Another wave of proinflammatory compounds, these known as chemotactic factors, activates the white blood cells to begin attacking pathogens and digesting damaged cells and circulating immune complexes. As pathogens are destroyed, their cell walls and internal components leak out, triggering still another phase of immune defense. In this phase, B cells produce antibodies specific to the pathogen or cell under attack and also alert macrophages, the "vacuum cleaners" of the immune system, that invaders are present.

Natural Therapies for Calming the Immune System

- Oral tolerization
- Auto-sanguis dilution therapy
- Urine therapy
- Herbal remedies

The oxidizing chemicals released by white blood cells to destroy pathogens can inadvertently affect normal cells. The healthy cells surrounding an inflammatory response attempt to protect themselves by secreting anti-inflammatory prostaglandins, antioxidants, antichemo tactic chemicals, and enzymes. All of these chemicals attempt to counter the destructive substances released by white blood cells.[1] When the body is functioning normally, proinflammatory chemicals are soon suppressed by the anti-inflammatory chemicals secreted by neighboring cells. The inflammatory response subsides: Suppressor T cells stop the production of antibodies, blood vessels return to their normal size, and the repair process begins to mend damaged tissues.

Uncontrolled Inflammation: The Autoimmune Response

When a person has an autoimmune disease, their immune system fails to recognize that the acute danger of infection has passed, and the immune response continues unabated. Researchers have yet to determine the sequence of events that leads to the immune system turning against the body, but they have identified the following suspects: proinflammatory agents including prostaglandins, autoantibodies (immune cells produced by lymphocytes that attack body cells), and defective suppressor T cells (see "The Major Players in the Immune System," page 184).

One of the chemicals released during the inflammatory cascade is nuclear factor kappa beta (NFkB). This substance increases the production of cytokines, which activate white blood cells, command the inflammatory response, and communicate messages to other cells. These messages are varied; some act to recruit and train other white blood cells to join in the fight, while others act as down-regulators, signaling that the fight is over. NFkB is an important modulator of the inflammatory response in many disease processes, including diabetes,[3] cellular aging,[4] and autoimmune illnesses.[5]

T-helper cells are divided into two subsets: T-helper cells type 1 (Th1) produce inflammatory compounds including tumor necrosis factor alpha (TNF-alpha), gamma interferon, and interleukin-2 (IL-2). TNF-alpha amplifies the immune response, and this has important ramifications in autoimmune arthritis. Gamma interferon encourages the presentation of foreign antigens to T-helper cells, while IL-2 stimulates the replication of T cells, which are programmed for attack. T-helper cells type 2 (Th2), respond to immune stress by releasing cytokines that downregulate autoimmunity, particularly such interleukins as IL-4, IL-5, and IL-6. The balance between the activity of Th1 and Th2 cells can be a contributing factor in the progression of RA. Patients with autoimmune disease often have an elevated Th1 level and a low Th2 level.[6] Specific treatments to enhance Th2 cells and their anti-inflammatory

The Major Players in the Immune System

The immune system is extremely complex, with many "players" and myriad feedback mechanisms that interact continuously.[2] There are two major categories of immune response: antibody-mediated immunity, also called humoral immunity, and cell-mediated immunity. In antibody-mediated immunity, antigen particles bind to antibodies, initiating an immune response. Antibodies, also called immunoglobulins, are protein molecules produced by B cells against a specific antigen. Antibodies are usually formed within three days after the first encounter with an antigen. In cell-mediated immunity, specialized white blood cells bind to the antigen, which again triggers a series of responses by various immune modulators.

The immune system is made up of millions of "workers" that have specific roles in guarding the body. The most abundant and varied workers are the white blood cells, comprised of neutrophils, eosinophils, basophils, macrophages, and lymphocytes. Neutrophils, or granulocytes, make up 50% to 70% of the white blood cells circulating in the bloodstream. They engulf invading particles, especially bacteria and fungi. Eosinophils make up about 5% of all the white blood cells and are involved in allergic reactions and the suppression of parasites. Basophils account for less than 1% of the white blood cells. Basophils that reside in body tissues are called mast cells, and these combat specific parasites and fungi. They're also involved in the release of histamines caused by allergic reactions.

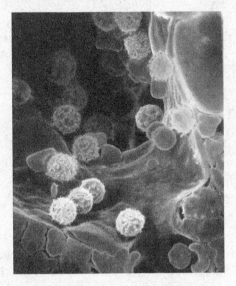

Macrophages swallow foreign proteins, then release an enzyme that chemically damages, kills, or neutralizes whatever is ingested. Macrophages ingest antigens and the by-products of inflammation (damaged cells and tissue debris). They comprise 5% of the circulating white blood cells.

Lymphocytes make up 20% to 40% of the white blood cells and serve as the immune system's security guards, migrating between the blood and tissues. Lymphocytes can live up to 20 years and have two subsets, T and B cells. About 70% of the lymphocytes are T cells. They specialize their function to become helper, suppressor, or natural killer cells.

T-helper cells organize the immune sys-

cytokines while dampening the number of Th1 cells along with their proinflammatory cytokines could be of benefit in the treatment of these illnesses.

Patients with RA often have elevated levels of proinflammatory prostaglandins.[7] Although a certain amount of these prostaglandins is tem's function: They facilitate the production of antibodies by the B cells, direct other defender cells to an area, and monitor the attack. Two functionally distinct T-helper cell subsets have been identified. One type, T-helper cells type 1 (Th1), produce inflammatory compounds such as tumor necrosis factor alpha (TNF-alpha), gamma interferon, and interleukin-2. T-helper cells type 2 (Th2) release anti-inflammatory compounds, particularly such interleukins as IL-4, IL-5, and IL-6, which down-regulate the immune response.

Suppressor T cells suppress the production of antibodies by B cells so that an attack doesn't get out of control. Natural killer cells are nonspecific, free-range cells armed with 100 different biochemicals to kill foreign proteins upon first encounter. T cells also function as the immune system's memory. They remember foreign substances and alert other immune components upon future exposure to those substances.

B cells, which account for 10% to 15% of all lymphocytes, produce antibodies to neutralize specific foreign cells. B cells don't survey the body for foreign invaders as do the T cells; instead they wait for the T cells to signal for the production of a particular antibody. The antibody then binds tightly with the invader, creating a circulating immune complex (CIC).

Other chemical components of the immune system prepare the body to attack the foreign substance. Cytokines are hormone-like substances, such as interleukins and interferons, which are responsible for

heightening an immune response. Prostaglandins are complex fatty acids that affect inflammatory processes and constriction and dilation of blood vessels. Essential fatty acids (EFAs) in the diet (both omega-3s and omega-6s) provide the raw material for prostaglandin production. Once ingested, these essential fatty acids can be converted to prostaglandins by nearly any cell in the body. Prostaglandins derived from omega-6s are the most common type and can either promote or inhibit inflammation, while most prostaglandins converted from omega-3 fatty acids help reduce pain and inflammation.

The complement system, made up of approximately 30 proteins, is dormant until activated by a series of enzymatic reactions initiated by circulating immune complexes (antibodies attached to antigens) or certain bacteria and viruses. Once activated, the complement system stimulates the release of inflammation-enhancing chemicals, clears away immune complexes, and kills bacteria. The complement system is very powerful and is carefully controlled by inhibitors to keep it from damaging the body.

 For **other factors and causes in immune system dysfunction**, see chapter 2, What Is Arthritis? pages 18–38.

part of the normal immune response, excessive amounts cause swelling and pain. Defective lymphocytes promote the production of autoantibodies—antibodies that attack the body's own cells. There are different types of autoantibodies that attack specific cells. Antinuclear antibodies (ANAs) target the nucleus of cells, and elevated ANA levels are often

Know Thyself

How does the immune system distinguish between friend and foe? All cells have cell membranes with chains of glycoproteins (sugar-protein complexes) that coat the cell membranes like the fuzz on a tennis ball. These glycoproteins are configured in various patterns that identify their function and type. For example, joint cells display a certain pattern that differs from that of the heart or other organ tissues. Similarly, some bacteria and viruses have specific glycoprotein patterns that identify them as foreigners in the body.

We inherit genetic markers that determine the glycoprotein pattern of our cell membranes. These markers, known as the major histocompatibility complex or HLA (human leukocyte antigen), are divided into three classes that are expressed, respectively, on all cells with a nucleus, certain immune cells, and genes typically involved in autoimmune diseases. In 1973, it was discovered that ankylosing spondylitis fre-

quently occurs in individuals with the genetic marker HLA-B27. Further research determined that over 100 diverse types of diseases are associated with specific types of HLA markers. Researchers have theorized that HLA-associated diseases, particularly autoimmune diseases, are induced by molecular mimicry, wherein bacteria and viruses are able to cloak themselves in a cellular pattern similar to one in normal body tissues and thus escape detection by the immune system. Once the invader is detected, a vigorous immune response ensues against the invader, which also unfortunately attacks the normal body cells with the similar cellular pattern.

Genetic testing can ascertain the presence of particular genetic markers, such as HLA-DR4 (associated with RA) and HLA-B27 (associated with ankylosing spondylitis). However, these diseases also occur in individuals without these markers.

present in autoimmune illness. The immune system differentiates between friend and foe via patterns on the outside of cell membranes. When healthy cell membranes are torn apart, the cell's internal components leak out, and as a result, the immune system becomes confused, no longer recognizing the cell as part of the body, Thus confused, the immune system begins to attack healthy tissues, leading to autoimmune disease.

Measuring the Autoimmune Reaction

Standard blood tests can determine the activity of different immune components and help determine if a patient has an autoimmune disease.

- Erythrocyte sedimentation rate (ESR) measures blood levels of fibrinogen, a protein that makes the red blood cells clump together. The level of fibrinogen varies with the degree of inflammation in the body, and an elevated ESR indicates inflammation. RA patients typically have an elevated ESR.

- Antinuclear antibodies (ANAs) are antibodies that attack the nucleus of a person's own cells; they are often present in auto-immune diseases. The distinctive speckled pattern of ANAs can be viewed under a microscope.

- C-reactive protein is produced in the liver and involved in stimulating white blood cell activity. This inflammation marker is often elevated in RA patients.

- Rheumatoid factor (RF) is an autoantibody present in 70% of people with RA. It may also be positive in people with tuberculosis, parasitic infections, leukemia, or connective tissue disorders. In some cases, RF renders joints more susceptible to damage by other immune cells.

Natural Therapies for Calming the Immune System

The most common allopathic treatment for autoimmune disease is immunosuppressant drugs called disease-modifying antirheumatic drugs, or DMARDs. Although these drugs work quite well for many people in terms of controlling pain, they have many serious side effects. DMARDs include auranofin (oral gold), gold sodium thiomalate (injectable gold), azathioprine, chlorambucil, cyclophosphamide, cyclosporine, hydroxy-chloroquine sulfate, leflunomide, and methotrexate.

Knowledge of the importance of the ratio of Th1 to Th2 in healthy immune function was used to develop a line of medications for RA called biologic response modifiers (BRM). (Recall, people with autoimmune diseases often have elevated levels of Th1 and depressed levels of Th2.) These drugs inhibit Th1 and its inflammatory cytokines by binding to TNF-alpha, thus inhibiting its inflammatory interaction with receptors in the joints. BRMs include adalimumab, etanercept, infliximab, and anakinra. They are often prescribed along with DMARDs.

Like many conventional drugs, BRMs quickly mask the immune system's aggressive behavior. But their inhibiting effects are not localized to rheumatic joints. If used for long periods of time, they affect all cells throughout the body that reproduce rapidly—specifically, the cells located in the gastrointestinal tract, reproductive organs, and bone marrow, as well as white blood cells. Prolonged use has deleterious results, including gastrointestinal problems, increased susceptibility to infection, sterility, and injury to the kidneys, liver, spleen, and bone marrow.[8]

Unlike conventional methods, natural therapies balance the immune system without suppressing normal immune function. Instead, they

> Unlike conventional methods, natural therapies balance the immune system without suppressing normal immune function. Instead, they promote the immune system's own regulating components and encourage them to turn off the abnormal auto-immune response.

promote the immune system's own regulating components and encourage them to turn off the abnormal autoimmune response. These therapies include oral tolerization, auto-sanguis dilution therapy, urine therapy, and herbal remedies.

Several of these therapies are based upon homeopathy's main principle of "like cures like," meaning that a substance that causes particular symptoms in large doses can cure those symptoms when given in small doses. Examples of this principle can be found in modern immunization, which uses trace amounts of infectious agents to invoke the body's immune defenses, and in the treatment of allergies, where minute levels of the suspected allergen are used to bolster the body tolerance. When treating RA, the body's immune response can be modulated through therapies drawing upon homeopathic principles.

Equally important is homeopathy's holistic model, which treats illness as a unique experience for each individual. A homeopathic practitioner carefully reviews all symptoms of the patient, using seemingly unrelated complaints build an individual profile that can then be matched to a remedy specifically suited for that profile.

For more on the **connection between allergies and arthritis**, see chapter 9, Allergies and Arthritis, pages 166–180.

When treating the autoimmune response of RA, the practitioner's job is simplified because the patient's own bodily fluids (blood or urine) contain the causes and agents involved in the disease and therefore can be used to easily identify the patient's specific profile.

Homeopathic treatment is not a simple, short-term procedure, however. It involves a step-by-step program instituted over a period of months or years, depending on the individual's response. The first focus is on decreasing pain and swelling by using nontoxic pain-relieving and anti-inflammatory modalities, as well as identifying and treating underlying causes (intestinal imbalances, nutritional deficiencies, toxicity, allergies, and so on). After relieving discomfort with natural pain relievers and beginning to reverse the disease process by addressing the underlying disorders, patients are often able to decrease or discontinue their prescription drugs (but only with the consent of their rheumatologist). Then, after the patient stops taking all conventional pain medications, immune-regulating therapies are pursued.

Oral Tolerization

Oral tolerization is an adaptation of a common immunological procedure in which a highly allergic person is exposed (usually through injections) to the substances causing the allergies. In oral tolerization, the offending substance is ingested rather than injected. A specific type of collagen cell, the most abundant protein in cartilage, is considered to be the allergenic substance in autoimmune diseases, and is ingested via the use of chicken cartilage or cockscomb.

In one study, researchers at Harvard Medical School gave oral doses of collagen to patients with RA for one month. The patients showed a substantial response: improvement of swollen and tender joints, less morning stiffness, better grip strength, and a reduction of inflammatory indicators in their blood. No adverse reactions were reported.[9] Researchers suspect that orally ingesting collagen may alter or reprogram T-cell function, either by desensitizing T cells to collagen antigens or by triggering the production of suppressor T cells that migrate to joints and block inflammation mediated by T cells. Cartilage derived from bovine, shark, and chicken sources are available as nutritional supplements.

Auto-Sanguis Dilution Therapy

In auto-sanguis dilution therapy, small doses of the patient's blood are prepared as a homeopathic remedy. The effectiveness of this therapy is rooted in the homeopathic principle that small doses of a substance reverse symptoms caused by large doses of the same substance. People who suffer from an autoimmune disease have elevated levels of pro-inflammatory agents, antibodies, and circulating immune complexes in their bloodstream, all of which are involved in the abnormal immune response. A homeopathic mixture containing minute traces of these substances can reduce or even completely eliminate the autoimmune response, as exemplified by the following case history.

Success Story: Auto-Sanguis Therapy Calms the Autoimmune Reaction. Yvonne, 13, developed symptoms of juvenile RA shortly after a visit to the dentist. When she came to our clinic, we performed our standard diagnostic tests, which included screening for infectious organisms (viruses, bacteria, and parasites). The results of the streptozyme titer (a test measuring specific antibodies to streptococcus bacteria) were very high, indicating an immune response against streptococcus.

She also had the genetic marker HLA-DR4, which is commonly associated with RA. This means that the structure of Yvonne's cell membranes exhibited a pattern easily mistaken for the streptococcus bacteria. Through molecular mimicry, streptococcus has evolved a cell membrane pattern so similar to the body's own cell membranes in those with the HLA-DR4 marker that the immune system treats the invader as one of its own cells.

> **CAUTION** The specific process outlined in this case history should only be attempted while working with a knowledgeable, licensed health-care practitioner trained in these procedures.

But once the invading bacteria are discovered, the immune system attacks all cells with this pattern (both streptococcus and the body's own cells) and an autoimmune response ensues.

In order to reverse Yvonne's arthritis, we had to eradicate her strep infection and modify her autoimmune response. This was achieved through two autoimmune therapies: auto-sanguis oral nosode therapy and injectable auto-sanguis dilution therapy. First, we prescribed the homeopathic remedy Streptococcinum 200C; three sublingual pellets were to be taken once a day between meals for one month. We also prepared an oral auto-sanguis nosode (SEE QUICK DEFINITION) using the following method: An extraction of a small amount of Yvonne's blood was placed in a centrifuge for 20 minutes. One part serum was mixed with nine parts purified water, and the mixture was shaken vigorously 100 times. This process produces a homeopathic nosode at 1X potency. The process was repeated six times, rendering the remedy at a potency of 6X. We added 15% ethyl alcohol to stabilize the solution. Yvonne placed 10 drops of this solution under her tongue three times a day. Upon her second visit, we increased

 QUICK DEFINITION A **nosode** is a homeopathic remedy made as an energy imprint from disease-causing microorganisms, such as bacteria or viruses that cause tuberculosis, measles, bowel infections, influenza, or any of about 200 other substances. The nosode, which contains no physical trace of the disease, stimulates the body to remove all taints or residues it holds of a particular disease, whether it was inherited or contracted. Only qualified practitioners may administer a nosode.

the potency of the original nosode to 12X potency; it was increased to 30X potency on her third visit, and finally to 60X potency.

In addition, Yvonne was treated with an injectable auto-sanguis dilution by extracting 3 cc (cubic centimeters) of her blood and emptying the syringe until only a microscopic film of blood remained in the cartridge. We then mixed into the same syringe 1 cc of the homeopathic nosodes for streptococcus and 1 cc of homeopathic remedies designed for trauma, inflammation, and degenerative processes. The mixture was agitated 20 times, rendering a solution at 1X potency, and was injected into her buttock. The process was repeated to produce a remedy at 2X potency and injected as well.

Sulfur and the Immune System

Two sulfur-containing substances, dimethylsulfoxide (DMSO), derived from wood pulp or garlic oil, or as a by-product of petroleum, and methylsulfonylmethane (MSM), a sister compound derived from food sources, can be helpful in modulating autoimmunity. DMSO can help to decrease the activity of an over-zealous immune system.[11] When used topically, these substances have the added benefit of relieving joint pain with minor skin irritation as the only possible adverse effect.[12]

Yvonne returned for treatment once a week for one month, during which time the injections reached a potency of 4X.

Two weeks after Yvonne's last treatment, we repeated all the blood tests we had initially done and found that her body was no longer producing streptococcus antibodies. She also no longer had positive blood factors for autoimmune reactions (RF and ANA), and she experienced complete relief of her arthritis symptoms. We suspected that Yvonne's recent visit to the dentist explained how she was infected by the strep bacteria. During her routine dental cleaning, strep cell fragments in her teeth or gums translocated to other regions of her body, prompting an immune response and leading to autoimmunity. We suggested that in the future, Yvonne should receive preventive homeopathic treatments with Streptococcinum 200C before visiting the dentist. We advise all patients to pay strict attention to oral health care, because translocation of organisms found in the mouth is routinely linked to health problems, including joint inflammation and heart disease.[10]

Urine Therapy

Many patients are surprised to find that urine has a broad spectrum of health benefits. We normally think of it only as a waste product that's unhealthy and unclean. But in actuality, when it is first passed from the body, healthy urine is completely sterile and rich in nutrients. Early on, drug manufacturers discovered that urine contains many important chemical compounds. Urine is routinely collected from humans, horses, and other animals for the purpose of isolating and condensing desirable components. For instance, estrogen for hormone replacement therapy is generally derived from the urine of pregnant mares. Urokinase, a drug commonly used to treat patients with advanced atherosclerosis (calcified fatty deposits on the arterial walls), is manufactured from urine collected from portable toilets. Most shampoos and cosmetics contain urea, a component of urine.

Urine is made up of water, urea (a breakdown product of proteins and amino acids), hormones, enzymes, minerals, and salts. Its precise composition is specific to the individual, and the chemical components of a person's urine reflect the individual's health profile. This physiological fingerprint contains evidence of infectious agents, specific types of antibodies used to combat them, circulating immune complexes, substances that have initiated an immune response, hormones and other natural chemicals used to regulate and control the body's functions, vitamins, and other nutritive substances.[13]

The urine of people with autoimmune illnesses contains autoantibodies involved in the immune response. When their urine is reintroduced into their body, it acts as homeopathic signaling agent, which helps to turn off the autoimmune response. Although science has not yet deciphered the mechanism of this action, we've witnessed many patients experience a marked reduction in symptoms after initiating urine therapy. The concentration of urine is so dilute that the substances it contains don't pose a threat to the body.

Doctors trained in urine therapy often prepare an injectable solution, but it can also be very effective if taken orally.[14] People with an aversion to drinking their own urine can start off very slowly, following this procedure: in the morning, catch a small amount of urine in a clean cup; have another cup of filtered water available. Then, use a clean glass eyedropper and add just two drops of urine to the cup of water. Every few days, increase the amount of urine by one drop. Go slowly, adding a drop each morning. The ideal dosage is 10 drops of urine to four ounces of water. Once this amount is reached, maintain it indefinitely. Urine tastes like salty water, but you can add a drop of peppermint oil to disguise the taste if you wish.

For more on **homeopathic remedies for arthritis**, see chapter 13, Supplements for Arthritis, pages 257–294.

Herbs for Inflammation

High levels of inflammatory agents spur the immune system into constant activity, initially against foreign substances but later against the body's own tissues. Herbs that reduce inflammation can help calm the immune system. Please note that herbs and other nutritional supplements often have potential interactions with pharmaceutical drugs. They may decrease or increase the activity of the drug. Both situations may warrant a change in your prescription drug regimen. If you're taking any prescription drugs, consult with your health-care provider before using any herbs or nutritional supplements. Helpful information on this topic is available at www.supplementinfo.org and www.med .umich.edu/1libr/aha/umherb01.htm, and in *Mosby's Handbook of Drug-Herb & Drug-Supplement Interactions* by HealthGate Data Corporation and Mosby.

Boswellia (Boswellia serrata). The *Boswellia serrata* tree grows in the arid and mountainous regions of India. The tree's gum resin has been used for centuries in Ayurvedic medicine as a tonic for a variety of health conditions. The medicinally active extract of this resin acts as a natural anti-inflammatory and is particularly helpful for OA and RA. Research has shown *Boswellia serrata* to be both safe and effective, and several mechanisms of action that lead to boswellia's positive effects for arthritis have been discovered. Boswellia limits the infiltration of leukocytes into arthritic joints, and boswellic acid, the biologically active component of boswellia extract, reduces the number of leukotrienes by inhibiting the activity of the enzyme needed for their formation. Boswellia also inhibits Th1 cytokines and increases Th2 cytokines, which favorably balances the Th1 to Th2 ratio, reducing inflammation.[15] Boswellia is found in a variety of products, including both oral supplements and topical creams that can be applied directly to stiff or sore joints.

Ginger (Zingiber officinale). Ginger's high concentration of proteolytic enzymes (which break down proteins) is responsible for its ability to subdue pain and inflammation. Proteolytic enzymes block the action of several inflammatory substances, including prostaglandins and leukotrienes.[19] Ginger has been shown to decrease pain in arthritis[20] and has been tested specifically for arthritis that effects the knees it has been shown to be beneficial.[21]

Ginger can be ingested or used topically. Try adding a 1/2-inch slice of

A Spot of Tea for Arthritis

Green tea and black tea are actually derived from the same plant (*Camellia sinensis*). Green tea isn't oxidized, so it maintains its original green color and is higher than black tea in active medicinal constituents, such as antioxidants, polyphenols, theanine, and a wide variety of vitamins and minerals. Catechins, a specific category of polyphenols, include epigallocatechin gallate (EGCG), which has antioxidant activity about 25 to 100 times more potent than vitamins C and E. It has also been shown to help fight arthritis. The substance is anti-inflammatory due to its inhibition of inter-leukin-1,[16] cyclooxygenase-2 and nitric oxide synthase-2[17], and it inhibits the breakdown of cartilage in the joints.[18]

ginger to vegetable juice. Or use ginger to make a hot tea: Add 1 teaspoon of grated fresh ginger root to 1 cup of boiling water, cover to prevent the escape of important essential oils and aromatics, and steep 15 minutes; add honey or stevia if you wish. Ginger can also be used as a hot compress: Grate fresh ginger root, place it on a warm washcloth, and apply it to sore muscles or joints. Keep the cloth warm with a hot water bottle. Try this on a small area to observe your skin's reactions, as fresh ginger may irritate delicate skin. Powdered ginger can also be effective in a compress.

Turmeric (*Curcuma longa*). Turmeric is a bright yellow spice used in preparing curries. It's powerful anti-inflammatory properties are credited to the chemical component curcumin. Research suggests that turmeric suppresses nuclear factor kappa beta[22] and interleukin-8, while enhancing synthesis of glutathione.[23] In one study, curcumin was found to be better at reducing acute inflammation than either cortisone or phenylbutazone, two commonly prescribed drugs.[24] Use turmeric in combination with ginger as a flavorful food seasoning. Turmeric can also be used as a poultice for aching joints.

Cayenne Pepper (*Capsicum annuum*). Cayenne pepper contains capsaicin, a chemical component useful for pain relief. Capsaicin depletes body reserves of substance P, which is believed to be responsible for intensifying and prolonging muscle and joint inflammation and pain.[25] Substance P, a group of several amino acids bonded together, is normally present in minute amounts in the nervous system and intestines. Typically involved in the pain response, substance P expands and contracts smooth muscles in the intestines and other tissues. In patients with fibromyalgia, substance P has been found in abnormally high levels and is regarded as one of the most potent compounds affecting smooth muscle contraction and inflammation. For arthritis relief,

 For more **herbs helpful for inflammation**, see chapter 13, Supplements for Arthritis, pages 257–294.

capsicum, an active constituent of cayenne is usually used as a topical cream that's rubbed into painful joints and muscles.[26]

Stinging Nettle *(Urtica dioica).* The leaves of the stinging nettle have been used as a medicine and food since ancient times. "Nettle" originated from the Anglo-Saxon word *netel* or *noedl,* meaning "needle." It refers to the tiny needlelike hairs of the plant, which are coated with formic acid, histamine, serotonin, and acetylcholine and cause a localized swelling and rash when touched. Historically, treatment of the pain and swelling of arthritic conditions with nettles focused on its topical use. People rubbed the stingers of the plant directly over the painful joint and experienced an analgesic (pain-relieving) effect.

Medical studies have provided astonishing validation of this ancient practice. In a randomized, controlled, double-blind crossover study, patients with osteoarthritic pain in their thumb or index finger applied stinging nettle leaf daily for one week to the painful area. The effect of this treatment was compared with that of a placebo, white dead nettle, a variety that looks similar but has no stinging hairs. After one week's treatment with stinging nettle, score reductions on both pain and disability were significantly greater than with placebo.[27]

Stinging nettle is also useful for arthritis when taken orally. This action may be due to nettle leaf's ability to lower body levels of the inflammatory compound TNF-alpha.[28] Nettle leaf also alters the genetic transcription of another inflammatory compound, nuclear factor kappa beta (NFkB), thereby decreasing inflammation of synovial tissue in the joints.[29] Additionally, nettle leaf extract has a suppressive effect on the development of dendritic cells, which stimulate T cells to release inflammatory chemicals. This may contribute to the therapeutic effect of nettle leaf extract on inflammatory diseases mediated by T cells, such as RA.[30] There are various preparations of nettle leaf extract on the market. These are not to be confused with standardized nettle root extracts, used in the treatment of certain prostate problems.

Herbs for Autoimmune Disease

Immunological researchers have discovered several important plants that seem to have pharmacological action against aggressive autoimmune responses.

Chinese Thunder God Vine *(Tripterygium wilfordii). Tripterygium wilfordii* grows wild in remote areas of southern China and has been used in traditional Chinese medicine for 2,000 years. Clinical trials have found it effective in treating autoimmune diseases (RA and ankylosing spondylitis) and other types of arthritis. It contains chemical components called glycosides, which have immune-suppressing, anti-inflammatory, and analgesic properties. This herb has been found to have a wide array of immunosuppressive chemical constituents,[31] which accounts for its many mechanisms of action effective against arthritis and inflammation. These include inhibiting the production of inflammatory cytokines and blocking the activity of TNF-alpha, cyclooxygenase-2 (COX-2), and nuclear factor kappa beta (NFkB).[32]

While the results obtained with the use of this herb are promising, there are related side effects with *Tripterygium wilfordii*. Adverse reactions include skin rashes, dry mouth, poor appetite, menstrual disturbances, and hormonal disturbances in men.[33] Researchers have also found that it causes a temporary reduction of sperm count in men and so have begun to develop a male contraceptive drug from the plant's active ingredients. However, fertility is restored upon cessation of use.[34] The side effects of *Tripterygium wilfordii* are reduced when it's administered in combination with other Chinese herbs.

Indian Sarsaparilla Vine (*Hemidesmus indicus*). Indian sarsaparilla vine is not a true sarsaparilla; it's actually closely related to American milkweed and European pleurisy root. It's traditionally used for snakebites, chronic skin diseases, and autoimmune illnesses such as RA. Its active chemical constituents include coumarins and triterpenoid saponins, which work in a manner similar to immunosuppressing drugs but with a lower incidence of adverse effects, probably due to the

 Because of the possible side effects of *Tripterygium wilfordii*, use this herb only under the care of a licensed health-care professional.

plant's kidney-protective qualities.[35] *Hemidesmus indicus* down-regulates the activity of proinflammatory agents (interferons, interleukins, and prostaglandins) and other immune cells (T and B cells, antibodies, and cytokines) involved in the inflammatory process, and acts as a powerful tissue-protective antioxidant.[36]

Sarsaparilla (*Smilax* spp.). Though sarsaparilla grows throughout the world, the tropical varieties found in the Caribbean, South America, Mexico, and Central America are most prized for their medicinal value. It is particularly useful for illnesses caused by spirochetes, such as syphilis, leptospirosis, and Lyme disease. Sarsaparilla was included in the *United States Pharmacopoeia* as a treatment for secondary syphilis until 1950.[37] In

China, the herb has been used in combination with other botanicals for chronic syphilis and leptospirosis.[38] We have experienced excellent clinical success using sarsaparilla for patients with Lyme disease. Our protocol combines Jamaican or Honduras sarsaparilla (5:1 solid extract), cat's claw (*Uncaria tomentosa*), standardized olive leaf extract, and a combination of Chinese botanicals including *Lonicera japonica*, *Glycyrrhiza uralensis*, *Dictamnus dasycarpus*, *Portulacae oleracea*, *Taraxacum mongoli*, and *Dipsacus japonicus*. These herbs are used as part of a comprehensive holistic protocol with other modalities to address the ravages of Lyme disease.

Many illnesses, including RA, psoriasis, gout, and acne have been associated with increased levels of endotoxins, and the saponins found in sarsaparilla emulsify and bind to endotoxins in the gastrointestinal tract, aiding in their elimination. Sarsaparilla also has anti-inflammatory properties that aid in arthritis. This has been linked to its ability to inhibit TNF-alpha-induced NFkB activation.[39]

Rehmannia glutinosa. Popular in Chinese medicine, the root of *Rehmannia glutinosa* has shown promise in bringing balance to aggressive autoimmune states. Referred to in Chinese medical literature as *ti huang*, it's one of the most effective blood and kidney (adrenal) yin tonics. In Western terms, yin properties are related to anti-inflammatory and reproductive hormones, such as the glucocorticoids produced by the adrenal cortex. This herb has mild immunosuppressive effects without entirely inhibiting the healthy action of the immune system.[40] Therefore, it has less adverse effects than disease-modifying antirheumatic drugs (DMARDs), which suppress the immune system to such a degree that they increase susceptibility to infectious illnesses.

In traditional Chinese medicine (TCM), rehmannia is used to cool the blood (reduce inflammation), purify the blood (remove circulating immune complexes), and decrease sweating (increase glucocorticoid production), the latter a common symptom in many inflammatory autoimmune diseases. Modern pharmacological research has isolated various components in rehmannia that may be responsible for its immunomodulatory and anti-inflammatory effects and its ability to tonify the adrenals. Rehmannia also reduces allergic reactions by decreasing histamine release caused by tumor necrosis factor alpha.[41]

Rehmannia, like most TCM herbs, is almost always used in a time-honored formulation with other items from the TCM pharmacopoeia. One classic TCM formula, Ren Shen Yang Rong Tang, contains rehmannia, ginseng, dong quai, atractylodes, hoelen, licorice, astragalus, cinnamon, schizandra, citrus, and polygala. It has been shown to regulate the imbalanced Th 1 to Th 2 ratio often seen in auto-immune diseases.[42]

Stephania (Stephania tetrandra). In Chinese medicine, stephania is called "Han-Fang-Ji," and has an extensive record of medicinal use for inflammation, a variety of disorders involving the kidneys and cardio-vascular system, and red, hot, swollen joints. By relaxing both the smooth and skeletal muscles, and inhibiting fibrosis (painful scar tissue deposition in muscles), stephania relieves the pain and stiffness associ-ated with rheumatic ailments and fibromyalgia. The active component, tetrandrine, has been used to treat patients with silicosis (an autoimmune disease of the lungs triggered by silica dust), RA, and hypertension. Tetrandrine has a wide variety of immunomodulating effects, including inhibiting tumor necrosis factor alpha,[43] as well as the formation of anti-type 2 collagen antibodies, which are directly responsible for the destruc-tion of cartilage and are involved in autoimmune arthritis.[44]

Reishi Mushroom (Ganoderma spp.). The reishi mushroom has been called the mushroom of immortality. It is a member of the Polyporaceae fam-ily and is commonly found growing in a shelflike form on decaying trees. Ancient Chinese medical texts list it as an immune regulator and blood tonifier, with calming, pain-relieving action.[45] While illnesses such as can-cer and viral infections require an increase in immune function, allergic reactions and autoimmune diseases call for a down-regulation of the immune system. Reishi is a true amphoteric herb, meaning it can up-regulate (increase the activity of) or down-regulate the immune system, as needed. Although there are several natural herbal remedies that have been shown to have this dual action, no pharmaceutical drugs can accomplish this feat. Reishi is rich in polysaccharides, immunomodulat-ing proteins, and steroidal saponin glycosides that influence the adrenal-hypothalamic-pituitary axis feedback loop, which regulates inflammation. Ling zhi-8, an amphoteric protein isolated from *Ganoderma* spp. was shown to be both mitogenic (causes white blood cells to multiply) and immunosuppressive (reduces TNF-alpha and the formation of antibod-ies) in autoimmune disease, depending on the need of the individual.[46]

Chinese Quince Fruit (Chaenomeles lagenaria). The Chinese quince, or *mu gua*, is a delicious fruit with immunomodulating, anti-inflammatory, and antispasmodic effects. It increases blood circulation and qi (vital energy), which directly relaxes muscles.[47] This relieves spasms, normalizing bio-mechanical activity of the joints, and also decreasing the stress on

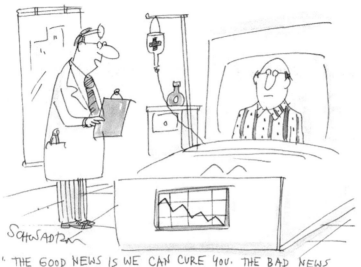

" THE GOOD NEWS IS WE CAN CURE YOU. THE BAD NEWS IS THE CURE IS WORSE THAN THE DISEASE.

cartilage formation, which is common to both RA and OA. Studies have discovered that steroidal glucosides found in Chinese quince fruit modulates TNF-alpha and blocks interleukin-1, the foremost cytokine involved in the destruction of cartilage.[48] We recommend combining quince with dong quai (*Angelica sinensis*), peony (*Paeoniae lactiflorae*), cinnamon (*Cinnamomum cassia*), and *Erythrina variegata* to help joint pain and muscle spasms, especially if the condition becomes worse with overexertion or exposure to wind, cold, and dampness. You can enjoy quince by adding this delicious fruit to your diet. Concentrated extracts are also available.

eleven

Mind-Body Approaches to Arthritis

Stress is a common part of everyday life, but it can become harmful to the body when it is prolonged or chronic. It affects the body in very real, physical ways by influencing the immune and hormonal systems. For people with arthritis, this can mean an increase in pain and inflammation. In this chapter, we examine how stress, suppressed emotions, and lifestyle choices can contribute to arthritis. We also explore a number of therapies that can help you reprogram negative thought patterns into more healthful ones, deal with stress in a positive way, and incorporate habits for relaxation into your life.

Success Story: Mind-Body Therapies for Rheumatoid Arthritis

Prue, 42, developed RA seemingly overnight. The pain and stiffness hit her feet first, then spread to her wrists and hands, and finally affected her neck and back. Synovial cysts had formed on her carpal bones (which connect the wrists to the hands), and were aggravated by the repetitive motions of typing, which was required for her job. Like many of our arthritis patients, Prue first pursued conventional medical treatment with rheumatologists, who prescribed prednisone, Plaquenil, and other NSAIDs. After two years on these drugs, Prue experienced very little pain relief and eventually developed gastrointestinal problems (gas, bloating, irritable bowel, and occult blood in the stool indicating gastrointestinal bleeding). To offset the pain caused by her pain medication, Prue took an average of 12 aspirin per day, which caused yet more side effects. Frustrated and feeling hopeless, Prue came to see us six years after the onset of her arthritis.

Mind-Body Therapies for Arthritis

- Meditation
- Cognitive therapy
- Neuro-linguistic programming
- Biofeedback
- Hypnotherapy
- Guided imagery and visualization
- Restricted environmental stimulation therapy (REST)
- Flower remedies
- Aromatherapy

We ran a battery of tests that showed a number of underlying physical problems contributing to Prue's arthritis.

- Intestinal permeability or leaky gut syndrome: Intestinal permeability means that toxins and incompletely digested food particles leak into the bloodstream through the intestinal lining. Once they enter the bloodstream or become absorbed by connective tissues, they can trigger inflammation.

- An overburdened liver: Prue's liver was overwhelmed by the increased levels of toxins entering her bloodstream from her intestines. It was unable to filter these toxins, and they reentered the bloodstream. From there, they were absorbed into her tissues, leading to inflammation and putting additional stress on her immune system.

- Bacterial infection: *Enterobacter taylorae*, a harmful bacteria present in Prue's stool sample, contributed to her maldigestion and intestinal permeability. Harmful bacteria can alter the pH of the stomach, which shuts down the sequential phases of digestion. As a result, food is not properly digested and nutrients are not absorbed.

- Mineral deficiencies: A hair trace mineral analysis found that Prue had inadequate levels of calcium, magnesium, zinc, chromium, as well as selenium, germanium, and molybdenum, nutrients

> Stress is a common part of everyday life, but it can become harmful to the body when it is prolonged or chronic. It affects the body in very real, physical ways by influencing the immune and hormonal systems. For people with arthritis, this can mean an increase in pain and inflammation.

important in the liver's detoxification processes. Also, her copper level was too high.

- Food allergies: Prue had sensitivities to bananas, beans (green, kidney, and yellow wax), cheese, eggs, cow's milk, mushrooms, black and white pepper, sugar cane, wheat, and baker's and brewer's yeast.

Our first goal was to help Prue solve these underlying problems and achieve better control of her pain and inflammation without depending on prescription drugs. We initiated a program of dietary changes, vitamin and mineral supplements, and other therapies to alleviate her condition.

Once this was accomplished, Prue wanted to focus on the psychological and emotional elements of her arthritis. She was frustrated at work because she found it difficult to say no to additional tasks, even if she was too busy to handle it. People, especially her immediate supervisor, took advantage of her pleasant and good-natured disposition and never considered the physical limitations of her arthritis. Hiding behind an artificial smile, Prue felt angry at herself for not expressing her true feelings. Her silence toward her coworkers eventually grew into resentment and jealousy. She was jealous of their self-confidence, a quality that she didn't possess, which she compensated for by trying to please everyone. Prue's silence didn't help improve her self-esteem; instead, it only fed her unexpressed anger and diminished her ability to stand up for herself.

We explained the psychological effects of holding in anger, as expressed in her body by the freezing up of her joint mobility. The effects of suppressed emotions can extend beyond the psyche and into the physiological realm, where the body responds to pent-up anger by slowly breaking down. Prue turned all of her frustrations in on herself, contributing to the onset of her arthritis, ultimately a self-destructive disease.

We often see emotional problems such as anger in correlation with liver imbalances. This connection is clearly elucidated in traditional Chinese medicine, which recognizes correspondences between areas of the body and different emotional states. In Prue's case, this connection was the major contributor to her onset of arthritis. The problems with her coworkers weren't isolated incidents, but an example of a long-term pattern of behavior that contributed to her history of chronic illness. Another effect of Prue's internalized anger and subsequent low self-esteem could be found in her poor lifestyle choices, which undermined her health. Prue had uncontrollable chocolate cravings that she succumbed to daily. The amount of sweets (pies, ice cream, and cookies) that she ate in a week outnumbered the amount of fruits or vegetables. In addition, she rarely exercised. These are lapses that even conventional doctors wouldn't condone for a RA patient.

To support Prue's recovery, we had to redirect the way she perceived herself and her emotions and help her make wiser choices in both behavior and health. We used a technique called neuro-linguistic programming (NLP), a question-and-answer exchange that detects unconscious patterns of thought and behavior and provides ways to alter negative patterns. We asked Prue about her identity, personal beliefs, and life goals. She considered her disease part of her identity, as if she wouldn't be herself without arthritis. Based on this first NLP session, we designed affirmation tapes that would help her regain control of her identity. She listened to these tapes during hydrotherapy in a flotation REST (restricted environmental stimulation therapy) tank, which we recommended to reduce her stress levels.

In NLP, the patient envisions being healthy and happy. If Prue could imagine herself healthy, then her body could respond to this positive stimulus by triggering the necessary immunological responses for healing. Without positive visualizations of health, Prue might have dutifully taken the supplements that we prescribed yet not believed that they would make a difference. She would be stuck thinking that she wasn't worthy of being healthy. Her body would have believed her defeatist attitude, and she would have remained sick.

We also used visual imagery sessions to teach Prue how to relax in stressful situations. We asked her to hold in her mind a picture of a distressing or emotion-provoking situation (such as a conflict with a coworker or supervisor) and to focus on relaxing her body in that situation. Imagery is like a dress rehearsal, allowing the patient to learn to feel more relaxed when a stressful situation occurs in real life.

After 12 weeks on this program, Prue was pleased by her improved physical health. She no longer suffered stiffness and pain in her joints, and her digestive problems had cleared up shortly after discontinuing conventional drugs and changing her diet. The cysts along her wrists were no longer painful, but an MRI scan showed evidence of fluid in the synovial sheaths (membranes lining the cavity of a bone through which a tendon moves). Examination by an orthopedic surgeon determined that aggressive surgery to remove the fluid was not necessary since Prue had no pain from the increased fluid and hadn't lost strength in her grip. And Prue found that she had more self-confidence, as well. She actually said no to a coworker's request to take on an additional project and felt like her response generated a more respectful attitude from that coworker.

For more information on **neuro-linguistic programming,** see this chapter, pages 214–216.

Stressed-Out: A Pervasive Problem

Although the concept of stress—being stressed-out or under constant stress—may be commonly discussed today, its role as a contributing factor in many diseases is underappreciated. Estimates suggest that as much as 70% to 80% of all visits to physicians' offices are for stress-related problems.[1] Chronic stress directly affects the immune system and, if not effectively dealt with, can seriously compromise a person's health.

Stress is a pervasive problem among Americans, according to a 1996 poll of corporate executives. For example, 44% of employees polled said their workload is excessive (compared to 37% in 1988); 43% are bothered by excessive job pressure; 55% worry considerably about their company's future; 25% of both men and women feel stressed-out at work every day, another 12% feel it almost every day, and another 38% feel it once to several days a week.[2]

Stress can be defined as a reaction (to any stimulus or interference) that upsets normal functioning and disturbs mental or physical health. It can be brought on by internal conditions, such as illness, pain, emotional conflict, or psychological problems, or by external circumstances, such as bereavement, financial problems, loss of a job or spouse, relocation, food allergies, and electromagnetic fields. Stress, when it becomes chronic, is often unrecognized by the person whose body is experiencing it; they begin to accept it as a fact of life, without being aware of how it is actually compromising all their bodily functions and laying the foundation for illness.

More specifically, research confirms that high levels of emotional stress increase a person's susceptibility to illness. Unrelieved chronic stress begins taxing and eventually weakening or even suppressing the immune system. Stress can also lead to hormonal imbalances, which in turn interfere with immune function. Of all the body's systems, the one most damaged by stress damages is immune function. This is because stress overly activates the sympathetic part of the autonomic nervous system, the part that controls the fight-or-flight response and initiates adrenaline and cortisol release.

Common Causes of Stress

- Illness
- Pain
- Emotional conflict
- Financial problems
- Death of a family member or close friend
- Job or career pressures
- Allergies
- Poor diet
- Substance abuse
- Environmental pollution

Research in psychoneuroimmunology (PNI) has shown that the immune and nervous systems are linked by extensive networks of nerve endings in the spleen, bone marrow, lymph nodes, and thymus gland (a primary source of T cells). Additionally, receptors for a variety of chemical messengers—catecholamines, prostaglandins, thyroid hormone, growth hormone, sex hormones, serotonin, and endorphins—have been found on the surfaces of white blood cells. Such connections serve to integrate the activities of the immune, hormonal, and nervous systems, enabling the mind and emotional states to influence the body's resistance to disease.[3]

Fight-or-Flight Response

Pioneering stress researcher Hans Selye, M.D., a Canadian physiologist, noted a consistent pattern of response to stress and termed this the general adaptation syndrome, commonly referred to as the fight-or-flight response. This response occurs in three stages: the initial alarm reaction, resistance, and exhaustion.

Initially, the body's biochemistry tends to react to stress in an orderly fashion. Stimulation of the sympathetic nervous system (part of the autonomic nervous system) activates secretion of hormones from the endocrine glands and constricts both the blood vessels and the involuntary muscles. When the endocrine glands (pancreas, thyroid, pituitary,

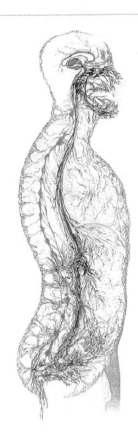

Think of the autonomic nervous system (ANS) as your body's automatic pilot. It keeps you alive by controlling your breathing, heart rate, and digestion, without your being aware of it or participating in its activities. The ANS has two divisions: the sympathetic nervous system, which expends body energy, and the parasympathetic nervous system, which conserves body energy. The sympathetic nervous system is associated with arousal and stress; when you perceive a threat or challenge, it prepares you physically by increasing your heart rate, blood pressure, and muscle tension. The parasympathetic nervous system slows heart rate and increases activity of the intestines and most glands.

sex glands, and particularly the adrenals) are stimulated, heart rate, glucose metabolism, and oxygen consumption increase. The parasympathetic nervous system is also stimulated, which begins a process of relaxation. The pituitary gland responds by releasing a variety of hormones throughout the body; these hormones influence the defensive and adaptive mechanisms. Endorphins, the body's own natural painkillers, are also released.

Dr. Selye points out, however, that eventually chronic stress depletes the body's resources and impairs its ability to adapt. If stress continues and remains unattenuated for a long period, coping functions will be compromised and illness will result.[4]

Stress, the Adrenal Glands, and Arthritis

The adrenal glands, part of the body's endocrine system, are located atop the kidneys. They're composed of two types of tissue: the adrenal medulla and the adrenal cortex. The adrenal medulla, comprising 10% to 20% of the gland, is located in the interior portion and is responsible for production of the hormones epinephrine (adrenaline) and norepinephrine (noradrenaline). These hormones are released in direct response to the sympathetic nervous system, which is responsible for the fight-or-flight response to stress or physical threats. The adrenal cortex, the outer layer, surrounds the medulla and accounts for 80% to 90% of the gland. It is responsible for the production of corticosteroids (also called adrenal steroids). Over 30 different steroids have been isolated from the adrenal cortex, including cortisol and cortisone.

Secretion of cortisol (as well as the adrenal gland's other steroids, DHEA, adrenaline, and aldosterone) occurs in daily cycles, peaking in the morning and having the lowest values at night. Cortisol promotes protein building, regulates insulin and glycogen synthesis, and helps produce prostaglandins (hormonelike fatty acids involved in inflammatory processes). Under conditions of stress, high amounts of cortisol are released. Imbalances in cortisol secre-

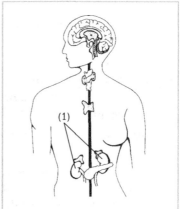

The adrenal glands (1) are two triangular-shaped glands above the kidneys. They release adrenaline and other hormones in the fight-or-flight response to stress.

tion are linked with low energy, inflammation, muscle dysfunction, impaired bone repair, thyroid dysfunction, immune system depression, sleep disorders, and poor skin regeneration.

When stress is prolonged, chronic pain sets in as the adrenals become exhausted and supplies of cortisol and other adrenal hormones plummet and eventually run out. One function of cortisol is to act as a potent anti-inflammatory hormone. If you have arthritis, the pain and inflammation in your joints will worsen as your adrenal glands stop producing cortisol. This results in fatigue, muscle weakness, depression, and a magnification of arthritic symptoms.

Based on our clinical experience with hundreds of patients, we find that people with both OA and RA are typically in a moderate to advanced state of adrenal exhaustion. Researchers are also beginning to find evidence of a connection between stress and arthritis. A recent study found that in 86% of cases, the onset of RA was preceded by stressful events in the patients' lives. In addition, there was a correlation between arthritis flare-ups and stressful events in 60% of patients.[5] When people with psoriatic arthritis are questioned, a correlation between a stressful life event and the initial onset of the condition is often found.

In conventional medicine, those suffering from adrenal exhaustion are typically given pharmaceutical drugs similar to cortisol (corticosteroids) for their pain and inflammation. But these allopathic drugs are often much stronger than the body's own hormones. Prednisone, for example, is 30 times as potent as endogenous cortisol.[6] Many practitioners of natural medicine feel that, while the judicious use of corticosteroids is helpful for a short period of time to stabilize the patient, long-term use of and reliance on these powerful drugs is devastating. They can suppress immunity, interfere with sleep cycles, and increase bone and collagen breakdown. They can also suppress the production and proper functioning of adrenal hormones and further diminish the functioning of the adrenal glands.

The Arthritis Personality

The most critical aspect of stress is not the event itself, but your response to or interpretation of the situation. Do you respond with hope or despair? With helplessness or commitment to resolve the situation? With pent-up anger or tranquility? How you respond, to some degree, reflects your personality type.

Human behavioral patterns are commonly broken down into two basic personality types, type A and type B. Type A personalities are described as aggressive and competitive, easily angered, always in a hurry, and hostile. Type B personalities, on the other hand, are more deliberate, thinking through a situation and formulating a plan of action. Studies have shown that personality type can have a profound influence on your health. One study followed 3,000 middle-aged men over an eight-and-a-half year period and found that type A's were twice as likely to develop heart disease as type B's.[7] A study of air traffic controllers found that type A's had three and a half times more job-related injuries and 38% more illnesses than type B's.[8]

Health-care practitioners report that certain common personality characteristics are exhibited by those with arthritis. One observation is that arthritis frequently develops in people who have a constant pattern of criticism of themselves and others.[9] The critical tendency doesn't have to be overt: It might be completely internal—an inner voice that keeps telling the person that things are not okay, that they could be better.

However, it's generally not in the nature of the arthritis personality to express their feelings or attempt to creatively change the situation that disturbs them. This is the second trait of the arthritis personality: They are more likely to appear to accept change, but actually have an internal resistance to it. Researchers at Ohio State University, in Columbus, conducted a study to evaluate the personality traits of people with rheumatoid disease. Their findings indicate that "patients with rheumatoid diseases are likely to be excessively conscientious, fearful of criticism yet critical of themselves and others, frequently depressed, and have a poor self-image." The study group exhibited characteristics that led them to try to be overly nice to other people at the expense of their own well-being, to be stoic, and to conceal their emotions (especially anger). "Many rheumatic disease sufferers have a situation of long-standing tension or anger in their lives, yet would assert when questioned that everything was okay, even though it was furthest from the truth. They were remarkably conforming to these traits, which seemed to precede their disease, not be caused as a result of it."[10]

In these individuals, unfulfilled expectations lead to a sense of increased frustration and even anger that they keep to themselves, perhaps eventually turning the immune system against itself.[11] From this perspective, arthritis can be seen as a form of frozen impulse. Those with the arthritis personality, due to their critical nature, want things to be different, but their impulse to change is constantly suppressed by an unwillingness or inability to change. Biochemically, this may manifest itself by the accumulation of stress hormones in the body, particularly in the joints, the area of the body representing the greatest flexibility and mobility. Stiffness and rigidity are the dominant states of mind, and they are also the dominant conditions of an arthritic joint.

Those traits seem related to a third one we've noted in our work with arthritis patients: a pronounced tendency to cling to the status quo. They tend to be very rigid and structured in their dietary routines, sedentary or overly active lifestyle, and even dependence on medications. We've found it extremely difficult to persuade arthritis patients to adopt the

Emotional Tissues

The particular area of the body affected by arthritis reveals emotional issues related to it:

- The arms represent the capacity to embrace life.
- Elbows represent flexibility in changing directions.
- Legs represent the ability to move ahead in positive directions.
- Joints represent changes and directions in life and the ease of these movements.
- Old emotions are stored in the joints.
- Inflammation indicates suppressed anger and frustration.
- Swelling represents clogging and stagnation in emotional thinking.
- Stiffness in the body represents stiffness in the mind: inflexible attitudes and beliefs, feeling stuck or trapped, repressed anger, and other strong emotions.[12]

> Those with the arthritis personality, due to their critical nature, want things to be different, but their impulse to change is constantly suppressed by an unwillingness or inability to change. Stiffness and rigidity are the dominant states of mind, and they are also the dominant conditions of an arthritic joint.

lifestyle changes needed for recovery, sometimes in spite of their severe pain.

Are You Stressed-Out?

If you answer yes to more than five of the questions below, it indicates that you have too much stress in your life. In parentheses after each question are some potential underlying causes for the problem.

- Do you often grind your teeth? (digestive dysfunction, parasites)
- Is your breath shallow and irregular? (low metabolic energy, food allergies)
- Are your hands and feet cold? (hormonal imbalance, adrenal or thyroid weakness)
- Do you have trouble sleeping or tend to wake up tired? (liver dysfunction, food allergies)
- Do you often have an upset stomach? (food allergies)
- Do you get mad or irritated easily? (liver dysfunction)
- Do you feel worthless? (low metabolic energy, chronic fatigue)
- Do you constantly worry? (hormonal imbalance)
- Do you have problems concentrating and articulating your thoughts? (low metabolic energy, digestive or hormonal imbalance)
- Do you frequently fidget, chew your fingers, or bite your nails? (food allergies, digestive disturbances)
- Do you have high blood pressure? (food allergies, digestive disturbances)
- Do you eat, drink, or smoke excessively? (low metabolic energy, poor diet)

- Do you sometimes turn to recreational drugs just to get away? (low metabolic energy, poor diet)

Are Your Adrenal Glands Stressed?

The Adrenal Stress Index (ASI) can pinpoint whether an imbalance in the adrenal glands might be contributing to stress and arthritis. This test evaluates how well a person's adrenal glands are functioning by tracking hormone levels over a 24-hour cycle. Four saliva samples taken at intervals throughout the day are used to reconstruct a person's adrenal rhythm in the laboratory. Saliva has been shown to closely mirror blood levels of hormones, and is easy to collect at home. These samples are used to determine whether two primary stress hormones (cortisol and DHEA) are being secreted in proper proportion to each other and at the right times. Based on the results, a physician can prescribe the appropriate treatment to restore the balance of hormones and correct the circadian rhythm.

Symptoms Associated with Stress

- Anxiety
- Indigestion
- Weight loss or gain
- Depression
- Premenstrual syndrome (PMS)
- Bad breath or body odors
- Muscle spasms

Mind-Body Therapies for Arthritis

Whether a person experiences stress as a positive motivational force or as a negative, detrimental one depends on their perception of the stress.[13] People who feel as though they are in control of their lives and generally feel good about themselves will use life's stressors in a positive fashion. However, those who feel that outside forces and other people control their life circumstances tend to react negatively to stress. The perception of stress can be consciously shifted by deliberately reprogramming the mind with positive instead of negative thoughts through meditation, cognitive therapy, and neuro-linguistic programming. Relaxation therapies, such as biofeedback, hypnotherapy, guided imagery, flower remedies, and aromatherapy, can also help reduce your stress levels and relieve arthritis pain.

Meditation

Meditation is a safe and simple way to balance your physical, emotional, and mental states. It's easy to learn and can be useful both for treating

A Simple Meditation Exercise

The first step to practicing meditation is learning to breathe in a manner that facilitates a state of calmness and awareness. The following exercise is recommended for achieving a sense of calmness. Find a quiet place where you won't be disturbed and practice for several minutes each day.

1. Assume a comfortable position lying on your back or sitting. If you choose to sit, keep your spine straight and let your shoulders drop.

2. Close your eyes if it feels comfortable to do so.

3. Bring your attention to your belly, feeling it rise or expand gently as you inhale and fall or recede as you exhale. Keep your focus on your breathing.

4. When your mind wanders away from your breath, notice what thoughts took you away and then gently bring your attention back to your belly and the feeling of your breath moving in and out. When your mind wanders away from your breath, don't judge or criticize yourself, simply bring your mind back to the breath every time, no matter what it has become preoccupied with.

Practice this exercise for 15 minutes every day, whether you feel like it or not, for a week and see how it feels to incorporate a disciplined meditation practice into your life.

stress and in pain management. In the broadest sense, meditation is any activity that keeps your attention focused in the present. When the mind is calm and focused in the present, it is neither reacting to past events nor preoccupied with future plans, two major sources of chronic stress. There are many forms of meditation, but they can be categorized into two main approaches: concentration meditation and mindfulness meditation.

Concentration meditation focuses the lens of the mind on an object, sound (mantra), thought, image (mandala), or the breath to still the mind and allow greater awareness or clarity to emerge. The breath is one of the most common objects of focus in this type of meditation. As the person focuses on the ebb and flow of their breath, their mind is absorbed in the rhythm and becomes more placid, tranquil, and still.

Mindfulness is the simple act of truly paying attention. It is a keen awareness of each moment. The idea is to hone your focus and your five senses on every detail of an experience: the smell and texture of a flower, the taste and feel of food in your mouth, the colors and sounds experienced on a walk in the park. Mindfulness teaches people to slow down, to be aware of their surroundings, and to connect with themselves. It can be practiced just about anywhere while doing just about anything.

Transcendental Meditation (TM), a popular form of concentration meditation, is the most well-documented regarding the physiological effects of meditation, with over 500 clinical studies conducted to date.[14] Research shows that during TM practice the body gains a deeper state of relaxation than during ordinary rest or sleep.[15] Brain wave changes indicate a state of enhanced awareness and coherence, and TM has been found to increase intelligence, creativity, and perceptual ability and reduce blood pressure and rates of illness by 50%.[16] TM also causes decreased blood levels of cortisol, a hormone responsible for many of the deleterious physiological changes seen with stress.[17] When cortisol levels are reduced, the adrenal glands are allowed to heal, which mitigates pain and inflammation.

A direct effect of meditation on arthritis is the reduction of pain. In one study, 72% of the patients with chronic pain achieved at least a 33% reduction in pain after participating in an eight-week period of mindfulness meditation, and 61% of the patients achieved at least a 50% reduction in pain and perceived their bodies as being less problematic, suggesting an improvement in self-esteem.[18]

Cognitive Therapy

It has been estimated that the average human being has around 50,000 thoughts per day. Unfortunately, many of these thoughts are negative—angry, fearful, pessimistic, or worrisome. Up to 85% of the thinking we regularly engage in is negative and self-defeating.[19] The basis of cognitive therapy is to identify—through maintaining a journal and by introspection—the negative, self-defeating inner dialogue of thoughts (what cognitive therapists refer to as automatic thoughts) and use positive, coping thoughts to counter the negative thoughts. The goal is to pull yourself out of reflexive self-destructive mental behavior that may be exacerbating your illness and to bolster the positive, self-reliant aspect of your personality.

Cognitive therapy doesn't focus on the root causes of psychological problems; rather, it seeks to support health by interrupting the flow of negative thoughts. Actually listing negative thoughts on paper and generating a list of positive responses to each problematic thought enables the mind to reframe the situation. For arthritis sufferers, replacing negative thoughts with positive ones can help facilitate

How to Stop a "Thought Attack"

One technique to stop a "thought attack" involves keeping a rubber band around your wrist. When you become aware of a negative thought, snap the rubber band in order to snap your consciousness out of its negative pattern. Then replace the negative thought with a positive affirmation that means something to you personally. "I am making progress in treating myself as a friend," for instance. This coping technique helps you become aware of your automatic thoughts and begin to change them consciously.

Success Story: Cognitive Therapy Relieves Stress-Induced Arthritis

Ray came to our office suffering extreme pain due to chronic psoriatic and gouty arthritis. It was clear that he had a very stressful life: He was in bankruptcy, was contemplating divorce, had very low self-esteem, and had problems with his teenage children. He was so depressed that he had even contemplated suicide. Not surprisingly, he felt like he was caught in a downward spiral, with little he could do to improve his situation.

The first thing we realized about Ray was that his sense of hope was low and his sense of helplessness was high. His team of rheumatologists hadn't offered much beyond higher doses of medication and opiates to control his pain. We explained to Ray that chronic pain is a complicated mixture of physical, perceptual, cognitive, emotional, environmental, and other factors— that pain is actually an individual experience and is real, regardless of whether an organic cause can be found.

We stabilized Ray's depression with a combination of kava (*Piper methysticum*) and an herbal supplement for muscles and joints that includes white willow bark, licorice, and boswellia, DL-phenylalanine (an amino acid helpful in pain management), and cognitive therapy. We made a list of his negative thoughts and brainstormed with him on positive coping thoughts to replace them. Every time Ray caught himself in the act of a negative thought, he would snap a rubber band he kept on his wrist as a reminder, then repeat his coping thoughts in the form of personal, positive affirmation stated in the present tense.

The combination of naturopathic arthritis treatment, diet changes, and cognitive therapy that we recommended helped Ray tremendously. He began to transform himself into a positive thinker and became less critical of himself and others. He felt strong enough emotionally to manage his pain and cure himself of arthritis. He ended his dysfunctional marriage (a major component of his constant stress) and began to work from his home again. He smiled more and became angry less frequently. He occasionally slipped back into his old habit of worrying, but when he became conscious of doing it, he would snap the rubber band, then go for a walk or interrupt his downward-spiraling vortex of negative thoughts in some other way. After 10 months, Ray was not only completely out of pain but also in possession of a different self-image. "Not only is my arthritis better but I've learned to manage my emotions, and I've become a better, happier person," he said.

---

healing. Cognitive therapy may also be helpful for dealing with pain. The intensity of pain is partly determined by how you perceive it—if you "catastrophize" the pain, you may actually make it worse. Cognitive therapy can be used to gain control of your thought processes and allow you to alter your perception of pain.

Neuro-Linguistic Programming

Similar to cognitive therapy, neuro-linguistic programming (NLP) helps people detect unconscious patterns of thought, behavior, and attitudes that contribute to their illness. These unconscious patterns are then reprogrammed in order to alter psychological responses and facilitate the healing process. "Neuro" refers to the way the brain works and how thinking demonstrates consistent and detectable patterns; "linguistic" refers to verbal and nonverbal expressions of thinking patterns; and "programming" refers to how these patterns are recognized and understood by the mind and how they can be altered.

NLP was developed in the early 1970s by a professor of linguistics and a student of psychology and mathematics, both at the University of California at Santa Cruz. They studied the thinking processes, language patterns, and behavioral patterns of several accomplished individuals. They found that body cues—eye movement, posture, voice tone, and breathing patterns—coincided with certain unconscious patterns of a person's emotional state. Based on their findings, they developed the NLP technique to help people with their emotional problems.

People who have difficulty recovering from physical illness have often adopted negative beliefs about their recovery. They perceive themselves as helpless, hopeless, or worthless, as expressed in statements like "I can't get healthy" or "There's no hope." NLP tries to move the person from their present state of discomfort to a desired state of health by helping reprogram these beliefs about healing.

NLP practitioners ask questions to discover how the person relates to issues of identity, personal beliefs, life goals, and their health. Then they observe the person's language patterns, eye movements, postures, muscle tension, and gestures. These relay information about how the person relates to their condition in both conscious and unconscious ways, revealing what limiting beliefs may exist. These belief structures can then be altered using NLP. The practitioner will ask people to see themselves in a state of health. By doing so, an outcome is set that facilitates the healing process. The brain's natural response is to duplicate whatever

Stress Management Helps Rheumatoid Arthritis

A study at the Harry S. Truman Memorial Veterans Hospital, in Columbia, Missouri, showed that stress management techniques produced clinical benefits for RA patients. In this study of 141 patients, one group received stress management training while the other received standard medical care without additional psychological counseling. The training consisted of a 10-week course on stress management techniques followed by a 15-month maintenance phase. At the end of this period, the researchers found that the stress management group showed statistically significant improvements in measures of self-efficacy, coping, feelings of helplessness, pain, and overall health status.[21]

images or beliefs are created about getting better.[20] The brain then triggers the necessary immunological responses to guide the body toward health. NLP has proved successful in treating people with chronic illnesses, such as AIDS, cancer, allergies, and arthritis.

Biofeedback

Biofeedback training is a method that uses simple electronic devices to teach people how to consciously regulate normally unconscious bodily functions (such as breathing, heart rate, and blood pressure). Biofeedback is particularly useful for learning to reduce stress, eliminate headaches, reduce muscle spasms, and relieve pain. Biofeedback can help people with arthritis by relaxing tight muscles, correcting muscular imbalances, and providing muscular re-education, which can prevent and correct abnormal joint biomechanics. It can also intercept a chronic fight-or-flight response and aid in revitalizing adrenal gland functions. By teaching patients both relaxation techniques and control over their muscle spasms, biofeedback helps them reduce or eliminate pain.[22]

Biofeedback devices give immediate feedback, or information, about the biological systems of the person being monitored so that they can learn to consciously influence that system. For example, a person seeking to regulate their heart rate would train with a biofeedback device set up to transmit one blinking light or one audible beep per heartbeat. Electrodes are placed on the skin (a simple, painless process), and the patient is instructed to use various techniques such as meditation, relaxation, and visualization to affect the desired response (muscle relaxation, lowered heart rate, or lowered temperature). The biofeedback device reports the person's progress by a change in the speed of the beeps or flashes. By learning to alter the rate of the flashes or beeps, the person would be subtly programmed to control their heart rate.

When a patient suffering from pain understands the causes, nature, mechanisms, and role of their pain, they've taken an important step in successfully handling their problem. Developing some degree of control over the situation further empowers the person and helps alleviate any sense of hopelessness. [23] Biofeedback helps a person take this critical step in controlling arthritis pain.

Hypnotherapy

Hypnotherapy has applications for both psychological and physical disorders. A skilled hypnotherapist can facilitate profound changes in respiration and relaxation to create positive shifts in behavior and an enhanced sense of well-being. A physiological shift can be observed in a hypnotic state, as can greater control of autonomic nervous system functions normally considered to be beyond a person's control. Stress reduction is a common benefit, as is a lowering of blood pressure.

Hypnosis can be used to alleviate many varieties of pain, such as back, abdominal, and joint pain, as well as headaches and migraines. It works by accessing the unconscious mind and training it to react in a positive way to the experience of pain, such as inducing an immediate sense of relaxation. Hypnotherapy can be a nurturing and highly relaxing experience. Certified hypnotherapists don't attempt to control your mind or take you into a state so deep that you don't have control over yourself. Most people are aware of everything that transpires during a hypnotherapy session, yet they are able to mobilize deeper levels of their mind to facilitate healing.

Hypnotherapy is currently taught in several allopathic medical programs and has been approved by the American Medical Association as a clinical adjunct in the management of chronic pain.[24] Some states certify the profession of hypnotherapy by requiring a certain level of training. Other types of practitioners, such as psychotherapists and bodyworkers, may also use hypnosis as a tool to help their patients relax.

Guided Imagery and Visualization

Using the power of the mind to evoke a positive physical response, guided imagery and visualization can modulate the immune system and reduce pain. Guided imagery uses the imagination to elicit positive physiological responses. By directly accessing emotions, imagery can help an individual understand the needs that may be represented by their illness and can help develop ways to meet those needs. Imagery is also one of the quickest and most direct ways to become aware of emotions and their effects on health, both positive and negative.

Imagery is simply a flow of thoughts that one can see, hear, feel, smell, taste, or otherwise experience internally, in the mind. While the sensory phenomenon experienced in the mind may or may not represent external reality, it always depicts internal reality. What this means is that the sensations in the body that imagery creates are very real; they can be measured via laboratory devices. Research using brain scans indicates that imagery activates parts of the cerebral cortex and centers of the primitive brain. During visualization, the visual (optic) cortex is active, and when sounds are imagined, the auditory cortex is active. It appears that the cortex can create imaginary realities and that the lower centers (and perhaps every cell in the body) respond to this information.

Imagery is a proven method for pain relief, helps people tolerate medical procedures, reduces side effects of treatments, and stimulates the body to heal. Patients who are constant worriers are especially good candidates for guided imagery because the internal process involved in worrying is very similar to the process of "imagining yourself well."[25]

Imagery has been used to treat people with autoimmune arthritis as well as systemic lupus. Studies show that depression and other psychiatric symptoms often precede the development of lupus and RA.[26] In order to reverse the disease, the patient must access and reverse their recurring negative thought patterns. In one case, a patient was instructed to use two sets of visual images to rid herself of RA, which had developed after a life of depression and destructive self-criticism. She was first instructed to visualize and compare the difference between what a bacteria looks like and what normal cells look like. This would help inform her immune system of the difference between "self and nonself" and the mistake her immune cells were making in killing normal cells. The second set of visual images were developed to relieve her arthritic symptoms: She pictured little dragons carrying ice to put out the arthritic "fire" in her joints. In less than three weeks, 75% of her arthritic pain was gone and she was able to discontinue medication.[27]

Restricted Environmental Stimulation Therapy

Restricted environmental stimulation therapy (REST), a therapeutic tool that has been researched for over 35 years, is known to aid in relaxation. The key technique in this therapy is to isolate the person from sensory input in their external environment by using a flotation tank.

In REST, you customarily float for one hour in a small, shallow flotation tank or pool. The water is 18 inches deep and supersaturated with 1,000 to 1,500 pounds of Epsom salts (magnesium sulfate). This makes the water so buoyant that it is impossible to sink. You just float effortlessly on the surface and experience something that only astronauts usually experience—the feeling of weightlessness. In addition, the environment of the flotation tank is specifically designed to reduce the perception of all external stimuli, which can lead to powerful healing effects on the body and mind. The water and air are kept at a constant temperature of 93 to 94°F; this allows the patient to lose the ability to discern where their body ends and the outer environment begins.

Flotation provides the most reliable induction of deep relaxation attainable without medication or years of training in meditation or biofeedback. REST has been scientifically documented to produce myriad psychological and physiological responses conducive to relaxation. The following are particularly beneficial to those with arthritis: decrease in pain,[28] diminished response to stress,[29] decline in cortisol levels in the blood,[30] and increase in magnesium levels.[31] Magnesium is important because it helps muscles relax; low levels of magnesium can contribute to muscle spasms. People with arthritis often have a deficiency of magnesium.

One person with arthritis who used flotation described it this way: "My health status followed my mind. If I can use computer jargon to illustrate the point, flotation helped me erase my old mental software and install new programs. This enabled me to print out a new, disease-free prototype of my body. The pain is completely gone and all lab tests that were previously positive for arthritis indicators have now been normal for five years. I am truly cured of arthritis."[32]

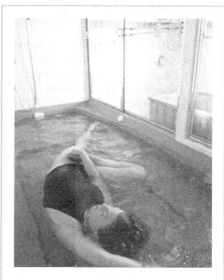

Flotation provides the most reliable induction of deep relaxation attainable without medication or years of training in meditation or biofeedback.

Flower Remedies

Flower remedies directly address a person's emotional state in order to facilitate both psychological and physiological well-being. By balancing negative feelings and stress, flower remedies can effectively remove the emotional barriers to health and recovery. Flower remedies comprise subtle liquid preparations made from the fresh blossoms of various plants, even trees, to address emotional, psychological, and spiritual issues underlying physical and medical problems. The approach was pioneered by British physician Edward Bach, who introduced the 38 Bach Flower Remedies, based on English plants, in the 1930s.

The Placebo Effect

The power of the mind is acknowledged in conventional medicine, where it is called the placebo effect. A placebo is an inactive substance, such as

The Spiritual Connection to Healing

Spirituality and a feeling of connection to a divine presence can cultivate a hopeful attitude and a sense of meaning in a person's life, which may help promote healing and recovery even with an illness as serious as arthritis. The particular way spirituality is expressed, whether through a specific religious practice or simply time spent in nature, is not the important issue. Additionally, over 250 studies have shown that prayer (of any kind whatsoever) has health benefits and can be used as an effective means of promoting physical wellness and healing.[33]

A study at the University of Michigan, in Ann Arbor, found that people who attended religious services at least once per month lived significantly longer than those who didn't. The national survey followed 3,617 Americans over a seven-year period. The nonchurchgoers were about one-third more likely to die over the study period. Churchgoers tended to be more physically active, at a healthy weight, and nonsmokers. Even eliminating these healthier lifestyle factors, the nonchurchgoers still had a 25% greater likelihood of dying. Researchers speculated that the community involvement and religious rituals might promote feelings of hope, serenity, and optimism, all helpful in prolonging life. Attending religious services "extends the life span about as much as moderate exercise or not smoking," the researchers concluded.[34]

a sugar pill, which is often used alongside an active substance, such as a drug, to see how much effect the drug actually has. The famous 'double blind placebo control trial' has been the gold standard for proving the efficacy of certain pharmaceutical agents. The well-documented placebo effect collaborates the power of the mind in healing. The placebo effect is thought to work through three mechanisms:

1. conditioning
2. endorphin release
3. expectation

For instance, if people are given sugar water and told it is a pain killer, they will often experience a decrease in pain. The placebo response rate can be quite high—up to 80% in some experiments![35] Rather than relating to this well-documented phenomena as an annoyance that interferes with drug research, perhaps we should honor and extol this effect, and use it to its maximum potential in self-healing.

The Power of Intention

Intentionality research is a new area of science that is investigating how human intention can be directed to influence specific biological processes. An exciting paper delivered by Dr. Glen Rein clearly demonstrates that focusing your conscious mind can either cause DNA strands to wind or unwind. Dr. Rein concluded that when test subjects were able to synchronize their heart and mind, determined by measuring EKG and EEG patterns, they could successfully wrap or unwrap DNA strands at will![36] Further research in this area will lead to our understanding more about the unlimited healing capacity we all have available to us. Meanwhile, it is encouraging to know that science is collaborating what ancient healers have honored for centuries—that the healing potential of the human mind is powerful.

Rather than considering the placebo effect as irrelevant, many physicians and scientists consider it to be critical to understanding the body-mind connection to health and wellness. The placebo effect is being repositioned as a powerful tool that can be used to initiate a meaningful therapeutic response.[37] Most of the understanding of the neurobiological mechanisms of the placebo effect have been studied through experiments with pain control, which have discovered that the physiological pain relieving effects initiated by drug therapies, are often replicated within the body when a placebo is ingested.[38] Arthritis patients can immediately put this powerful tool to work by recognizing the self-healing potential available and learning to focus positive energy through the use of techniques described in this chapter.

Today, an estimated 20 different brands of flower remedies, based on plants native to many landscapes, from Australia to India to Alaska, offer about 1,500 different blends for a diverse range of psychological conditions. Each flower remedy addresses a particular emotional issue. For example, Vine helps increase feelings of self-worth, Impatiens is recommended for feelings of impatience with others and yourself, and Aspen is for feelings of fear. An individual formula can be made by combining four to six of the remedies and taking them orally or rubbing them into the skin. They can be taken for a short time to cope with a crisis or for a period of months.

 For **dietary recommendations for arthritis**, see chapter 12, The Arthritis Diet, pages 225–256.

Amanda, 52, came to our office in severe pain. She described her arthritis as being out of control: Her joints were swollen and stiff, she was suffering from chronic fatigue, and she felt hopeless. After blood tests and food allergy assessments, we reviewed her life situation. She had been through a terrible divorce over the past year and her arthritis symptoms had increased during that time. Along

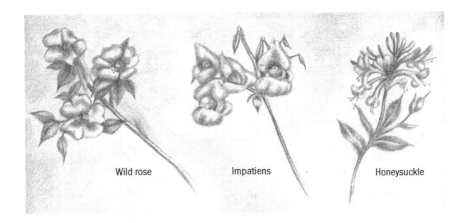

Wild rose   Impatiens   Honeysuckle

with recommending initial dietary changes (switching to the arthritis diet), we put together a Bach flower remedy combination to help with her emotional issues: Cherry Plum (for feeling a loss of control), Crabapple (for cleansing), Rock Rose (for terror), and Water Violet (for more self-reliance). Amanda was instructed to take ½ teaspoon of this combination four times daily. "I can't believe it," she said after three days on the therapy. "The feeling of hopelessness has lifted. It feels like a veil of confusion was covering my head, and now it's gone. Best of all, these flower remedies don't have any of the side effects, like drowsiness, that I got from the antidepressant medications I used before."

Aromatherapy

Aromatherapy is a unique branch of herbal medicine that utilizes the medicinal properties found in the essential oils of various plants. Through a process of steam distillation or cold-pressing, the volatile constituents of the plant's oil (its essence) are extracted from its flowers, leaves, branches, or roots. The immediate and often profound effect that essential oils have on the central nervous system also makes aromatherapy an excellent method for stress management.[39] The term "aromatherapy" was coined in 1937 by the French chemist Rene-Maurice Gattefosse, who observed the healing effect of lavender oil on burns.

 For information on **nutrients and herbs to support the adrenal glands and reduce stress**, see chapter 13, Supplements for Arthritis, pages 257–294.

Essential oils have a number of pharmacological properties: antibacterial, antiviral, antispasmodic, diuretic, and vasodilating (widening blood vessels). They are able to energize or pacify, detoxify, and help digestion. Their therapeutic properties also make them effective for treating infections, interacting with the various branches of the nervous system, modifying the immune response, and harmonizing moods and emotions. Aromatic molecules that interact with the nasal cavity give off signals that travel to the limbic system, the emotional switchboard of the brain.[40] There they create impressions associated with previous experiences and emotions that involved similar aromas. The limbic system is directly connected to those parts of the brain that control heart rate, blood pressure, breathing, memory, stress levels, and hormone balance.

The effects of aromatherapy on brain wave patterns when essential oils are inhaled or smelled have been studied. The findings show that oils such as orange, jasmine, and rose have a tranquilizing effect, altering the brain waves into a rhythm that produces calmness and a sense of well-being.[41] Essential oils of citronella and *Eucalyptus citriodora* can be diffused in the air or rubbed on the wrists, solar plexus, and temples for quick and effective relaxation. Lavender oil added to a bath or sprayed on bedsheets reduces tension and enhances relaxation.[42] Roman chamomile (*Anthemis nobilis*) is recommended to calm an upset mind or body; a drop rubbed on the solar plexus can bring rapid relief of mental or physical stress.

There are several different methods for using essential oils.

- Diffusion: Diffusers disperse microparticles of essential oils into the air. They can be used to benefit respiratory conditions or simply to charge the air with the mood-lifting or calming qualities of the fragrance.

Aromatherapy to Soothe Arthritis Pain

Place 2 ounces of almond oil in a small bowl, then add four drops each of lavender, birch, cypress, and juniper oils. Mix thoroughly and apply the oil to any painful or tense joint or muscle area. Place some of the same mixture in a diffuser or directly on a lightbulb and leave the light on. This will fill the room with a relaxing, stress-reducing fragrance. You can experiment with different combinations of the following essential oils recommended for relieving arthritis pain: nutmeg, lavender, helichrysum, ginger, fir, cedar, and Roman chamomile.

 In their pure state, certain oils such as clove and cinnamon can cause irritation or even burn the skin. These oils require careful and expert application. Dilute them with a less irritating essential oil before applying them to the skin. Essential oils can cause toxic reactions if ingested, so consult a physician before taking oils internally.

- External application: Oils are readily absorbed through the skin. Convenient methods of external application are baths, massages, hot and cold compresses, or a simple topical application of diluted oils. Essential oils in a hot bath can stimulate the skin, induce relaxation, or energize the body. In massage, the oils can be worked into the skin and, depending on the oil and the massage technique, can either calm or stimulate. When used in compresses, essential oils soothe minor aches and pains, reduce swelling, and treat sprains.

- Floral waters: These can be sprayed into the air or sprayed on skin that is too sensitive to the touch for massage with essential oils.

- Internal application: For certain conditions (such as organ dysfunction), it can be advantageous to take specific oils internally. However, some oils can be toxic when taken internally, so it's essential do so only with proper medical supervision.

twelve

The Arthritis Diet

Dietary practices have a major impact on arthritis. In fact, if you eat the standard American diet (SAD), it could be making your arthritis worse. Among the offenders are saturated fats (found in cooking oils and fried foods), white flour and sugar, red meat, chemical additives, yeast, and milk and dairy products. These foods can increase inflammation, invoke allergies, and interfere with hormone production, cellular integrity, and the function and mobility of the joints.

Changing the way you eat will change the way you feel. The right foods can keep you free of stiff joints, swelling, and fatigue, while also promoting longevity and overall health. If you adhere to only one therapy from this book, choose to eat right by eliminating problematic foods and increasing your daily intake of vegetables, fruits, and whole grains. In this chapter, we explain which foods are arthritis-friendly and which foods should be avoided. We also look at the different types of dietary fats and their effects on inflammation. Finally, we provide recipes tailored to OA and RA to give you easy and delicious ways to incorporate these dietary changes and relieve your arthritis symptoms.

IN THIS CHAPTER

- The Arthritis Diet
- The Fats Connection to Arthritis
- Success Story: Diet and Detoxification Defeat Gout
- Arthritis Recipes

The Arthritis Diet

What we call the arthritis diet is primarily a vegetarian, whole foods diet consisting of fruits and vegetables, grains, raw seeds and nuts and their butters, fermented bean products, and fish—all considered arthritis-friendly foods. (See "Friendly and Unfriendly Arthritis Foods," pages 230–232.) These foods are high in dietary fiber, which helps move food and wastes through the digestive tract before they have a chance to form toxic substances. Many degenerative illnesses, including arthritis, are related to a diet low in fiber.

Whole (unprocessed) foods are rich in the nutrients needed to fight destructive free radicals; promote skin and tissue health; repair bones, muscles, and tendons; and promote regularity. In addition, being more nutrient dense, whole foods are more filling and decrease the likelihood of overeating and subsequent weight gain. Since being overweight puts stress on weight-bearing joints, losing weight or maintaining a healthy weight is crucial to recovering from arthritis. Whole foods also put less overall stress on the body because they're more easily digested and contain fewer toxic substances than processed foods.

Dietary fats are an important consideration for anyone with arthritis. The wrong kinds of fats can increase inflammation in joints, while the "good" fats will help keep inflammation in check. As a percentage of calories, most vegetables contain less than 10% fat and most grains contain 16% to 20% fat. By comparison, whole milk and cheeses contain 74% fat (even low-fat milk contains 38% fat on a percentage-of-calories basis). Most animal foods contain large quantities of fat, mostly saturated, which raise levels of inflammatory compounds in the body and increase arthritic symptoms. Shellfish and commercially produced dairy products and corn-fed meat are also high in arachidonic acid, which is converted into powerful proinflammatory compounds by the body. Whole foods, however, are typically high in healthy fats, including the essential fatty acids, which help decrease inflammation and improve the health of people with RA, psoriatic arthritis, and OA.

 For more on **types of fat and their effect on arthritis**, see "The Fats Connection to Arthritis" in this chapter, pages 229–233.

People with arthritis commonly have a high level of acidity (a urine pH lower than 6.3) (SEE QUICK DEFINITION), which increases the potential for developing inflammatory conditions. Acidity can be decreased by reducing your intake of acid-forming foods and increasing intake of

> Changing the way you eat will change the way you feel. The right foods can keep you free of stiff joints, swelling, and fatigue, while also promoting longevity and overall health.

alkaline-forming foods. The most acid-forming foods are sugar, alcohol, vinegar, coffee, meat, and dairy products. Foods known to increase the alkalinity of the body include all vegetables (except tomatoes), aloe vera, and "green" foods, such as chlorella, barley grass, wheatgrass, chlorophyll, parsley, and alfalfa. As a general rule of thumb, the greener the vegetable, the more it will help increase alkalinity in the body.

We suggest that you keep a food diary, recording what you eat each day and any changes in your arthritis symptoms (including joint stiffness, swelling, tenderness, and fatigue). A food diary

 The abbreviation **pH** stands for "potential hydrogen," and is a scale for measuring the relative acidity or alkalinity of a solution. A pH of 7.0 is neutral; 0.1 to 6.9 is acidic; and 7.1 to 14 is alkaline. The numbers refer to how many hydrogen atoms are present compared to an ideal or standard solution. Normally, blood is slightly alkaline, at 7.35 to 7.45; urine pH can range from 4.8 to 8.0 but is usually somewhat acidic, with a normal reading between 5.0 and 6.0.

can help you determine which foods are most beneficial for reducing your arthritis symptoms. If symptoms worsen, use your food diary to locate potential problem foods. The next day, experiment with those particular foods to identify the triggering agent and then eliminate it from your diet.

Tips to Ease the Shift to Healthier Foods

Making changes in diet can be difficult. Since eating is often a social activity, in addition to changing the foods you eat, you'll also face some complications in how to handle meals with others. Here are a few tips on simple ways to change your eating habits and ease into the arthritis diet.

- Begin by changing one meal a day to be more healthful. This makes shopping and cooking more manageable while you adjust to the new lifestyle. Maintain this for about a month, then tackle the next meal. Within three months, your habits will be transformed.

- Stop buying snack foods such as sodas, chips, and cookies. Substitute trail mix, popcorn, and herb teas as an interim step.

- Cook large quantities of main dish recipes so you'll have leftovers for lunch or the next day's dinner. Avoid freezing foods, as this process may destroy important nutrients.

- Do not insist that children or other family members eat your diet. Simply serve an increasing number of healthful choices with each meal. This approach, combined with weaning family members from sugar and refined flour products, will produce a hunger for good food.

- When dining at other people's homes, eat lightly, focus on what you can have, and pass up the allergenic foods. Avoid debates about diet. Soon your improved health may prompt a great deal of positive interest in your diet.

- Choose restaurants that offer healthful choices. Ask if the chef will modify a dish (skip the cream sauce, for example) to fit your new diet. If that's not possible, you can eat beforehand at home and just sip a beverage or eat a salad while enjoying the social occasion. Be positive, keep the focus off your diet, and, above all, don't be self-righteous.

The Arthritis Diet Daily Menu Plan

Here's an example of how you might eat on a typical day when following the arthritis diet.

General tips. Avoid simple sugars; include plenty of onions or garlic, five or more servings of fruits and vegetables (including 4 ounces of blueberries or blackberries), and 3 ounces of soy products; substitute green tea for coffee.[1]

Breakfast. Eight ounces of filtered water with freshly squeezed lemon juice. One piece of fresh fruit, such as pineapple, pear, papaya, or apple. Protein shake: In a blender, mix the recommended amount of protein drink powder and water, along with 1/4 cup to 1/2 cup organic berries (fresh or frozen) and 1 tablespoon flaxseed oil.

Lunch. Green Goodness Salad with Herb Dressing (see recipe). One to two medium bowls of steamed vegetables, such as squash (butternut, summer, or spaghetti), kale, collard greens, beets, broccoli, and carrots. Or one sheet of nori seaweed (available in Asian grocery stores and health food stores) filled with sliced avocado, shredded carrots, diced cucumbers, and sprouts, drizzled with Herb Dressing. If you're not pursuing a detoxification program, you may eat a small portion of free-range chicken, beef, or game. Buffalo, ostrich, venison, and emu are meats particularly high in omega-3 essential fatty acids.

Snack. Fresh fruit or vegetables and alkaline-forming nuts and seeds, such as almonds or sesame seeds. Soak seeds in filtered water to increase protein content and ease digestion.

Dinner. One or more of the main dish recipes (see pages 241–252) for your type of arthritis.

The Fats Connection to Arthritis

The kinds of fats in your diet directly affect the severity of inflammation and other arthritic symptoms. There are "good" and "bad" dietary fats, and if your diet contains too many of the bad fats, it may be making your arthritis worse or even helping to create it in the first place (see "A Quick Guide to Fats," page 234). The inflammatory process can become uncontrollable when certain dietary factors skew the delicate balance of inflammation-mediating substances. Prostaglandins, complex fatty acids that can either cause or decrease inflammation, are composed of different fatty acids. The type of prostaglandins manufactured by your body (anti-inflammatory or proinflammatory) depends upon the fats in your diet, as well as the presence of certain nutrients (vitamins C, B_3, and B_6, magnesium, and zinc).

Prostaglandins that cause inflammation are formed when the diet is high in animal fats, which contain high amounts of arachidonic acid. Arachidonic acid is a long-chain polyunsaturated omega-6 fatty acid found primarily in animal foods such as meat, poultry, and dairy products. When the diet is abundant in arachidonic acids, they are stored in cell membranes. An enzyme transforms these stored acids into prostaglandins and leukotrienes that instigate inflammation. If there is an overabundance of arachidonic acid or "bad" fats, more proinflammatory agents will be produced by the body.

Merely eliminating inappropriate fats from the diet can produce

Acid-Forming Foods

Alcohol, cocoa, coffee, and caffeinated teas; vinegar; meat and other animal proteins; sugar and all products that contain sugar; some fruit (especially cranberries, plums, and prunes); many fats and oils; some nuts and seeds (cashews, peanuts, pecans, hazelnuts, and Brazil nuts); cheese; white flour, baked goods, pasta, wheat, corn, and oats; many beans and legumes

Alkaline-Forming Foods

Fresh vegetables (except tomatoes); avocados and most fruit; some nuts and seeds (particularly almonds, chestnuts, coconut, flaxseeds, and pumpkin, sesame, and sunflower seeds); herbal teas (especially dandelion and ginseng); soy products

Friendly and Unfriendly Arthritis Foods

■ Nuts and Seeds

INCLUDE

Limited amounts of natural raw nuts, particularly walnuts, almonds, and pecans; raw nut butters; seeds, such as chia, sesame, pumpkin, and flax.

AVOID

Roasted or salted nuts and seeds; nuts with a high omega-6 fatty acid content, such as cashews, brazil nuts, pine nuts, and peanuts.

■ Oils

INCLUDE

Expeller-pressed unsaturated oils, such as organic, unprocessed coconut, flax-seed, sesame, walnut, soy, cod liver, and hemp seed. These oils should never be heated.

AVOID

Any oils containing hydrogenated fats, trans-fatty acids, or saturated fats, such as shortening, margarine, and cottonseed oil.

■ Fish

INCLUDE

Cold-water fish (trout, cod, salmon, halibut, bluefish, sardines, and smelts). Wild fish are better than farm-raised fish.

AVOID

All shellfish.

■ Vegetables

INCLUDE

Raw or steamed organic vegetables, such as artichokes, asparagus, beets and beet greens, broccoli, brussels sprouts, cabbage, carrots, celery, corn, cucumbers, endive, green and wax beans, green peas, kale, lentils, lima beans, onions, watercress, yams, lettuce, arugula, and radishes.

Sprouts, such as mung, lentil, alfalfa, radish, soy, and wheatgrass.

Wild greens and roots, such as burdock, dandelion leaves, chickweed, yellow dock root, wild alliums, purslane, lamb's-quarters, pigweed, and sorrel.

AVOID

Nightshade vegetables, including tomatoes, eggplant, peppers, and potatoes.

■ Spices and Seasonings

INCLUDE

Bragg Liquid Aminos, Celtic Sea Salt, gomasio (a combination of sesame seeds and salt), lemon juice.

Chives, cilantro, garlic, parsley, bay leaves, marjoram, sage, thyme, savory, kelp, and other vegetable or herb seasonings.

AVOID

Pepper, refined table salt, products that contain yeast (such as soy sauce and tamari), vinegar, mustard, mayonnaise, chemical additives such as monosodium glutamate (MSG).

■ Grains

INCLUDE

Organic whole-grain breads made from millet, quinoa, rye, or buckwheat (free of yeast gluten, and preservatives).

Millet, wild rice, brown rice, and egg-free pasta made from buckwheat, rice, quinoa, soy, or vegetable flours.

Cereals made from millet, oatmeal, brown and wild rice, buckwheat groats, barley, quinoa, amaranth, and teff.

AVOID

Processed grain products such as white flour, white bread, and white rice, as well as commercial products labeled "whole wheat."

Processed cereals that are puffed or flaked.

■ Fruits

INCLUDE

Fresh organic fruits, such as apples, apricots, berries, cherries, currants, guavas, grapefruit, lemons, mangoes, melons, nectarines, oranges, papaya, peaches, pineapple, pears, plums, persimmons, and tangerines (use citrus fruits sparingly).

AVOID

All dried fruits.

■ Meat

INCLUDE

Small amounts of wild game, free-range beef, or organic chicken, except when undergoing a supervised fast or detoxification program.

AVOID

Nonorganic meat products.

(continued)

Friendly and Unfriendly Arthritis Foods *(continued)*

■ Beverages

INCLUDE

Filtered water, using a certified water filter.

Herb teas containing mint, spearmint, licorice root, eucalyptus, dandelion leaves and roots, red clover, or ginger.

Pero, Roma, Caffix, and Postum (coffee substitutes).

Fresh, unsweetened juice from organic lemons, oranges, pears, pineapple, prunes, beets, carrots, cucumber, celery, garlic, onions, radishes, red cabbage, and turnip; dilute all juices by 50% to 75% with filtered water. If you have candidiasis, avoid all fruit juices (and other foods containing naturally occurring sugars).

Milk substitutes such as soy, almond, or tahini milk (you can find recipes for tahini milk on the Internet). Use nut milks sparingly and dilute them with water.

AVOID

Alcohol, cocoa, coffee (regular and decaffeinated), all dairy-based beverages, soft drinks, all juice concentrates, and canned or frozen apple, orange, berry, cherry, grape, and grapefruit juices.

■ Eggs and Cheese

INCLUDE

Soy, rice, or almond cheese.

AVOID

Eggs and all dairy, goat, or sheep cheeses.

■ Desserts and Sweeteners

INCLUDE

Desserts containing fresh fruits, natural fruit gelatin (available at health food stores), or whole tapioca sweetened with moderate amounts of sorghum, raw honey, maple syrup, or stevia (a natural sugar alternative).

AVOID

Foods containing white sugar, yeast, bleached flour, and dairy products; canned fruits, ice cream, custards, an candy. If you've tested positive for candida, klebsiella, have hypoglycemia or diabetes, avoid all sugar except fresh fruit and stevia.

immediate benefits for arthritis sufferers. Doctors at the Karolinksa Institute in Stockholm, Sweden, found that when 14 RA patients fasted for seven days, their joint pain and inflammation decreased. The researchers explained that cessation of fat intake reduced leukotriene formation and favorably altered the fatty acid balance, thereby reducing inflammation.[2] Researchers at the National Hospital in Oslo, Norway, reported that both fasting and long-term vegetarian diets can reduce arthritic symptoms, concluding that "dietary treatment can reduce the disease activity in some patients with rheumatoid arthritis."[3]

Increase Your Intake of the "Good" Fats

Essential fatty acids (EFAs), which are derived only from the diet and not manufactured in the body, help control inflammation and maintain the integrity of cell membranes. EFAs are the building blocks of prostaglandins, hormonelike substances that either encourage inflammation (prostaglandins of the 2 and 4 series) or discourage inflammation (prostaglandins of the 1 and 3 series). In healthy individuals, the body maintains these prostaglandins in a strict ratio to ensure adequate immune function and to limit inflammatory responses.

The two principle types of essential fatty acid are omega-3 and omega-6. Deficiencies in EFAs, particularly the omega-3s, are quite common in the United States because of modern food-processing techniques. Humans evolved on a diet that contained small but roughly equal amounts of omega-3s and omega-6s. About a century ago, when processed foods began to increasingly dominate the U.S. food supply, the amount of omega-3s in many commercial products declined. At the same time, the domestic livestock industry began to use feed grain, which happens to be rich in omega-6 fatty acids and low in omega-3s. Because of these changes, the American diet now has 20 to 25 times more omega-6s than omega-3s, rather than the ideal 1 to 2 ratio. When a person is deficient in EFAs, their levels of anti-inflammatory prostaglandins (1 and 3 series) tend to decline and they also tend to develop food sensitivities (allergies) as well as increased inflammation. All of these can lead to joint damage and other symptoms of arthritis.

People with arthritic conditions should avoid foods high in omega-6 fatty acids (such as most vegetable oils, including safflower, corn, peanut, and sesame) because the body converts them into proinflammatory prostaglandins as well as arachidonic acid and leukotrienes (which both cause inflammation). Instead, boost your dietary intake of omega-3

A Quick Guide to Fats

Fats or oils (lipid is the biochemical term) are one of the six basic food groups. Fats and oils are made of building blocks called fatty acids. Structurally, a fatty acid is a chain of carbon atoms with a certain quantity of hydrogen atoms attached. The more hydrogen atoms attached to the carbon atoms, the more saturated the fat. Fats come in three natural forms—saturated, monounsaturated, and polyunsaturated—and one man-made form—hydrogenated, or trans fats.

Saturated fats: These are composed of fatty acids that have their full quota of hydrogen atoms. Saturated fats are solid at room temperature and are primarily found in animal foods and tropical oils, such as coconut and palm oil. The body produces saturated fats from sugar, which is one reason many low-fat diet foods don't decrease body fat: They're often high in sugar, which is converted into fat and stored in the body. Although a high fat intake from animal sources has been associated with heart dis-

ease, some amount of saturated fat in the diet is necessary to help the body's cells remain healthy and resistant to disease.

Unsaturated fats: These tend to be liquid at room temperature. Most vegetable oils are unsaturated (coconut and palm oil are exceptions). "Unsaturated" means some of the carbon molecules are not attached to as many hydrogen atoms as they could be.

- Monounsaturated fats: Fatty acids lacking only two hydrogen atoms are referred to as monounsaturated. Monounsaturated fats are considered healthier than polyunsaturated fats because they can lower blood levels of "bad" cholesterol and maintain or raise levels of "good" cholesterol. Canola oil and olive oil are naturally high in monounsaturated fats. Olive oil is the best oil for cooking, because it doesn't break down easily into singlet oxygen molecules (free radicals) like most fats and oils do when heated. Olive oil is also the best choice due to its anti-inflammatory properties.

fatty acids (which are anti-inflammatory) by eating more green leafy vegetables; flaxseed, hemp seed, soy, and walnut oils; pumpkin seeds, sesame seeds, walnuts, and almonds; and the wild plants chia, cattail, and purslane.

The primary omega-3 fatty acid is alpha-linolenic acid (ALA), which is abundant in flaxseed oil. Unheated flaxseed oil can be put on salads, steamed vegetables, or other foods. Purchase oils that are expeller-pressed, not just cold-pressed. Check the expiration date and adhere to it; flaxseed oil can rapidly turn rancid and should be stored in the refrigerator. The seeds themselves can also be used to add a nutty flavor to cereals, vegetables, or casseroles; place a few tablespoons of organic whole flaxseeds in a coffee grinder to make the seeds more digestible and to release their oils. Purslane (*Portulaca oleracea*), often considered a weed, is actually a nutritious vegetable high in omega-3 fatty acids. Less than 1 cup provides a full day's supply of ALA. Purslane also contains

Choose a high-grade, organic extra virgin olive oil.

- Polyunsaturated fats: Fatty acids lacking four or more hydrogen atoms are referred to as polyunsaturated. They can be found in both healthy and unhealthy fats and oils. Oils high in polyunsaturated fats include flaxseed and canola oils, as well as oils made from pumpkin seeds, purslane, hemp seed, walnuts, and soybeans, all of which contain both omega-3 and omega-6 essential fatty acids.

Hydrogenated and trans fats: These terms refer to fats manipulated by a synthetic process in which they are transformed into semisolid fats by adding a hydrogen atom to an unsaturated fat molecule. This process is widely used to make margarine and to prolong the shelf life of commercial baked goods, packaged foods, and most dressings. Avoid all commercial cooking oils and baked goods that contain them. The molecules that make up these fats, called transfatty acids, are known to interfere with the

healthy functioning of our bodies due to their unusual molecular shape.

Essential fatty acids (EFAs): Unsaturated fats required in the diet are called essential fatty acids. Omega-3 and omega-6 are the two principle types of essential fatty acids. A balanced intake of EFAs is necessary for good health. Fats in fish such as salmon, cod, trout, and mackerel are rich in omega-3 fatty acids. Linoleic acid, the main omega-6 fatty acid, is found in vegetable oils, including safflower, corn, peanut, sunflower, soybean, and sesame oils. For those who have arthritis and other inflammatory conditions, the most important concern is to increase intake of omega-3 fatty acids since an adequate amount of omega-6 oils is usually present in the diet. Decrease intake of "bad" fats. Once in the body, omega-3 and omega-6 fatty acids are converted to prostaglandins, complex hormonelike fatty acids that affect smooth muscle function, inflammatory processes, and constriction and dilation of blood vessels.

vitamin E, a potent antioxidant necessary for formation of the anti-inflammatory prostaglandins, as well as vitamins A and C.

Other types of omega-3 fatty acids include eicosapentaenoic acid (EPA) and docosahexaenoic acid (DHA), which are chemically closer to becoming prostaglandins than ALA. Food sources high in EPA and DHA include salmon, bluefish, bass, trout, organ meats, and brown and red algae. High cooking temperatures can destroy the EFA content in certain foods and oils, so baking or grilling fish is a preferable cooking method to frying. For arthritis, we recommend supplementing with all three forms of omega-3s (ALA, EPA, and DHA).

Fish and Fish Oils as Sources of EFAs. Fish consumption can benefit arthritis, but be cautious, particularly of farmed fish, as many fish species contain high toxicity levels. Increased use of fish, both as a whole food and as fish oil supplements, can be a sound beginning in reversing arthritis.

Assess Your Fatty Acid Intake

The first step in looking at your dietary fats is to assess your intake of essential fatty acids. We generally rely on two approaches. First, we have the patient complete a food diary detailing their food choices over a one- to two-week period, enabling us to evaluate the levels of good and bad fats they're receiving through their regular diet. We then perform a darkfield microscopic analysis of their blood, which reveals physiologic problems due to a poor diet. For example, poor formation of red blood cell membranes reflects a fatty acid deficiency, usually of omega-3s.

Second, we may use red blood cell membrane fatty acid analysis. This test determines the composition of the fatty acids in the patient's body, which can be used to adjust their diet to increase levels of deficient fatty acids and decrease levels of detrimental ones. It usually takes six months of supplementation before we see a change in the fatty acid composition of a patient's cell membranes. Then there is commonly a remarkable correlation between a change in fatty acid status—an increase in anti-inflammatories—and the abatement of the joint pain and swelling associated with arthritis.

Research shows that fish oils can block the activity of arachidonic acid, which otherwise produces inflammation. Rheumatologists at the Royal Adelaide Hospital in South Australia found that RA patients who took fish oil supplements (18 grams daily) for 12 weeks had a 30% reduction in leukotrienes (proinflammatory agents).[5] In another study, 49 RA patients took either fish oil (rich in DHA) or olive oil in varying dosages for 24 weeks. Both fish oil and olive oil reduced the number of tender and swollen joints, but a high dose of fish oil proved most effective.[6]

But while fish, especially salmon and other cold-water fatty fish, have high levels of beneficial EFAs, there are also a few problems associated with eating fish. Increasingly, the salmon reaching the North American market are farm raised rather than caught from oceans, rivers, and streams. Farmed fish have a less desirable fatty acid profile than wild fish; specifically, researchers have found that farmed fish are lower in omega-3s.[7] Additionally, fish and other seafood harvested from the wild are becoming increasingly less healthy. As water temperatures rise, some microorganisms mutate into forms that can cause disease. When these microorganisms are ingested by seafood or fish, and subsequently by humans, they present a threat to human health.[8] High levels of heavy metals are yet another contamination issue associated with fish consumption.

Eating fish that is boiled or baked is preferable to eating it fried. Fried foods have high levels of polychlorinated phenols, toxic by-products created by heating oils to high temperatures. These phenols increase inflammation and worsen arthritis symptoms.[9]

Finding Healthy Oils

All vegetable oils contain both unsaturated and saturated fats. Generally, those with a higher percentage of unsaturated fats and a lower percentage of saturated fats are more healthful.[4]

Oil	Monounsaturated	Polyunsaturated	Saturated
Canola	62%	32%	6%
Corn	24%	59%	13%
Flaxseed	72%	19%	9%
Hemp seed	80%	12%	8%
Olive	72%	9%	14%
Peanut	46%	32%	17%
Pumpkin seed	57%	34%	9%
Safflower	12%	75%	9%
Sesame seed	40%	40%	18%
Soybean	23%	59%	14%
Sunflower	20%	66%	10%

(Percentages generally don't add up to 100% because most oils contain small amounts of other fatty substances that are neither saturated nor unsaturated.)

Dietary Recommendations. The following recommendations can help you increase the level of "good" fats in your diet:

- Eat foods rich in the three types of omega-3 fatty acids.
  - *Alpha-linolenic acid (ALA):* The oils of flaxseed (58%), chia seed (30%), poppy seed (15%), pumpkin seed (15%), canola (7%), walnut (5%), and soy (9%); purslane; cattail; and dark green leafy vegetables (50%)[10] (Percentages reflect how much of the total fat content is comprised of the given EFA.)
  - *Eicosapentaenoic acid (EPA):* Cold-water fish, salmon, mackerel, halibut, and Chinese snake oil
  - *Docosahexaenoic acid (DHA):* Cold-water fish
- Obtain an adequate supply of niacin, vitamins B_6, E, zinc, and magnesium to enhance fatty acid metabolism. Beans (especially lima, soy, great northern, kidney, and navy), poultry, and fish contain these important nutrients as well as omega-3 fatty acids. Be sure to check for food allergies first.
- Reduce your carbohydrate intake and avoid all refined sugars, processed foods, margarine, hydrogenated oils, and gluten-containing foods, such as wheat, oats, and barley.

- For better mineral density, increase your consumption of raw nuts and seeds, seaweeds, fish, tempeh, tofu, and legumes.

- Incorporate certain spices and herbs into your diet, including fresh mint leaves, thyme, and ginger; these foods contain substances that will help stabilize fats in the cell membranes.

- Avoid all fats and oils containing very-long-chain fatty acids, such as mustard, peanut butter, peanut oil, and canola oil.

Avoid the "Bad" Fats

Hydrogenated fats and trans-fatty acids can directly contribute to inflammation and the destruction of joint tissues. We recommend avoiding foods that contain these fats, which are, unfortunately, a common ingredient in most processed foods. Read the labels of packaged foods before you buy to determine if they contain hydrogenated fats. In the list of ingredients, you will see them described as either hydrogenated or partially hydrogenated oils. The Nutrition Facts label will also provide you with amounts of saturated and unsaturated fats.

The membrane of every cell is a thin envelope of fats that encases and protects the internal biochemical components. Within this fatty envelope are thousands of proteins that act as a gate and facilitate communication and transport across the cell membrane. The ability of the cell wall to change shape, so that life-sustaining nutrients can be absorbed and wastes expelled, is dependent upon fatty acids.[11] Normal fatty acids have a rounded shape and help form a strong yet flexible membrane surface. But trans-fatty acids have a straight shape that forms a weak, brittle cell wall that can't efficiently transport nutrients and wastes. A weak cell wall can break or become distorted, leaving it vulnerable to free radicals and other processes that break down cell membranes, which leads to cell destruction.[12] When this process of cell destruction occurs in joint tissues, it causes pain, inflammation, and the degenerative process leading to arthritis.

Studies have connected abnormal fatty acid levels with the beginning of arthritic symptoms. Researchers at the University of Verona in Italy studied the fatty acid composition of 25 patients with psoriatic arthritis and found significant direct correlations between levels of fatty acids, specific red blood cell factors, incidence of morning stiffness, and the duration of illness.[13]

The "fake" fats, olestra being the most well-known, pass through the digestive tract without being absorbed. When olestra is in the digestive tract, it mixes with and absorbs fat-soluble vitamins (A, D, E, and K), carotenoids (coenzyme Q_{10}, lycopene, and lutein) and other essential nutrients and antioxidants—all nutrients in which people with arthritis tend to be deficient.[14] These absorbed nutrients pass right through the digestive tract along with the olestra and are eventually excreted. As a result, fake fats appear to be potentially detrimental to those with arthritis.

Success Story: Diet and Detoxification Defeat Gout

Ramsey, 56, came to us complaining of fatigue, fever, and severe pain in the big toe of his left foot. The pain in his toe had begun suddenly and without warning two days earlier. A blood test revealed high levels of uric acid (a waste product of urine metabolism), and darkfield microscopic examination of his blood showed elevated numbers of sharp crystalline structures and overactive white blood cells (indicative of an inflammatory response). Ramsey was diagnosed with an acute attack of gout.

Ramsey had just returned from a two-week vacation. During his trip, he had indulged in rich foods, including large quantities of steaks and other meats, rich desserts, and alcoholic beverages. We often see attacks of gout preceded by a dietary change such as Ramsey's vacation indulgences. The body, overwhelmed by these rich and strange foods, is unable to process the uric acid as it normally would. Sodium urate crystals then build up in the joints or skin, leading to inflammation.

We immediately recommended dietary changes for Ramsey, both to reduce his exposure to foods that would aggravate his gout and to help his body detoxify. He was to avoid meat, alcohol, coffee, sugar, bread, and wheat. We recommended he eat a soup made from organic cabbage, onion, garlic, carrots, zucchini (yellow and green), Jerusalem artichokes, and kale. To this, he was to add an amino acid supplement to provide a source of protein. Ramsey could eat as much of this soup as he wanted but was to have no other solid food.

We also recommended black cherry juice, which is specifically helpful

Common Foods That May Contain Bad Fats

- Margarine
- Diet foods
- Mayonnaise
- Crackers and chips
- Cookies, cakes and cake mixes, pastries, and doughnuts
- Candy
- Commercial breads
- Canned creamed soups and gravy
- Breakfast cereals and frozen waffles
- Microwave popcorn
- Frozen entrees, French fries, fish sticks, and chicken nuggets

for gout due to its high bioflavonoid content and its ability to block the enzyme xanthine oxidase (which increases uric acid in the body). Ramsey was to drink six to eight 4-ounce glasses of black cherry juice throughout the day. He was also to drink two to three 8-ounce glasses daily of a vegetable juice made from carrots, beets, ginger, cucumber, and zucchini, with a generous amount of turmeric powder. In addition, we recommended a detoxifying tea made by combining 2 teaspoons each of burdock, dandelion, prickly ash, milk thistle, yellow dock, and red clover and steeping in 6 cups of steaming hot water; the entire 6 cups was to be drunk (hot or cold) over the course of each day.

Ramsey was to stay on this mostly liquid diet for five days. We also recommended folic acid (10 mg daily) and quercetin (300 mg, three times daily), both of which help control the buildup of uric acid, along with homeopathic remedies for liver and kidney support during the detoxification process. Another support therapy we included was hydrotherapy: Ramsey soaked his foot in warm, salted water two to three times per day. Ramsey also prepared an herbal poultice containing a mixture of one white potato (grated), 1 teaspoon of turmeric powder, and half a cucumber (grated). He covered his toe with this mixture and wrapped it in gauze, changing the dressing two to three times per day.

After three days on this protocol, Ramsey called to say that his toe was completely better; additionally, he felt more energetic and clearheaded. When we retested his blood after one week, his uric acid levels had returned to normal. As an extra benefit from the cleansing diet, Ramsey's cholesterol levels had dropped and he'd also lost 5 pounds.

Arthritis Recipes

The recipes on the following pages are divided into two major categories, those most appropriate for OA and those for RA, but these recipes can be used by anyone, regardless of arthritis type. They are also quite healthy even if you don't have arthritis.

In general, the recipes in this chapter eliminate foods that aggravate or escalate arthritis symptoms, particularly the common culprits such as eggs, dairy, wheat, and fried foods. Our chef, Elieth Ameni Harris, has developed and written these recipes specifically for people with arthritis so that they can begin to eat healthfully without sacrificing flavor. Most ingredients are available in local supermarkets, health food stores, or farmers' markets. All produce should be purchased just prior to use to ensure freshness and should be organic and nonirradiated. If certain vegetables or herbs are difficult to find in your area, consider planting a small garden and raising your own.

Osteoarthritis Recipes

Main Dishes

■ **Black Bean and Textured Vegetable Protein Soup**

12 cups vegetable stock
4 cups cooked black beans
2 cups TVP (texturized vegetable protein)
2 cups chopped green cabbage
1 1/2 cups diced carrots
1 1/2 cups chopped celery
1 large onion, chopped
2 large bay leaves
1/4 cup miso
1/4 cup chopped parsley
4 cloves garlic, minced
1/2 teaspoon ground cumin
2 tablespoons arrowroot powder
1/4 cup cold water
1/4 cup liquid amino acid supplement
Sea salt and freshly ground black pepper

In a large soup pot, combine the stock, beans, TVP, cabbage, carrots, celery, onion, and bay leaves. Bring to boil over medium-high heat, then lower the heat to a simmer and cook for 20 minutes. Meanwhile, dissolve the miso in about 1 cup of the vegetable stock (removed from the soup pot). Add the dissolved miso, parsley, garlic, and cumin and continue to simmer for an additional 5 to 7 minutes, stirring occasionally; don't allow the soup to boil, as this will destroy some of the nutrients in the miso. Dissolve the arrowroot in the cold water, then pour the mixture into soup pot while stirring. Allow to simmer for 5 minutes before seasoning with the liquid aminos and salt and pepper to taste.

Rice, Lentil, and Vegetable Salad

2 cups cooked long-grain brown rice
1 cup cooked lentils
1/2 cup finely chopped purple cabbage
1/2 cup diced carrots
1/2 cup diced zucchini or cucumber
1/4 cup chopped parsley
1/4 cup chopped scallions
2 tablespoons liquid amino acid supplement
6 tablespoons extra virgin olive oil
2 tablespoons lemon juice
1 tablespoon raw honey (optional)
1/2 teaspoon dried marjoram
1/4 teaspoon dried oregano
Sea salt and freshly ground black pepper

In a large bowl, combine the rice, lentils, cabbage, carrots, zucchini, parsley, and scallions and mix well. In a smaller bowl, whisk together the liquid aminos, olive oil, lemon juice, honey, marjoram, and oregano. Drizzle the dressing over the rice mixture while stirring, then season to taste with salt and pepper. Chill for at least 1 hour before serving.

Green and Purple Cabbage Rolls with Shiitake Mushroom–Red Onion Sauce

3/4 cup brown rice
1/4 cup wild rice
2 cups water
1 large green cabbage
1 large purple cabbage
1/4 cup sesame oil
1 cup peas, steamed
1 cup diced carrots
1 1/2 cups chopped shiitake mushrooms
1/2 cup minced shallots
1 teaspoon minced fresh ginger
2 cups cooked chickpeas, mashed
1/2 cup chopped parsley
1 tablespoon chopped cilantro
1/2 teaspoon ground cumin

¼ cup liquid amino acid supplement
Sea salt and freshly ground black pepper

Shiitake Mushroom – Red Onion Sauce

2 tablespoons cold-pressed olive oil
2 cups sliced mushrooms
1 cup coarsely chopped red onion
2 tablespoons white miso
2 cups vegetable stock
2 tablespoons cold water
¼ cup liquid amino acid supplement
2 tablespoons mirin
1 tablespoon arrowroot powder
Sea salt and freshly ground black pepper

Combine the brown rice, wild rice, and water in a saucepan and bring to a boil over high heat. Lower the heat, cover, and simmer for 45 minutes. Meanwhile, remove the stems of the cabbages by coring them with a paring knife. Steam the whole cabbages for 10 to 15 minutes, or until the leaves are pliable but still firm to the touch. Allow the cabbages to cool so that the leaves can be handled.

While the cabbage is cooling, heat the sesame oil in a large saucepan over medium-high heat and sauté the peas, carrots, mushrooms, shallots, and ginger for 5 minutes. Add the mashed chickpeas, parsley, cilantro, cumin, and liquid aminos and continue cooking for an additional 3 minutes, stirring constantly. Season with salt and pepper to taste, then remove from the heat and add the rice. Mix well and set aside to cool.

To make the sauce, heat the olive oil in a saucepan over medium-high heat and sauté the mushrooms and red onion for 3 to 5 minutes. Dissolve the miso into the vegetable stock, then add to the mushrooms and simmer for 5 minutes. Combine the water, liquid aminos, and mirin, then whisk in the arrowroot. Add the arrowroot slurry to the mushroom mixture while stirring and cook for an additional 3 minutes. Season with salt and pepper to taste.

Preheat the oven to 350°F, then assemble the cabbage rolls. First separate all of the cabbage leaves. Place a leaf in the palm of one hand, fill the lower end of the leaf (where the rib of leaf is thickest) with 3 to 4 heaping tablespoons of the rice mixture. Tightly roll the leaf around the filling to form a log. Holding one end of the log in your palm, stuff the edges of the cabbage leaves into the end of the log, then stuff in the edges of the leaves on the opposite end.

Place the cabbage rolls in a 12 by 18-inch baking dish and drizzle with the sauce. Cover and bake for 30 minutes.

▪ Saffron Rice and Peas

The peas need to be soaked overnight, so plan ahead before making this dish. Crushing the scallions releases their flavor but you can remove them before serving the dish. Scotch bonnet peppers are extremely hot, so only use one (or omit them altogether) if you don't tolerate spicy foods well. *Makes 6 servings*

1 1/2 cups pigeon peas (black-eyed peas may be substituted)
2 cups brown basmati rice
3 1/2 cups water
2 cloves garlic, crushed
1 cup lite coconut milk
6 scallions, crushed
2 Scotch bonnet peppers (optional)
4 sprigs thyme
1 teaspoon saffron
1 teaspoon sea salt

Soak the peas overnight, then cook until they yield to firm pressure, about 30 minutes. Combine the partly cooked beans, rice, water, and garlic in a saucepan and bring to a boil over medium heat. Add the coconut milk, scallions, peppers, thyme, saffron, and salt. Decrease the heat to medium-low, cover, and simmer for 45 minutes. Carefully remove the peppers without breaking their skin, and also remove the scallions and thyme. Fluff up the rice and mix so that the peas are evenly blended in. Serve hot.

▪ Vegetable Biriyani

Substitute other nuts for the cashews if you have candidiasis.

1 1/2 cups brown basmati rice
3 cups plus 2 tablespoons water
1/2 teaspoon sea salt, plus more for seasoning
3 tablespoons sesame oil
1 tablespoon chopped cilantro
1/4 cup chopped scallions
1/2 teaspoon saffron threads
1 cup frozen mixed vegetables, steamed for 10 minutes and drained

^{1}/$_2$ cup whole cashews (substitute other nuts if you have candida)

^{1}/$_4$ cup raisins

Freshly ground black pepper

Combine the rice, 3 cups water, and ^{1}/$_2$ teaspoon salt in a saucepan and bring to a boil over high heat. Lower the heat, cover, and simmer for 45 minutes. Heat the oil in a large saucepan over medium-high heat, add the cilantro and scallions, and sauté for 5 minutes. About 15 minutes before the rice is done, soak the saffron in the 2 tablespoons water. When the rice is cooked, add the saffron and its soaking water and mix well. Then stir in the mixed vegetables, cashews, raisins, and the sautéed cilantro and onions. Cook for an additional 5 to 10 minutes over medium heat, stirring until heated through.

▪ Curried Cauliflower and Bean Stew

This dish makes a nice accompaniment to Vegetable Biriyani. Since the chickpeas must be soaked overnight, plan ahead before making this dish.

1 ^{1}/$_2$ cups dry chickpeas

4 cups vegetable stock

^{1}/$_2$ cup yellow split peas, washed

^{1}/$_2$ cup red lentils, washed

^{1}/$_4$ cup barley

^{1}/$_4$ cup cold-pressed olive oil

^{3}/$_4$ cup coarsely chopped onions

^{3}/$_4$ cup coarsely chopped celery

1 large cauliflower, broken into florets

2 tablespoons minced fresh ginger root

1 ^{1}/$_2$ tablespoons ground coriander

2 teaspoons ground cumin

1 tablespoon turmeric

1 pound fresh spinach, stems removed, washed, and coarsely chopped

2 teaspoons sea salt

^{1}/$_2$ teaspoon freshly ground black pepper

Soak the chickpeas overnight, then cook in about 5 cups water until tender. Combine the vegetable stock, split peas, lentils, and barley in a saucepan and simmer over medium heat for 25 minutes, until tender. Meanwhile, heat the oil in a large skillet over medium heat.

Add the onions, celery, and cauliflower and sauté over medium-high heat for 10 minutes, stirring continuously. Add the ginger, coriander, cumin, and turmeric and continue cooking for 5 minutes. Stir in the spinach and the cooked chickpeas, split peas, lentils, and barley. Simmer for 3 to 5 minutes, then season with salt and pepper before serving.

▧ Scrambled Tofu

1 pound soft tofu
1 teaspoon turmeric
1 teaspoon basil
1 teaspoon sea salt
1/4 teaspoon freshly ground black pepper
2 tablespoons oat flour
2 tablespoons cold-pressed olive oil
3 tablespoons finely chopped onion
2 cloves of garlic, minced
3 tablespoons chopped parsley, plus more for garnish
Radishes, cut into flowers, for garnish

Mash the tofu in a bowl, then add the turmeric, basil, salt, pepper, and oat flour and combine thoroughly. Heat the oil in a skillet over medium heat, then add the onions, garlic, and parsley and sauté for 3 minutes. Add the tofu mixture and cook 5 to 7 minutes longer. Garnish with parsley and radish flowers.

Beverages

▧ Dr. Zampieron's Zingiber Zing

The stevia is optional; add it if you prefer a sweeter beverage. More ginger can be added for more bite.

1-inch slice of fresh, organic ginger root
1 organic Granny Smith apple
1 2-ounce piece of organic pineapple
Seltzer or sparkling water
1 to 2 drops of stevia extract (optional)

Juice the ginger, apple, and pineapple. Dilute with seltzer to taste and add the stevia, if desired.

Very Berry Banana Shake

Those with candidiasis shouldn't consume this shake.

1 cup blueberries
1 cup strawberries
1 large, very ripe banana
1 1/2 cups plain soy milk
3 tablespoons raw honey
1 cup ice cubes (optional)
1/4 teaspoon ground nutmeg

Combine all of the ingredients in a blender and blend until smooth.

Green Mobility Juice

1/2 cup organic green cabbage
1 cup organic broccoli
4 organic carrots
1 organic Granny Smith apple
2 bunches organic spinach
1 bunch organic parsley
1-inch organic ginger root
1/2 teaspoon vitamin C powder

Juice the cabbage, broccoli, carrots, apple, spinach, parsley, and ginger. Add the vitamin C powder and drink right away. If the juice tastes too strong, dilute by 50% with filtered water.

Juice for Gout Attacks

A juice made from the following combination is excellent for gout:

1 dandelion plant (roots, leaves, and flowers)
1 burdock root
1/2-inch piece yellow dock root
1 bunch parsley
1 bunch cilantro
1 bunch watercress
2 carrots

Dessert

Pineapple-Cherry Crisp

Many variations on this healthy and delicious snack are possible; for example, use chopped apples (Rome, Cortland, or Granny Smith), dried cranberries, and apple juice instead of pineapple and cherries. Reduce the amount of sugar in the topping if you have candidiasis. If you have wheat or gluten allergies, use oat flour instead of whole wheat flour. Dehydrated sugar cane juice is among the more healthful form of sugar; Sucanat is one of the most common brands. *Makes 12 servings*

Filling

3 cups crushed unsweetened pineapple (fresh or canned)

1 cup fresh or frozen cherries

1 teaspoon vanilla extract

$1/2$ teaspoon grated lemon zest

1 tablespoon agar flakes

1 teaspoon arrowroot powder

$3/4$ cup cold unsweetened pineapple juice

Crust

3 cups granola

$1/2$ cup safflower or sunflower oil

$3/4$ cup dehydrated sugar cane juice or maple sugar

$1/2$ cup whole wheat flour or oat flour

1 tablespoon ground cinnamon

$1/2$ teaspoon sea salt

To make the filling, combine the pineapple, cherries, vanilla, zest, and agar in a large saucepan and simmer over medium-low heat for 5 minutes, stirring often. Whisk the arrowroot into the pineapple juice, then pour the dissolved arrowroot into the fruit mixture and combine thoroughly. Cook 5 minutes longer, stirring often. Set aside to cool. Preheat the oven to 375°F.

To make the crust, coarsely chop the granola; pulsing a few times in a food processor works well. Combine the granola, oil, dehydrated sugar cane juice, flour, cinnamon, and salt in a large bowl. Spread half of the crust mixture evenly in a 9 by 12-inch baking dish, then spoon the fruit filling over the bottom crust. Top the fruit with the remaining crust mixture. Bake for 35 to 40 minutes, or until the fruit is bubbling hot. Allow to cool to room temperature before cutting into 3-inch squares.

Main Dishes

▦ Island Arthritis Recipes:
Pumpkin Soup with Herb Dumplings

Irish moss, available in many health food stores, is the source of carrageenan, a thickening and stabilizing agent used in many prepared foods. If you cannot locate Irish moss, substitute with agar-agar. When simmered in water, as in this recipe, Irish moss becomes mucilaginous and can bind ingredients together as egg whites do.

Island Pumpkin Soup
3 tablespoons cold-pressed olive oil
1 cup chopped onion
2/3 cup chopped celery
1/2 cup thinly sliced leeks
1/4 cup unbleached nonwheat flour
1/2 cup water
8 cups vegetable stock
4 cups cubed pumpkin, butternut squash,
    or buttercup squash, steamed
1 stick cinnamon
1 cup silken tofu
1 cup soy milk
1/2 cup liquid amino acid supplement
2 tablespoons chopped parsley
4 cloves garlic, minced
1 1/2 teaspoons sea salt
1 teaspoon ground cumin
1/2 teaspoon ground nutmeg

Herb Dumplings
1 tablespoon Irish moss or agar-agar
2 quarts water
2 1/2 cups spelt flour
1/2 teaspoon baking powder
1 teaspoon sea salt

1 cup soy milk
1 tablespoon extra virgin olive oil
2 tablespoons chopped chives
2 teaspoons chopped fresh thyme

To make the soup, heat the olive oil in a large soup pot over medium heat. Add the onion, celery, and leeks and sauté for 7 minutes. Whisk the flour into the water, then add it to the soup pot along with the vegetable stock, squash, and cinnamon stick and simmer for 15 minutes. Puree the tofu and soy milk in a food processor for 3 to 4 minutes, then whisk this tofu cream into the soup with a hand whisk. Stir in the liquid aminos, parsley, garlic, salt, cumin, and nutmeg and cook for an additional 10 minutes.

To make the dumplings, combine the Irish moss and water in a small saucepan and simmer over medium-low heat for 10 minutes minutes, until it thickens to a gummy consistency. Use a whisk to thoroughly blend the spelt flour, baking powder, and salt in a bowl. Add the Irish moss solution, soy milk, olive oil, chives, and thyme, and mix until homogenous. Make teaspoon-size dumplings, add them to the simmering soup all at once, and cook for an additional 10 minutes.

▪ Hearty Vegetable Stew

The Millet Pilaf makes an excellent accompaniment to this stew.

8 cups vegetable stock
2 1/2 cups cubed butternut squash
1 1/2 cups cubed carrots
1 1/2 cups cubed turnips
2 bay leaves
1 cup chopped celery
1 cup chopped onion
1/2 cup chopped parsley
1 1/2 cups cooked chickpeas
1/2 cup frozen peas
2 cups chopped Swiss chard
1/3 cup liquid amino acid supplement
1 1/2 teaspoons ground cumin
1/2 teaspoon ground turmeric
2 tablespoons arrowroot powder
1/4 cup cold water
Sea salt and freshly ground black pepper

Combine the vegetable stock, butternut squash, carrots, turnips, and bay leaves in a large pot. Cover and cook over medium heat for 10 minutes. Add the celery, onion, and parsley and cook for an additional 10 minutes. Next, add the chickpeas, peas, and chard and cook 5 minutes longer. Add the liquid aminos, cumin, and turmeric and simmer for 2 to 3 minutes. Dissolve the arrowroot in the cold water, then pour it into the soup and cook a few minutes longer to allow it to thicken. Season with salt and pepper to taste.

▪ Millet Pilaf with Baked Marinated Tofu

For a lighter dish or for easier preparation, you can omit the marinated tofu.

Marinated Tofu

1/4 cup sesame oil
2 teaspoons freshly squeezed lemon juice
1 tablespoon raw honey
1/4 cup mirin
1/2 teaspoon fresh thyme leaves
2 cloves garlic, minced
1 pound tofu, cut into 1/4-inch cubes

Millet Pilaf

3 tablespoons safflower or sunflower oil
2 cups millet
5 cups vegetable stock
Pinch of sea salt
1 cup cauliflower florets
1 cup diced celery
1/2 cup diced carrot
1/2 cup minced red onion
1/4 cup coarsely chopped fresh parsley
1 teaspoon dried marjoram
1 teaspoon dried oregano
2 tablespoons tamari
1/2 cup green peas
1/2 cup slivered almonds, for garnish

To prepare the tofu, whisk together the oil, lemon juice, honey, mirin, thyme, and garlic. Put the tofu in a small, shallow baking dish, pour the marinade over, and let stand at least 1 hour.

Preheat the oven to 375°F and lightly grease a baking sheet. Drain the tofu (discarding the marinade) and spread it evenly over the prepared baking sheet. Bake for 30 to 35 minutes, or until slightly brown. Meanwhile, prepare the millet. Heat 1 tablespoon of the oil in a heavy pot over medium heat and toast for 5 to 7 minutes, stirring often. Add vegetable stock and a pinch of sea salt, bring to a boil, then decrease the heat to low and simmer for 20 to 25 minutes.

While the millet cooks, heat the remaining 2 tablespoons oil in a skillet and sauté the cauliflower, celery, carrot, and onion for 3 minutes. Add the parsley, marjoram, oregano, and tamari, cook 2 minutes longer, and set aside. Bring a small saucepan of water to a vigorous boil. Add the peas and cook for 5 minutes.

To assemble the pilaf, gently combine the millet, sautéed vegetables, peas, and tofu. Garnish with the almonds before serving.

■ Poached Salmon in Creamy Asparagus Sauce

Use a rich, creamy soy milk for this recipe, not a lite version.

Salmon

1 medium red onion, sliced 1/4 inch thick
1 pound salmon steak (two steaks)
1 cup vegetable stock
1/2 teaspoon freshly ground black pepper
1/2 teaspoon sea salt
2 tablespoons chopped parsley
Sprig of thyme
1/2 cup vegetable stock

Creamy Asparagus Sauce

1 cup chopped asparagus
2 tablespoons sesame oil
2 tablespoons oat or barley flour
3/4 cup soy milk
3/4 cup stock (fish stock, vegetable stock, or a combination)
1 tablespoon minced shallot
1/2 teaspoon sea salt
1/4 teaspoon white pepper
1/4 teaspoon celery seed
1 tablespoon white miso
3 tablespoons water
2 tablespoons mirin

To prepare the salmon, preheat the oven to 375°F. Scatter the onion rings in the bottom of a 9 by 12-inch baking dish. Season the salmon with the salt and pepper and place the steaks atop the onions. Add the parsley, thyme, and vegetable stock, cover the baking dish, and poach in the oven for 20 to 30 minutes, or until it flakes easily with a fork. To make the sauce, steam the asparagus for 3 to 5 minutes, or until just tender. Rinse briefly under cool water to stop the cooking and set the green color. Heat the oil in a saucepan over medium heat, whisk in the flour, and cook, whisking continuously, for 2 minutes. Add the soy milk and stock and simmer for 8 minutes, stirring often. Stir in the shallot, salt, white pepper, and celery seeds and cook for an additional 5 minutes, then remove from the heat. Dissolve the miso in the water, then stir the dissolved miso and mirin into the sauce. Remove sauce from heat and stir in mirin and miso paste. Combine the sauce and steamed asparagus in a food processor and puree until smooth. Spoon the warm sauce over the salmon and serve right away.

Salads

Green Goodness Salad with Herb Dressing

If you won't be using all the salad in one meal, just serve the dressing on the side; the leftover salad will keep better if it's not dressed.

1 bunch romaine lettuce, torn into pieces
1 bunch arugula, chopped
2 bunches watercress, leaves only
1 bunch Swiss chard or spinach, torn into pieces
1 head of endive, diced
6 scallions, chopped
1 cup sunflower sprouts

Herb Dressing

1/2 cup extra virgin olive oil, flaxseed oil, or hemp seed oil
1/4 cup freshly squeezed lemon juice (vinegar may be substituted if you're not allergic to yeast)
1/4 cup liquid amino acid supplement
1 tablespoon prepared mustard
1 teaspoon dried tarragon
2 teaspoons chopped fresh chives

4 sheets toasted nori seaweed, cut into strips, for garnish
1/2 cup roasted pumpkin seeds, for garnish

Toss the romaine lettuce, arugula, watercress, chard, endive, and scallions together in a large salad bowl.

To make the dressing, combine the olive oil, lemon juice, liquid aminos, mustard, and tarragon in a blender and blend until thoroughly emulsified. Stir in the chives.

Toss the salad with the dressing and sprinkle the seaweed and pumpkin seeds atop the salad before serving.

Quinoa – Black Bean Salad with Cilantro-Lime Vinaigrette

3 cups cooked quinoa
1 1/2 cups cooked black beans
1/2 cup dried cranberries
1 cup chopped yellow squash
1 cup chopped zucchini
6 scallions, chopped
1/4 cup finely chopped parsley

Cilantro-Lime Vinaigrette

Freshly squeezed juice of 2 large limes
1/3 cup water
1/4 cup liquid amino acid supplement
1/4 cup extra virgin olive oil
2 tablespoons honey
1 clove garlic, minced
2 tablespoons chopped cilantro
Sea salt and freshly ground black pepper

Combine the quinoa, black beans, cranberries, squash, zucchini, scallions, and parsley in a large bowl and mix until thoroughly combined. To make the dressing, combine the lime juice, water, liquid aminos, olive oil, honey, and garlic in a blender and blend until thoroughly emulsified. Stir in the cilantro and season with salt and pepper to taste. Drizzle the dressing over the salad, stir well, and chill for 1 hour before serving.

Exotic Tropical Fruit Salad with Citrus Sauce

If you have a candida or klebsiella infection, consult with your physician to determine if this is a good recipe for you. You can substitute pineapple for the star fruit.

2 large mangoes, peeled and cubed
1 large papaya, peeled, seeded, and cubed
3 kiwis, peeled and cut into 1/4-inch slices
1 pint of strawberries, hulled and cut in half
1 large star fruit, cut into 1/4-inch slices

Citrus Sauce

Freshly squeezed juice of 2 large oranges (approximately 1 cup)
2 tablespoons freshly squeezed lemon juice
1 tablespoon honey
1/2 teaspoon ground nutmeg
Fresh mint leaves, for garnish

Combine the mangoes, papaya, kiwis, strawberries, and star fruit in a bowl and mix gently.

To make the sauce, whisk together the orange juice, lemon juice, honey, and nutmeg.

Pour the citrus sauce over the fruit and stir gently until thoroughly combined. Chill for 1 hour, then garnish with fresh mint leaves before serving.

Beverages

Inflam-Aid Drink

You can also make this as a smoothie; see directions below. Avoid this recipe if candidiasis is a problem.

1/2 cup black cherry juice
1 cup organic pineapple juice
1 to 2 teaspoons fresh ginger root powder
1/2 cup filtered water
1 cup crushed ice

Combine the juices with the water and ice in a blender and blend until well mixed. For a smoothie, add silken tofu (1/2 cup) and puree all ingredients in blender for 3 minutes until smooth.

Apple Spice Cake with Cranberry Kanten Glaze

If you have candidiasis, decrease the amount of honey.

2 cups barley or spelt flour
1 1/2 teaspoons baking powder
1 teaspoon baking soda
1/2 teaspoon sea salt
1 teaspoon ground cinnamon
1/2 teaspoon ground allspice
1 cup unsweetened apple juice
1/2 cup soy milk
1/2 cup sesame oil
1/4 cup raw honey or maple syrup (decrease amount if
    you have candida)
1 teaspoon vanilla
1 teaspoon stevia extract
2 cups diced apple (1/4-inch pieces)
3/4 cup chopped walnuts

Cranberry Kanten Glaze

1 tablespoon plus 2 teaspoons arrowroot powder or cornstarch
1 1/2 cups cold unsweetened apple juice
1 tablespoon plus 2 teaspoons agar
1 1/2 cups fresh cranberries

Preheat the oven to 375°F. Lightly oil a 9-inch round cake pan.

Combine the flour, baking powder, baking soda, salt, cinnamon, and allspice in a medium bowl. In a separate bowl, whisk together the apple juice, soy milk, oil, honey, vanilla, and stevia. Pour the wet ingredients into the flour mixture and stir until well mixed. Fold in the apples and walnuts. Spread the batter into the prepared pan and bake for 30 minutes, or until a toothpick inserted in the center comes out clean.

Meanwhile, make the glaze. Whisk the arrowroot and apple juice together in a saucepan over medium heat, then stir in the agar. Cook for 5 minutes, then add the cranberries and simmer for 2 minutes without stirring. Cool to room temperature, then spread evenly over the cake before serving.

thirteen

Supplements for Arthritis

The concept of using food as medicine is particularly important for people who have arthritis, although it is good advice for anyone. Conventional medicine accepts that a nutrient deficiency exists when a person develops a specific deficiency disease, such as scurvy due to lack of vitamin C. In alternative medicine, we believe a deficiency could be present when there is even a slight breakdown of the body's optimum function.

Levels of many important nutrients have immediate and direct consequences on joint function and cartilage structure. For example, low levels of antioxidant vitamins (such as C and E) increase the potential for free radicals to attack and destroy sensitive joint tissues. Deficiencies in amino acids (the building blocks of proteins), vitamin C, iron, selenium, and manganese contribute to the breakdown of cartilage, leading to arthritic changes in the joints, loss of mobility, and bone deterioration. If cartilage breaks down as a result of inadequate nutrition, then other bodily functions dependent on similar nutrients, such as the immune system, suffer as well. We encourage all people with arthritis to adopt an

IN THIS CHAPTER

- Vitamins
- Minerals
- Cartilage-Building Supplements
- Herbs
- Amino Acids
- Antioxidants
- Bioflavonoids
- Enzymes
- Homeopathic Remedies

arthritis-friendly diet and pursue a supplement program tailored to their individual profile.

In this chapter we discuss the most common nutrient deficiencies associated with arthritis and offer suggestions for preventative and therapeutic dosages. We also give advice on how to obtain these nutrients from food sources, as well as supplements.

Please note that vitamins, minerals, herbs, and other nutritional supplements may have interactions with pharmaceutical drugs, decreasing or increasing the activity of the drug. Both situations may warrant a change in the amount of the prescription drug that should be taken. If you're taking any prescription drugs, consult with your health-care provider before using any nutritional supplements. Helpful information on this topic is available at www.supplementinfo.org and www.med.umich.edu/1libr/aha/umherb01.htm, and in *Mosby's Handbook of Drug-Herb & Drug-Supplement Interactions* by HealthGate Data Corporation and Mosby.

Vitamins

Vitamins that are useful for pain and inflammation include those with a high degree of antioxidant activity (vitamins C and E), those involved in bone structure and joint mobility (vitamins A and K), and those typically deficient in arthritis patients (vitamin B_3 and B_5). (DV stands for "daily value"; by law, this term has replaced RDA, for "recommended daily allowance," on food labels in the United States.)

Vitamin A and the Carotene Complexes

Vitamin A (retinol) is needed for the growth and repair of body tissues; it creates smooth and supple skin, protects all mucous membranes, and establishes stronger immune function.[1] Cortisone drugs, frequently prescribed for RA, decrease the amount of vitamin A available in the body. The body obtains vitamin A from food sources or manufactures it through the conversion of carotenes (alpha-, beta-, and gamma-carotene). Because high levels of vitamin A can be toxic, it's usually safer to boost your intake of carotenes, which your body will convert into sufficient amounts of vitamin A. The inflammatory compound (NFkB) is elevated in response to a vitamin A deficiency and is suppressed by a sufficient amount of vitamin A.[2]

Food sources of vitamin A: Fish oil, such as cod liver oil.
DV: 5,000 IU.
Therapeutic dose: 10,000–20,000 IU.

The concept of using food as medicine is particularly important for people who have arthritis, although it is good advice for anyone. Conventional medicine accepts that a nutrient deficiency exists when a person develops a specific deficiency disease, such as scurvy due to lack of vitamin C. In alternative medicine, we believe a deficiency could be present when there is even a slight breakdown of the body's optimum function. Levels of many important nutrients have immediate and direct consequences for joint function and cartilage structure.

Precautions: Very high levels of vitamin A can cause headaches and irritability and can be toxic; even moderately high levels should be avoided during pregnancy.[3]

Food sources of carotenes: All yellow and green vegetables, including carrots, beet greens, spinach, and broccoli.[4]

Supplements: Most broad-spectrum multivitamins contain beta-carotene and other carotenoids, including lycopene and lutein.

DV: None.

Therapeutic dose: 100,000–300,000 IU.

Vitamin B_3 (Niacin)

Vitamin B_3 maintains the integrity of the mucosal lining of the intestines, plays a role in nervous system function, and improves circulation. Low levels of B_3 can cause muscle weakness, fatigue, skin sores, irritability, and depression. Eating a diet high in refined sugar as well as prolonged use of antibiotics will deplete B_3 reserves in the body. The anti-inflammatory action of vitamin B_3 may be due to its ability to balance the Th1 to Th2 ratio in favor of Th2 by inhibiting IL-1, IL-12, and TNF-alpha production. In addition, vitamin B_3 helps protect the liver from damage caused by methotrexate, which is commonly prescribed for arthritis.[5] Besides being useful for arthritis, vitamin B_3 also helps to lower LDL (bad) cholesterol.[6]

Food sources: Meat, chicken, fish, peanuts, brewer's yeast, and wheat germ.

Supplements: Niacin is the natural form of vitamin B_3. When taken in dosages of over 100 mg, niacin can cause a very distinctive reaction known as a nitrogen flush. Flushing, tingling, and redness begin in the lower part of the body and move up to the face, hands, and head. This sensation typically subsides after 15 to 20 minutes and causes no harm. Niacinamide causes no flushing and is the niacin of choice in many modern supplements.

DV: 15–20 mg.

Therapeutic dose: 50 mg.

Precautions: Liver enzymes may be affected when utilizing high levels of B_3 or niacinamide. Inositol hexoniacinate, another form of B_3, has shown no toxicity and may be the best choice for this supplement.

Vitamin B_5 (Pantothenic Acid)

Vitamin B_5 is involved in the production of adrenal hormones and red blood cells and also helps metabolize fat and carbohydrates. Levels of vitamin B_5 are typically low in patients with RA.[7] This vitamin can be used therapeutically to help decrease pain and increase joint mobility.[8]

Food sources: Liver, meat, chicken, whole grains, and legumes; eating a variety of foods can ensure adequate levels of vitamin B_5.

DV: None.

Therapeutic dose: 10–2,000 mg.

Vitamin B_6 (Pyridoxine)

Vitamin B_6 helps form prostaglandins (pro- and anti-inflammatory agents) and red blood cells. It's also involved in the function of the nervous and immune systems. Deficiency of pyridoxine has been documented in inflammatory disease.[9] Vitamin B_6 can also help alleviate pain associated with arthritis and carpal tunnel syndrome. Low levels of vitamin B_6 can cause depression,[10] skin eruptions, and neurological problems. Deficiencies occur as a result of eating a diet high in fats and low in fruits and vegetables or from intake of synthetic food dyes (especially FD&C Yellow 5), the conventional drugs frequently prescribed for arthritis, or excessive amounts of protein.

Food sources: Whole grains, legumes, nuts, and seeds.

Supplements: There are two forms of B_6: pyridoxine hydrochloride and pyridoxal-5-phosphate (the most active form). For the body's efficient absorption of vitamin B_6, sufficient levels of riboflavin and magnesium should be present.

DV: 2 mg.

Therapeutic dose: 50 mg.

Precautions: High levels of pyridoxine (over 250 mg a day, long term) can cause toxic side effects.[11]

Vitamin C

Both an antioxidant and an anti-inflammatory, vitamin C helps repair and maintain healthy connective tissues. It is essential for collagen production and the maintenance of joint lining, helps tissue repair, and reduces the bruising and swelling often associated with arthritis. Vitamin C from food sources helps reduce the risk of cartilage loss and the progression of joint breakdown in osteoarthritis.[12]

Food sources: Most fruits and vegetables, especially oranges, grapefruit, kiwis, lemons, avocados, and parsley.

Supplements: The most cost-effective form of vitamin C is ascorbic acid, which is extracted from rosehips or acerola. Ester-C, another form of vitamin C is purported to stay in the body longer, thereby increasing absorption.[13]

DV: 60 mg.

Therapeutic dose: 500–5,000 mg (depending on bowel tolerance).

Vitamin D

Vitamin D, a fat-soluble nutrient, is considered to be both a vitamin and a hormone. It controls the absorption of calcium and phosphorus used in bone formation. The major diseases caused by vitamin D deficiency, rickets and osteomalacia, are now relatively rare in the United States, but mild deficiencies of vitamin D cause aches and pains in the hips and other joints, a symptom often found in arthritis. A deficiency of vitamin D has been linked to increased likelihood of hip fractures and osteoporosis-related bone problems. In addition, supplementation with D_3 has been shown to increase the production of healthy bone cells. It is interesting to note that the bone cells most damaged due to osteoarthritis have a higher response to vitamin D supplementation than normal bone cells.[14]

Vitamin D is naturally synthesized by the body through exposure to sunlight. About 20 minutes a day of sunlight is necessary, although older people and those with very dark skin may need an hour. The sun can hit any part of the body but has to contact the skin directly; it is not effective through clothing, glass windows, or a sunscreen. People who are sensitive to the sun are advised to cover areas that are very sensitive with a sunscreen but allow the sun to hit areas that are less sensitive. People who are housebound due to arthritis should attempt to be outside 20 minutes a day or at least a few hours a week to generate enough vitamin D for healthy bone repair.

Food sources: Cod liver oil, fatty fish such as salmon and mackerel, butter, and egg yolks.

Supplements: D_2 (ergocalciferol) is synthetically derived; D_3 (cholecalciferol) is the natural form from fish oils. Alfacalcidol (1-alpha-hydroxy vitamin D_3), a vitamin D analog, has demonstrated positive effects on bone mineral density, fracture rates, immune function, and autoimmune diseases, including RA.

DV: 400 IU.

Therapeutic dose: 400 IU.

Precautions: Vitamin D can be toxic if taken in high amounts: Over 1,000 IU per day of vitamin D on an ongoing basis could cause malaise, drowsiness, extreme thirst, nausea, and calcification of soft tissues.

Vitamin E

Vitamin E protects cell membranes from oxidative damage and acts as an anti-inflammatory, blocking the activity of an enzyme that provokes inflammation. It also maintains the elastic quality in cells, which in turn increases elasticity in muscles. Levels of vitamin E are typically low in those with RA. Several studies indicate that people given vitamin E report a decrease in pain and joint swelling. Many patients report that they are able to reduce their doses of NSAIDs while taking vitamin E.

Food sources: Cold-pressed oils such as sunflower and safflower, almonds, hazelnuts, avocado, and wheat germ.

Supplements: Vitamin E is actually a group of compounds called tocopherols. When purchasing vitamin E supplements, avoid products that contain vitamin E in the DL-alpha tocopherol acetate form, a petroleum-based synthetic form of the vitamin. The natural form of vitamin E will be designated with the letter D without the L. Research has shown that the natural form of vitamin E that occurs in foods and is sold as "mixed tocopherols" has better antioxidant properties than other forms.[16] Avoid taking iron supplements the same time of day as vitamin E supplements, as each prevents absorption of the other. Avoid chlorinated water and polyunsaturated fats, since these may destroy vitamin E.

DV: 30 IU.

Therapeutic dose: Up to 3,000 IU per day has shown no negative effects.

Vitamin K

Vitamin K is important for bone repair and collagen production. Deficiencies are common in people with osteoporosis and ankylosing spondylitis. Serum concentrations of vitamin K_1 (the natural form from plants) have been found to be significantly lower in patients who require hip replacement due to osteoarthritis.[17] Vitamin K can help the healing process in broken bones and provides joint support in OA.

Food sources: Green leafy vegetables (high in chlorophyll, a source of vitamin K), parsley, cabbage, and broccoli.

Supplements: There are three main kinds of vitamin K: K_1 is the natural form from plants; K_2 is produced from intestinal bacteria; and K_3 is synthetically produced.

DV: 50 mcg.

Therapeutic dose: 20–40 mg per day, with meals.

Folic Acid

Folic acid has a wide range of beneficial effects, including prevention of neural tube defects[8] and lowering elevated homocysteine levels.[19] High homocysteine interferes with normal bone structure. The active form of folic acid, 5-methyltetrahydrofolate (5-MTHF), has been studied for its ability to trap dangerous free radicals such as superoxides,[20] which cause tissue damage and joint breakdown.

Food Sources: Dark green leafy vegetables, brewer's yeast, liver, eggs, beets, broccoli, brussels sprouts, orange juice, cabbage, cauliflower, cantaloupe, kidney and lima beans, wheat germ, and whole grains. Friendly intestinal bacteria also produce folic acid.

DV: 400 mcg.

Therapeutic dose: 200–800 mcg daily.

A Quick Guide to Nutrients for Building Healthy Joints

Vitamins: Vitamins A, B_3 (niacin and niacinamide), C, D, E, and K

Minerals: Calcium, magnesium, manganese, copper, zinc, and boron

Cartilage builders: Glucosamine and chondroitin

Minerals

Minerals are essential cofactors for enzyme reactions, aid in the uptake of vitamins, and are structural components of the skeleton. Some minerals aren't manufactured by the body and must be obtained from the diet or nutritional supplements.

Boron

Boron helps maintain bone and joint function and activates the metabolism of vitamin D. Low levels of boron in the soil, and thus in foods, have been linked to increased incidence of osteoarthritis. [21] Boron supplementation helps reduce the excretion of calcium and magnesium, important minerals in bone structure and muscle function.[22] Boron can decrease joint pain and bone loss in osteoarthritis.[23]

Food sources: Organically grown fruits and vegetables (chemicals and artificial fertilizers tend to deplete boron levels).
Supplements: Sodium borate or sodium tetraborate decahydrate.
DV: None.
Therapeutic dose: 5–10 mg.
Precautions: Over 500 mg per day may cause nausea, vomiting, and diarrhea.

Calcium

Calcium is the most abundant mineral in the body. The main function of calcium (along with phosphorus) is to form a matrix that hardens bones and teeth. Calcium is also involved in muscle contraction, nerve function, and heartbeat regulation. It moderates acid-alkaline balance and regulates how nutrients cross cell membranes. Calcium absorption into the cells can be compromised by whole grains and cereals, spinach, tannins in tea, a high-protein diet, commercial sodas, refined sugar, and antacids that contain aluminum. Although calcium is found in dairy products, it isn't easily absorbed from those sources, especially by people with arthritis, who typically have deficiencies of stomach acid.[24]

Food sources: Broccoli, cabbage, almonds, hazelnuts, oats, lentils, beans, figs, currants, raisins, brussels sprouts, cauliflower, kelp, and green leafy vegetables, especially kale. Kale is very high in an easily absorbed form of calcium.[25]
Supplements: Calcium from bone meal, dolomite, and oyster shells has been found to have the highest levels of lead contamination and shouldn't be used as a supplement. Calcium citrate, calcium

gluconate, and microcrystalline hydroxyapatite have a much better absorption level.[26]

DV: 1,200 mg.

Therapeutic dose: 1,000–1,500 mg.

Precautions: Excessive intake of calcium oxalate may cause the formation of kidney stones, but this risk can be decreased by using calcium citrate or calcium gluconate. High calcium intake can interfere with iron absorption, cause chronic constipation, and may also increase blood pressure if taken along with NSAIDs. If heavy metal toxicity is present (often the case in arthritis), greater calcium intake may worsen arthritis symptoms; check for heavy metals through hair or urine analysis.

Copper

Copper, along with vitamin C and other nutrients, is important in the synthesis of collagen and elastin, the components of cartilage that provide support and structure. A copper deficiency can lead to joint degeneration, a general feeling of weakness, immune dysfunction, and fragile skin that's easily bruised or torn. A diet high in refined foods may block the body's absorption of copper, as will taking high levels of vitamin C, zinc, and iron. Note that high levels of serum copper have been correlated with an increased number of inflamed joints in juvenile arthritis, and therefore may be an issue in arthritis as well.[27]

Food sources: Beans, lentils, shellfish (especially oysters), liver, nuts, and green leafy vegetables.

Supplements: There are various forms of supplemental copper, such as copper sulfate, copper gluconate, copper picolinate, and others.

DV: 2 mg.

Therapeutic dose: 2–5 mg.

Precautions: Copper toxicity is seen more often than copper deficiency. Supplement with copper only after determining you have a deficiency by means of hair or urine analysis.

Iodine

Iodine is involved in the development and function of the thyroid gland, which is responsible for producing thyroid hormones important for energy production, mental processes, and speech. Iodine also is important in the synthesis of cholesterol and for healthy skin, nails, hair, and teeth. Deficiencies in iodine can cause thyroid dysfunction, which can lead to degenerative illnesses, including muscle weakness and arthritis.

Food sources: Seaweed, kelp, and fish. In the United States, table salt is iodized, which provides sufficient levels of iodine. Certain foods, called goitrogens, prevent iodine absorption. These include soybeans, turnips, cabbage, and pine nuts, especially if eaten raw.

Supplements: Supplements often contain iodine in inorganic forms, such as sodium iodide and potassium iodide. The elemental iodine found in iodine caseinate is absorbed well.

DV: 150 mg.

Therapeutic dose: 150 mg.

Precautions: Very high doses of iodine can cause acne and can down-regulate the thyroid gland, actually diminishing thyroid function.

Iron

Iron-deficiency anemia is common in RA.[28] Prolonged use of NSAIDs or commercial antacids, low levels of folic acid, or menstrual difficulties contribute to iron-deficiency anemia. Iron deficiency can also decrease hydrochloric acid in the stomach, impairing digestion and contributing to further nutritional deficiencies.

Food sources: Red meat, organ meat, shellfish, and egg yolks. Liver contains heme iron, which is very well absorbed by humans. Nonheme iron is found in vegetable foods such as oats, millet, parsley, kelp, brewer's yeast, and yellow dock root.

Supplements: Heme, the form of iron found in desiccated liver or liquid liver extract supplements is most easily absorbed and has fewer side effects. Of the nonheme forms of iron, ferrous fumarate and ferrous succinate are recommended.

DV: 10–15 mg.

Therapeutic dose: 10–15 mg.

Precautions: Ferrous sulfate, commonly used in conventional supplements, can cause the production of free radicals and should not be used. Elevated levels of iron in the blood are associated with an increased risk for heart attacks and other cardiovascular problems, as well as joint problems and lowered immunity.[29] Overdose in infants and small children can be serious or fatal, so be sure to keep your iron supplements out of the reach of children.

Magnesium

Magnesium is second only to potassium as the mineral most common within the cells. Magnesium helps form bones, relax muscle spasms, and decrease the pain involved in arthritis. It activates cellular enzymes, plays a large role in nerve and muscle function, and helps regulate the acid-alkaline balance.[30] Magnesium deficiency can cause anxiety, muscle tremors, confusion, irritability, and pain. Processed food or foods cooked at high temperatures are depleted of their magnesium content.

Food sources: Tofu, nuts, seeds, green leafy vegetables (especially kale), seaweed, and "green" foods, such as chlorophyll.

Supplements: Oral magnesium supplements are absorbed well and will increase the measurable levels inside red and white blood cells.[31] Epsom salts (magnesium sulfate), an old-fashioned remedy, are an excellent addition to a bath, but they have a strong laxative effect if taken as an oral supplement. We recommend using magnesium glycinate, magnesium fumarate, or magnesium citrate, all of which are usually better absorbed with less of a laxative effect.

DV: 400 mg.

Therapeutic dose: 500–1,000 mg.

Precautions: Very high doses of magnesium may be dangerous for those with kidney disease.

Manganese

Manganese has many functions in the body, including playing a role in normal growth and metabolism. It helps to activate enzymes, is used for normal bone development, and acts as an anti-inflammatory. Abnormalities in the gene that regulates the formation of the enzyme manganese superoxide dismutase (MnSOD) increase susceptibility to psoriatic arthritis.[32] Supplementation is recommended for people with RA, as they are usually significantly deficient in manganese.

Food sources: Nuts, egg yolks, dried fruits, whole grains, and green leafy vegetables.

Supplements: Forms that are not readily absorbed include manganese sulfate and manganese chloride; manganese picolinate and manganese gluconate are better absorbed.

DV: None.

Therapeutic dose: 150 mg.

Selenium

Selenium is an antioxidant with anti-inflammatory activities. This may be because selenium prevents the activation of nuclear factor kappa beta (NFkB).[33] Selenium works in conjunction with vitamin E in cell membranes to fight free radicals and protect against the absorption of heavy metals, such as aluminum, mercury, and lead.[34]

Food sources: Although the body needs only a very small amount of selenium, it may be difficult to get from diet alone, since industrial agriculture depletes soils of selenium. If grown in fertile soil, grains are a good source of selenium, as are liver, meat, and fish.

Supplements: Sodium selenite is not well absorbed. Organic selenium from yeast or the chelated form (selenomethionine) are better sources.

DV: 26 mcg.

Therapeutic dose: 200–1,000 mcg.

Precautions: Selenium toxicity is rare but possible, as the body needs only very small amounts. An overdose can cause hair loss, nail malformations, weakness, and slowed mental function.

Zinc

Zinc is found in the bones, nails, skin, and other organs. It helps synthesize protein, repairs wounds and fractures, and supports immune function. A zinc deficiency (often indicated by white spots on the fingernails) can cause painful knee and hip joints, especially in young men; this condition can often be misdiagnosed as arthritis.[35] Zinc levels have been found to be low in both adults and children suffering from arthritis.[36]

Food sources: Whole grains, nuts, seeds (especially pumpkin seeds), and shellfish.

Supplements: Zinc sulfate is not easily absorbed; zinc picolinate, zinc citrate, and zinc monomethionine are preferable.

DV: 15 mg.

Therapeutic dose: 50 mg.

Precautions: Zinc toxicity is rarely reported; however, prolonged use of over 150 mg a day can cause anemia.

Cartilage-Building Supplements

Healthy joints contain pliable cartilage that absorbs shock and ensures smooth motion. New cartilage cells are constantly replacing old, worn-out cells. However, several factors can alter this rebuilding cycle: Cartilage cells may dry out due to chronic dehydration; there may be a deficiency of one or more nutrients the cells require for normal rebuilding; or enzymes that break down dead cartilage may become inefficient or overly aggressive. Cartilage-building supplements provide the raw materials to rebuild damaged cartilage and stop the unnecessary destruction of healthy cells.

Glucosamine

Glucosamine is a building block of proteoglycans, the cells within cartilage that absorb water and make cartilage resilient to shock. Glucosamine is normally manufactured within the body and stimulates the production of glycosaminoglycans (GAGs), complex sugars in cartilage and the lubricating substance inside joints. The body's own production of glucosamine often decreases due to the aging process and other stresses on the body. This is a major cause of OA. Scientific research has shown that taking glucosamine orally over a period of time reestablishes the level of glucosamine available to the joints and significantly decreases the pain of OA.

Glucosamine has the distinction of being one of the few dietary supplements that has received positive support in mainstream medical journals, including the *Journal of the American Medical Association*,[37] and the *Cochrane Database Systematic Reviews*.[38] Articles published in both concluded that glucosamine was superior to placebo in the treatment of pain and functional impairment resulting from symptomatic OA. Perhaps even more important than its pain-relieving effect is that supplementation with glucosamine actually helps to increase the body's production of GAGs, leading to joint repair and decreasing further joint destruction.[39]

There are no known food sources of glucosamine. However, it can be derived from chitin, a compound extracted from the exoskeletons of shellfish, shrimp, lobster, and crabs. Glucosamine must be combined with some other component in order for the body to absorb it through oral ingestion. There are several forms of glucosamine currently on the market: The two most common are glucosamine sulfate and glucosamine HCl. Both of these forms have been used in scientific trials with positive results.[40]

The dosage of glucosamine sulfate needed for therapeutic benefits can vary from person to person, but we typically recommend starting with 500 mg, three times a day, on an empty stomach.

Precautions: Glucosamine isn't known to be toxic, even with long-term use, but some people occasionally experience gastrointestinal upset; this can be alleviated by taking it with food.

Glucosamine HCl versus Glucosamine Sulfate

PURITY

Glucosamine HCl is very stable and can be manufactured to a high level of purity (some manufacturers claim up to 99%). Glucosamine sulfate is an unstable compound that readily attracts water and starts to break down. It will turn from white to brownish tan when exposed to moisture. Therefore, either sodium or potassium is added as a stabilizer. This makes the supplement less concentrated in glucosamine, the active ingredient.

BIOAVAILABILITY

Either form must be broken down in the body to make it available to joint tissues. Hydrochloric acid in the stomach begins this breakdown process. After being broken down, glucosamine HCl yields more bioavailable glucosamine per dose because the supplement had less inert ingredients to begin with. The glucosamine is then transported first through the small intestines and then the bloodstream, through which it is carried to the joints, where it helps the body form GAGs and other compounds needed for healthy joints.

COST-EFFECTIVENESS

Since manufacturing glucosamine HCl requires fewer steps and materials, it is much more cost-effective than glucosamine sulfate. Less glucosamine HCl needs to be ingested to get the usually recommended dose of 1,500 mg of glucosamine.

THE ROLE OF SULFUR

Once glucosamine reaches the joints, the mineral sulfur must be present in order for it to function. One of the roles of glucosamine is to help the cartilage tissue incorporate sulfur, which is necessary for bone and cartilage development. Glucosamine sulfate, once broken down in the stomach, may provide a small proportion of the sulfur the joints need, but only if that sulfur, no longer attached to the glucosamine, also gets transported to the joint areas. However, at best, it can only provide a small amount of the needed sulfur. Sulfur is naturally present in every cell in the body and is widely available from food sources, including eggs, meat, fish, dairy products, and many vegetables, such as onions, broccoli, cabbage, and kale. Therefore, the important nutritional role of either glucosamine HCl or glucosamine sulfate is in providing the body with glucosamine, not with sulfur.

SUMMARY

	Glucosamine HCl	Glucosamine Sulfate
Proven effective in clinical trials	Yes	Yes
Purity	More	Less
Bioavailablity	High	Lower
Cost-effectiveness	More	Less
Provides Sulfur	No	Provides a small amount

Chondroitin Sulfate

Chondroitin sulfate is another important ingredient in proteoglycans (which fill in the space between collagen cells and hold water in the joints for shock absorption). Proteoglycans are shaped like bottle brushes, with the stem composed of proteins and radiating sugar chains that look like the brush's bristles. Located in the long sugar chains are GAGs, of which chondroitin sulfate is the most critical. Chondroitin seems to protect joints from breaking down and can speed the recovery of injured bones, especially when combined with glucosamine.[41]

The efficacy of chondroitin as a supplement is limited, with only 8–10% of the oral dose reaching the blood stream and joints. The injectable forms of chondroitin, however, have proven to be effective therapies for arthritis.[42] Thousands of patients in Europe, South America, and other countries have been successfully treated with various forms of injectable chondroitin, but such injections aren't not widely available in the United States. However, the Access to Medical Freedom Act, approved in several U.S. states, allows patients to receive this treatment if they sign a waiver indicating that they understand that the treatment isn't approved by the FDA. We recommend the use of injectable chondroitin products that have been clinically tested (outside the United States) with beneficial results; their benefits include reduction of pain and inflammation, improvement in joint mobility, and, in some cases, cessation of joint deterioration.

A Note about Chondroitin Sulfate

Chondroitin is a complex sugar or polysaccharide, while glucosamine is a disaccharide (containing only two sugars). This makes chondroitin a much larger molecule—200 times larger than glucosamine—and thus very difficult to absorb intact through the intestines. Oral supplements of chondroitin sulfate have not been shown to be as effective as oral supplements of glucosamine for rebuilding and supporting cartilage.

Hyaluronic Acid

Hyaluronic acid is a natural substance produced by the body. It lubricates cartilage within the joints, allowing for smooth movement. Hyaluronic acid levels decrease with age and are often quite low in people with joint pain and arthritis. When hyaluronic acid is lacking, joints tend to grind, causing further damage as well as pain and stiffness.

Hyaluronic acid is available in both oral and injectable forms, but benefits of oral supplementation are less well documented than those of injections. Soft-gel capsules are available at most health food stores, whereas injections are available only by prescription. When injected directly into a joint, hyaluronic acid often yields very positive effects.[43] In our clinical experience, we've seen some remarkable results using this therapy. One patient with OA, who'd had much of the cartilage in his right knee removed through surgery, was able to live without pain and resume normal activities after getting hyaluronic acid injections.

Cetyl Myristoleate

Harry W. Diehl, Ph.D., a researcher for the National Institute of Arthritis, Metabolism, and Digestive Diseases, stumbled upon cetyl myristoleate in 1962. He was assigned to inject an arthritis-inducing agent into laboratory mice for the purposes of testing a new synthetic drug. Dr. Diehl found that the mice were strangely resistant to developing arthritis symptoms and eventually identified that cetyl myristoleate, naturally present in the mice, was responsible for preventing arthritis.

Cetyl myristoleate occurs in only a few animal species: Swiss albino mice, sperm whales, and the male beaver. To make this useful substance available to the public, Dr. Diehl found that a mixture of myristoleic acid (from fish oils and butter) and cetyl alcohol (found in coconut and palm oils), rendered the same chemical substance found in the mice. Cetyl myristoleate appears to have three modes of therapeutic action that are helpful for both OA and RA: It acts as a lubricant, promoting smooth motion of joints and muscles; it modulates immune system function; and it has anti-inflammatory effects.

Therapeutic dose: Cetyl myristoleate is usually given orally for a one-month period at a dose of 10–15 grams. Topical application as a cream rubbed into painful joints has been documented to have positive effects on joint mobility and quality of life.[44]

Sulfur Compounds

The body uses sulfur-containing compounds to regenerate cartilage cells, maintain cellular functions, and produce the amino acid glutathione, which is used by the liver to process toxins. Food sources rich in sulfur include garlic, onions, brussels sprouts, and cabbage. Supplementation with sulfur-containing compounds helps arthritis by reducing inflammation, relieving pain, and rebuilding cartilage.

S-adenosylmethionine (SAMe). SAMe is a natural substance produced by the human body when the amino acid methionine combines with adenosine triphosphate (ATP), an energy source present in muscle cells. SAMe is a methyl donor, meaning it provides sulfur for important cellular activities such as rebuilding cell membranes, removing toxins and wastes, and producing mood-elevating brain chemicals (dopamine and serotonin). If the body is deficient in vitamin B_{12}, folic acid, or methionine, production of SAMe may decrease. Research has also found that levels of SAMe drop off with age and in people with OA, muscle pain, liver disease, and depression.

SAMe was initially used to treat depression in the 1970s. It has also been found to ease joint and muscle pain and contribute to cartilage regeneration. One study found that SAMe reduces pain in OA patients as effectively as the drug celecoxib, a COX-2 inhibitor, with fewer side effects.[45]

Therapeutic dose: 400 mg, four times a day.

Precautions: SAMe sometimes has side effects, such as nausea and gastrointestinal disturbances, but these usually don't occur if it's taken with a meal.

Dimethylsulfoxide (DMSO). DMSO, a source of sulfur derived from wood pulp, garlic oil, or as a by-product of petroleum, is a free radical scavenger with anti-inflammatory properties. DMSO acts as a carrier substance that increases absorption rates of other substances. Several forms of DMSO are available by prescription or over the counter: intravenous solutions, intramuscular injections, oral capsules, and topical lotions and ointments.[46]

Precautions: DMSO has shown great promise as a pain-relief therapy, but its side effects include occasional nausea, a strong sulfur smell on the skin and breath, and skin irritation.

Methylsulfonylmethane (MSM). MSM, a sister compound of DMSO, can be derived from food sources. MSM is also naturally produced in the body, but levels decrease with age, in degenerative illnesses such as arthritis, and in people with poor eating habits. Supplementing with MSM has been reported to reduce inflammation and scar tissue, relieve pain, increase blood flow (allowing for improved exchange of nutrients), reduce muscle spasms, promote peristalsis, increase cell wall flexibility, and reduce allergic reactions.[47] Of special relevance in RA, MSM can help normalize the immune system and reduce the autoimmune response. MSM is a source of biologically active sulfur, which plays many roles in the body. It's a component of amino acids, the building blocks of proteins, which in turn build cell walls, tissues, cartilage, bones, muscles, and organs. MSM doesn't have the unpleasant side effects associ-

Arthritis Help from the Sea

The **green-lipped mussel**, an edible shellfish native to New Zealand, is high in eicosatetraenoic acids (ETAs), a unique kind of fatty acid known to reduce inflammation.[48] This previously unidentified type of omega-3 fatty acid has more biological activity than other omega-3s. Green-lipped mussels also contain amino acids, trace minerals, and GAGs (glycosaminoglycans, a component of cartilage).

Therapeutic dose: A typical recommended dose is 500 mg, three times per day, with food.

Precautions: Side effects are rare and mild but include stomach discomfort, gas, nausea, fluid retention, and temporary aggravation of joint pain and tenderness. People with shellfish allergies should not use green-lipped mussel.

Sea cucumber (*beche-de-mer*) is a small marine animal related to starfish and traditionally used as an ingredient in Japanese and Chinese soups and stews. Health benefits of sea cucumber include relief of symptoms of RA, OA, and ankylosing spondylitis. Sea cucumbers also contain GAGs and chondroitins, important components of cartilage tissue.

Therapeutic dose: A typical recommended dose is 500 mg, twice a day.

Precautions: People with seafood or shellfish allergies should not take sea cucumber.

ated with DMSO. It's available in powder form, capsules, eye drops, and topical creams.

Therapeutic dose: Typically recommended dosage levels are 500–1,000 mg per day; under a doctor's supervision, therapeutic amounts may be prescribed.

Herbs

Bitter Melon (Momordica charantia)

Bitter melon, also called cerese root, has been used in traditional folk medicine for diabetes, worms, eczema, and arthritis.[49] It's also helpful for psoriasis and psoriatic arthritis because it acts to slow the rapid cellular proliferation that causes the scaly skin buildup so common with psoriatic conditions.

Boswellia (Boswellia serrata)

Boswellia serrata, commonly referred to as boswellia, has been used for centuries by Ayurvedic physicians for arthritic conditions. It contains boswellic acid, a powerful anti-inflammatory and analgesic that inhibits the production of inflammatory leukotrienes and also binds to and disables the enzyme 5-lipoxygenase.[50] In addition, boswellic acid inhibits other inflammation-causing agents, prevents interference with synthesis of GAGs, and improves blood and lymphatic circulation to the joints.

A standardized extract containing 60% boswellic acid is the most effective preparation for oral use. Boswellia is also well absorbed through the skin and can be added to topical preparations.

Therapeutic dose: 400 mg, three times daily.

Precautions: Boswellia contains high levels of gum resins, which can strain the kidneys when used for an extended period; supplement with boswellia only for a six-week period, then discontinue use for one week before resuming treatment.

Cat's Claw (Uncaria spp.)

Cat's claw is used by indigenous healers in the Amazon, where they refer to it as *uña de gato*. The plant is a liana (giant vine) named for its large hooklike thorns, which locals say resemble the claws of the jaguar. The two species that grow in the Amazon are *Uncaria tomentosa* and *Uncaria guianensis*; a third species that grows in West Africa, *Uncaria africana* (called parrot's beak), is utilized by healers.

Compounds isolated from cat's claw include 17 different alkaloids, quinovic acid glycosides, tannins, flavonoids, and sterol fractions.[51] Cat's claw contains several active compounds that give it both immune-stimulating and antimicrobial activities.[52] Although there is controversy as to which fraction of the cat's claw plant is most beneficial, researchers agree that the herb is valuable in the treatment of arthritis.[53]

Cat's claw is also useful for Lyme disease, but treatment must continue for an extensive period of time (perhaps several months). The spirochete that causes Lyme disease, *Borrelia burgdorferi*, passes through several life stages. Cat's claw is most effective against this organism during the transformation to the spirochetal form, so extended use guarantees that the herb is being taken during this stage. In our clinic, we have documented shedding of *B. burgdorferi* antigens (from dead spirochetes) in patients' urine with Lyme dot blot assays. This has been correlated with clinically documented Jarisch-Herxheimer (die-off) reactions, followed by symptom improvement following the use of standardized cat's claw.

Therapeutic dose: We recommend a 5:1 extract of cat's claw inner bark, 600–1200 mg per day, for a period of months to years depending upon the patient's degree of infection and severity of symptoms.

Cayenne Pepper (Capsicum annuum)

Cayenne pepper contains capsaicin, a chemical compound involved in pain relief. When applied topically, capsaicin enhances circulation to painful areas to help distribute nutrients, oxygen, and healing hormones to the afflicted area and remove waste products. Capsaicin also depletes body reserves of substance P (SEE QUICK DEFINITION), believed to be responsible for intensifying and prolonging muscle and joint inflammation and pain. Topically applied capsaicin, used repeatedly, brings about a long-lasting desensitization to pain and can increase the pain threshold.[54]

 Substance P, a neuropeptide that consists of several amino acids bonded together, is normally present in minute amounts in the nervous system and intestines. Typically involved in the pain response, substance P expands and contracts smooth muscles in the intestines and other tissues and muscles. It also suppresses serotonin, a precursor to melatonin, the hormone that regulates sleep-wake cycles.

Chinese Thoroughwax (Bupleurum spp.)

Modern scientific investigation has validated use of bupleurum as an anti-inflammatory.[55] The active components, saikosaponins, significantly increased blood levels of cortisone (a hormone that reduces pain) and ACTH (adrenocorticotropic hormone, a pituitary hormone that causes the adrenal glands to secrete cortisol).[56] Bupleurum also benefits the adrenal glands and protects them from the damaging effects of pharmaceutical drugs such as corticosteroids.

Therapeutic dose: Generally 500–2,000 mg bupleurum (dry root) are taken three times daily in capsules, or the root can be brewed into a tea.

Cinnamon (Cinnamomum cassia)

In Chinese medicine, cinnamon is one of the most widely used warming herbs for promoting circulation in joints and limbs. It's also helpful for indigestion, gas, and diarrhea. Cinnamon aids in blood sugar regulation,[57] which helps the body control inflammation. Hot topical application of cinnamon tea or cinnamon oil helps to improve circulation and ease the pain of fibromyalgia and arthritis.

Feverfew (Tanacetum parthenium)

Feverfew has been used traditionally to treat fevers and minor pain. Although one scientific study supports the use of feverfew for migraine headaches,[58] our clinic hasn't found it effective for all people who experience migraines. Parthenolide, one of the active constituents in feverfew, seems to block the inflammatory compound interleukin-6[59] and also slows the migration of certain white blood cells to the inflamed area, thus modulating inflammation and pain.

Therapeutic dose: 100–250 mg standardized to 0.2% parthenolide, one to three times a day.

Ginger (Zingiber officinale)

Ginger, an important culinary spice with an ancient ethnobotanical history, is rich in active anti-inflammatory components, including paradols, gingerols, shogaols, and gingerdiols.[60] NFkB is deactivated by gingerol, which is how ginger functions as a natural COX-2 inhibitor, and increases inflammation.[61] Studies have shown that ginger can inhibit inflammation by blocking synthesis of both prostaglandins and leukotrienes.[62]

Therapeutic dose: Research on the optimum dosage of ginger is conflicting. Additionally, the amount varies with the type of ginger preparation. In arthritis studies, patients taking crude fresh ginger were given from 1 to 4 grams per day for 3 months to 2.5 years; relief appeared to be dose dependent, with those consuming the most ginger achieving more rapid relief.[63] Ginger is also available as a standardized extract with a minimum of 4% volatile oils (gingerols and shogaols).

Jamaican Dogwood
(Piscidia erythrina and Piscidia piscipula)

The Jamaican dogwood tree grows in Jamaica, the Bahamas, Mexico, southern Texas, and Florida. Its active components, which have been traditionally used as an antispasmodic, are derived from the roots or outer bark. Jamaican dogwood eases painful cramping in both smooth and skeletal muscles.[64] In our clinic, we mix equal parts of Jamaican dogwood with kava, white willow bark, ginger, turmeric, boswellia, and other botanicals for a potent remedy for pain.

Precaution: Due to potential toxic neurological effects, do not use Jamaican dogwood except under the supervision of a licensed health-care professional.

Kava (Piper methysticum)

Kava is a powerful skeletal muscle relaxant and has been used traditionally for rheumatism and arthritis. It seems to function as a spinal, rather than cerebral, sedative. The mechanism of action of kava pyrones is unlike that of opiates, NSAIDs, or other pain relievers, as they don't bind to any of the body's normal receptors for pain-relieving substances.[65]

Therapeutic dose: For relief of arthritis pain and fibromyalgia, a typical dose of 100–150 mg of kava (depending on body weight) may be taken three times per day. For insomnia, a dose of 200–300 mg of kava, taken prior to bedtime, is recommended. When used properly, kava doesn't cause oversedation, nor does it affect reaction time, like alcohol does. Instead, kava improves sociability, reduces anxiety,[66] and eases depression.

Precautions: Because there is concern about long-term use of kava and its effect on the liver, we don't recommend taking this herb for extended periods of time, nor do we recommend it for anyone with compromised liver function. Kava causes drowsiness in some individuals, so when you first begin to use it, try it in the evening and when you won't be operating heavy machinery or driving.

Licorice Root (Glycyrrhiza glabra)

Licorice root is used to flavor candies and liqueurs, but it's also been used traditionally as a medicinal agent.[67] A common ingredient in Chinese medicinal formulas, licorice has significant antiviral and antibacterial activity. It stimulates interferon (a cytokine with antiviral activity) and enhances the body's production of cortisone (a natural painkiller).

Therapeutic dose: 250–500 mg standardized to 12%–20% glycyrrhizin, three times a day.

Precautions: Using high doses of licorice has been linked to elevated blood pressure in some individuals.[68]

Lignum vitae (Guaicum officinale and Guaicum sanctum)

Lignum vitae is a tree native to South Florida, the Caribbean, and South America. Gum from these trees (guaia-gum) contains therapeutic resins and oils used to relieve pain associated with arthritis, rheumatism, and gout.[69] An alcohol extract that dissolves the gummy resin is the preferred form for medicinal application.

Therapeutic dose: 5 ml of liquid extract, three times per day.

Oregon Grape Root (Berberis aquifolium)

Oregon grape root contains high levels of hydrastine and berberine, two alkaloids that have been shown to inhibit formulation of polyamines in the gut. Polyamines are bowel toxins that are abnormally high in individuals with psoriasis and psoriatic arthritis. They can also increase leaky gut syndrome, a factor in most cases of arthritis. This herb is particularly helpful for psoriasis and psoriatic arthritis.[70]

Therapeutic dose: Usually 1,000 mg.

Turmeric (Curcuma longa)

Turmeric, a bright yellow spice used in Indian cooking, has powerful anti-inflammatory properties credited to its chemical component curcumin.[71] Curcumin helps the liver detoxify by supporting the synthesis of glutathione, and it reduces inflammation by inhibiting the activation of nuclear factor kappa beta and interleukin-8.[72] Use turmeric in combination with ginger as a flavorful food seasoning and enjoy an inexpensive and accessible addition to your arthritis treatment. Turmeric can also be used as a poultice for aching joints.

Therapeutic dose: 100–300 mg standardized to 95% curcuminoids, three times a day with meals.

White Willow Bark (Salix alba) and
Black Willow Bark (Salix nigra)

Bark from both white willow and black willow has been used traditionally to reduce inflammation, fever, and pain. Its active chemical components are the herbal equivalents of synthetic aspirin and provide similar relief without the gastrointestinal side effects of most aspirin products.[73] Of the many species of willow, white willow contains the highest amount of salicin (the active component). The effectiveness of white willow bark may be reduced in people afflicted with dysbiosis (imbalance in the gastrointestinal microflora). This situation can be helped by taking probiotics, such as acidophilus. Standardized extracts at 15% salicin are recommended.

Therapeutic dose: 500–1,000 mg standardized to 15% salicin.

Wintergreen Oil (Gaultheria procumbens)

Purified wintergreen oil contains high levels of methyl salycilate, an aspirin-like compound that blocks prostaglandins, helps stop pain and inflammation, and has been used for arthralgia (nerve pain in the joints).[74] The application of wintergreen oil to joints or other afflicted areas can help relieve pain. Some people's skin becomes irritated when they use methyl salicylate, so try it on a small area before general use.

Chinese Herbal Formulas

Traditional Chinese medicine (TCM), practiced for over 5,000 years, is complex and often difficult for Westerners to understand. One important concept in Chinese medicine is the free-flowing motion of qi (SEE QUICK DEFINITION) and blood through channels, or meridians, in the body. Chinese medicine considers the flow of qi in a patient through close examination of the patient's pulse, tongue, body odor, voice tone and strength, and general demeanor, among other elements. Underlying imbalances and disharmony in the body are described in terminology analogous to the natural world (heat, cold, dryness, or dampness). The concept of balance, or the interrelationship of organs, is central to TCM. Disease arises when obstructions occur to impede the flow of qi and thus disturb the regulation of related organs and body systems. The primary symptoms of arthritis, according to TCM, are related to obstructions in the liver meridian, which governs the joints, tendons, sinews, ligaments, and muscles and oversees their proper function.

Kim Vanderlindine, N.D., from Vancouver, British Columbia, has documented the use of Chinese herbs for arthritis. Chinese herbs are classified by energetic functions (distinguished as cold, cool, warm, or hot) and the organs that their energies affect (lung, kidney, or liver). The diseases that affect the human body are classified accordingly—in terms of organ imbalances and excess or deficient energy. Inflammatory conditions are classified as an excess of hot, and after taking other factors into consideration, a cooling herb might be prescribed to balance the excess quality. Joint pain is characterized by wind or dampness, and therapeutic herbs to treat joint pain may dispel wind or damp. The following Chinese herbs are used, usually in combination with other herbs, to treat many aspects of a person's individual arthritic symptoms:

 Qi (pronounced CHEE) is a Chinese word variously translated to mean "vital energy," "essence of life," and "living force." In Chinese medicine, the proper flow of qi along energy channels (meridians) within the body is crucial to a person's health and vitality. There are many types of qi, classified according to source, location, and function (such as activation, warming, defense, transformation, and containment). Within the body, qi and blood are closely linked, as each is considered to flow along with the other. Qi may be stagnant (nonmoving), deficient (partially absent), or excessive (inappropriately abundant) in a given organ system. Qi has two essential qualities: yang (active, fiery, moving, bright, energizing) and yin (passive, watery, stationary, dark, calming).

Amino Acids

Amino acids are the building blocks of proteins. There are more than 22 amino acids, which are linked in various combinations to form 1,600 basic proteins necessary for the body's structures and for the formation of antibodies, hormones, enzymes, organs, and cell membranes. Some amino acids are manufactured in the body while others (the essential amino acids) must be obtained from dietary sources.

- Angelica family (dong quai, *du huo, chuan xiong, gao ben, qiang huo, fang feng*): These herbs are traditionally used to alleviate pain and to improve blood circulation. They work by dispelling wind and eliminating blockages to circulation. Herbs in the angelica family also relax smooth muscle cells and have been used to treat arthritis, uterine cramps, trauma, and headaches.

- *Bai shao* and *chi shao* (white peony and red peony): A cousin of the ornamental peony found in North American gardens, these medicinal peonies are frequently used to treat arthritis. They have an affinity for the liver and spleen meridians and invigorate the blood. Both peonies are often mixed with other Chinese herbs, such as cinnamon, bupleurum, dong quai, licorice, and Chinese lovage, for broad-spectrum arthritis formulas.

- Camphor (*Cinnamomum camphora*): Camphor is used in traditional Chinese medicinal balms and salves for the treatment of muscle pain (myalgia) and joint pain. Camphor is used topically to break up stagnant blood, warm the meridians, conduct qi, and dispel wind and damp. It has a warming, anesthetic effect on the skin that eventually feels like a cool sensation, and it's often mixed with menthol to expel wind and heat from the body. These essential oils are available in plasters, adhesive patches saturated with medicine that are applied to the affected area of the body for extended periods.

- Clematis (*Clematis chinensis*): A common ingredient in Chinese medicinal formulas, clematis expels damp wind and moves qi. An effective pain reliever, clematis is used to treat calcium deposits in the joints and calcium spurs in the synovial region of the joint, especially in gouty arthritis.

- Eleuthero root (*Eleutherococcus senticosus*): Formerly called Siberian ginseng, this all-purpose herb can enhance the body's production of cortisol, a hormone that reduces pain. It has a particular affinity for the extremities and removes excess fluid due to swelling. Thanks to its stress-reducing abilities, eleuthero root is also helpful for people coping with chronic pain and illness.

- *Niu xi* or ox knee (*Achyranthes bidentala*): Closely resembling a segmented joint, this herb was used traditionally to strengthen the ligaments, tendons, and sinews because of its tonic effect on both the liver and the kidneys. It is especially useful in treating swollen and painful knee joints and enhances the circulation of blood and qi. Research on this plant shows that it can dramatically relieve pain, particularly when it is combined with ligusticum, aconite, peony, ginseng, and licorice.

(continued)

When buying amino acids, look for USP pharmaceutical grade, L-crystalline, free-form amino acids. *USP* means that the product meets the standard of purity set by the reference book called *The United States Pharmacopeial. Free-form* refers to the highest level of purity of the amino acid. *L* refers to one of the two forms of most amino acids, designated D- and L- (for example, D-lysine or L-lysine). The L-form amino acids are proper for human biochemistry, as proteins in the human body are made from this form. The exception is phenylalanine, an amino acid that

Chinese Herbal Formulas *(continued)*

- *Sheng di huang* (*Rehmannia glutinosa*): Rehmannia promotes muscle growth, lowers blood sugar, and nourishes yin. It's used to treat damaged tendons and sprained joints. In Chinese medicine, rehmannia is prepared in several different ways (arranged here in descending order of potency): the fresh root, the dried root, and the root cooked and stir-fried in wine.
  PRECAUTIONS: Some people can develop edema (water retention) after using rehmannia. If you have high blood pressure, you should be monitored closely while using this herb.

- *Xu duan* (*Dipsacus japonicus*): This plant is also known as teasel. Commonly used in formulas for OA, the root of this herb tonifies the liver and kidneys, two of the organs most affected in arthritis. Teasel helps strengthen the bones and tendons and prevents damage from wear and tear. It also promotes the circulation of blood and helps lubricate the joints.

- *Yan hu suo* (*Corydalis ambigua*): One of the most powerful Chinese herbs for pain, *Corydalis ambigua* is a member of the poppy family. Corydalis is a sedative and is recommended for use at night when arthritis pains prevent sleep. It's often mixed with *chuan xiong* (*Ligusticum wallichii*) for body aches and pains, joint inflammation, headaches, toothaches, and stomachaches. Another common mixture includes corydalis, cinnamon, angelica, ligusticum, and lovage root. We recommend the patent medicine Yan Hu Suo Zhi Tong Pian (Corydalis Stop Pain tablets).

The Chinese herbs described above are typically sold in remedies combined with other herbs. Referred to as patent medicines, these remedies are standardized formulas based on recipes that have been used for over 2,000 years. Now available as pills, ointments, or tinctures, patent medicines are easier to take than the traditional tea beverages made from the same ingredients. It's important to find a reliable manufacturer of patent medicines—one who doesn't include artificial colorings, sugar coatings, or ingredients derived from endangered species. Reputable manufacturers provide a list of ingredients and the symptoms these ingredients benefit on the label of their product. Follow the directions carefully and consult with a health-care practitioner before beginning a course of Chinese herbs. Specific patent medicines that are useful in arthritis include Guan Jie Yan Wan (for joint inflammation), Kang Gu Zeng Sheng Pian (for OA and ankylosing spondylitis), Hong She Pills (for fibromyalgia and muscle aches), and Shang Shi Zhi Tong Gao (a topical plaster for pain).

consists of a combination of the D- and L- forms (thus its full name, DL-phenylalanine).

Below, we discuss the amino acids that are typically deficient in arthritis sufferers, and supplementing with them may improve symptoms. We do not, however, recommend taking individual amino acid supplements for indefinite periods, because this can create an imbalance among amino acids and may contribute to the development of other health conditions.

Cysteine

Cysteine is a sulfur-containing amino acid typically found in the protein complexes of hair, fingernails, and toenails. It acts as an antioxidant, shields the liver from toxic heavy metals, and helps prevent infections by augmenting the actions of vitamin C.

Food sources: Poultry, yogurt, oats, egg yolks, red peppers, broccoli, brussels sprouts, and wheat germ.

Therapeutic dose: Typically 1,000 mg a day in the form of N-acetylcysteine (NAC).

Glutamine

Glutamine, an essential amino acid that plays an important role in maintaining the integrity of the intestinal wall, can be very helpful in reversing leaky gut syndrome. It's used in the synthesis N-acetyl-D-glucosamine (NAG), an important nutrient that's fundamental in the production of the protective mucus that lines the entire digestive tract (and respiratory system). This lining is the first line of defense against leaky gut syndrome. Glutamine supplementation has also been shown to enhance levels of glutathione. NAG is critical in the formation of new cartilage.

Food sources: Cabbage and okra.

Therapeutic dose: 3–10 grams of glutamine per day, in divided doses between meals, can be very helpful for people with leaky gut syndrome.

Histidine

Histidine is essential for the growth and repair of tissues. It also maintains the fatty myelin sheaths that insulate nerves and is important in the production of red and white blood cells. During times of stress, histidine is needed more than any of the other amino acids because of its antioxidant and anti-inflammatory properties.

Food sources: Pork, poultry, cheese, and wheat germ.

Therapeutic dose: 1–5 grams. Supplementation should be monitored by measuring histidine levels in the blood and documenting any adverse reactions.

Phenylalanine

Phenylalanine is a building block of the mood-regulating brain chemicals dopamine and norepinephrine. Typically used for depression, phenylalanine may be helpful for people with arthritis who are depressed as a result of the pain caused by their illness. Phenylalanine can also be effective against pain associated with RA and OA due to its analgesic effect.[75]

Food sources: Meat, especially wild game.

Therapeutic dose: 3–5 grams daily of DL-phenylalanine, between meals on an empty stomach.

Precautions: People suffering from phenylketonuria (PKU), a genetic inability to metabolize phenylalanine, should not use supplements or eat foods high in this amino acid.

Antioxidants

An antioxidant is a natural biochemical substance that protects living cells from the damaging effects of free radicals. Free radicals cause oxidation, the same chemical process that causes metal to rust and apples to turn brown. In the body, if left uncontrolled, free radicals cause cell membranes to erode and die, leading to joint dysfunction and other degenerative conditions.

Produced as a by-product of cellular activities, free radicals are typically neutralized and rendered harmless by antioxidants. But when environmental and other toxins (poor diet, stress, cigarettes) introduce an increased burden of free radicals, the body's reserve of antioxidants is quickly exhausted. Many studies have found that people with arthritis have very low blood levels of antioxidants, and this may contribute to the onset and exacerbation of joint destruction and inflammation.

Bioflavonoids

The red of an apple or the many hues of peppers may seem only fanciful adornments, but the chemical pigments responsible for these colors can play an important role in fighting disease in the human body. Known as bioflavonoids, they boost the amount of vitamin C (an antioxidant) inside cells, strengthen capillaries, and fight damaging free radicals. They also have a unique ability to bind and strengthen collagen structures, which are vital for the integrity of connective tissue. Other beneficial effects on collagen include inhibition of enzymes that destroy collagen structures during inflammation and blocking inflammation-enhancing substances.

Health conditions that benefit from bioflavonoids include RA, periodontal disease, and other inflammatory problems. Bioflavonoids found in black cherries have been used to reduce uric acid levels and decrease tissue destruction associated with gout.[76] They also exhibit antimicrobial activity, which is helpful for arthritis linked to intestinal infections of microorganisms. In our clinic patients report a noticeable difference in pain levels after drinking 6 ounces of organic black cherry juice per day for one month.

There are over 4,000 bioflavonoid compounds found in different types of food. Anthocyanidin, which lends a deep red or blue color to blueberries, blackberries, cherries, grapes, and hawthorn berries, is the most effective of all the bioflavonoid compounds in providing collagen support. Boosting dietary intake of foods containing anthocyanidins helps relieve arthritis because they inhibit the release of pro-inflammatory mediators.[77] Other bioflavonoid compounds include citrus bioflavonoids, catechins, quercetin, hesperidin, and proanthocyanidins.

Types of Antioxidants

Amino acids: Cysteine, glutathione, methionine

Bioflavonoids: Anthocyanin bioflavonoids (in fruit, especially grapes, cranberries, and bilberries), citrus bioflavonoids (in grapefruit, lemons, and oranges), oligomeric proanthocyanidins (OPCs) in pycnogenol (from pine bark or grape seed extract)

Carotenes: Alpha- and beta-carotene (in red, yellow, and dark green fruits and vegetables), lycopene (in red fruits and vegetables, such as tomatoes and red grapefruit)

Spices: Cayenne pepper, garlic, turmeric

Herbs: Astragalus, bilberry, ginkgo, green tea, milk thistle, sage

Minerals: Copper, manganese, selenium, zinc

Vitamins: A, B_1, C, and E, coenzyme Q_{10}, NADH (nicotinamide adenine dinucleotide)

Enzymes: Catalase, glutathione peroxidase, superoxide dismutase

Hormones: Melatonin

Miscellaneous: Lipoic acid

Food sources: Fruits such as grapefruit, lemons, oranges, apples, apricots, pears, peaches, tomatoes, cherries, blueberries, cranberries, black currants, red grapes, plums, raspberries, strawberries, hawthorn berries, and other berries; vegetables such as red cabbage, onions, parsley, and rhubarb; herbs such as milk thistle and sage; grape skins, pine bark, red wine, and green tea.
Therapeutic dose: 500 mg of bioflavonoid complex, twice daily.

Green Tea (Camellia sinensis)

Green tea contains catechins, bioflavonoids that have anti-inflammatory and antioxidant properties and are helpful in treating RA by destroying free radicals that act on synovial membranes. Catechins also bind with heavy metals to decrease their harmful potential. Green tea contains other antioxidants, too, such as vitamins C and A (in the form of beta-carotene). Other benefits of green tea include a slight stimulating effect from its small amount of caffeine, as well as antimicrobial and cancer-fighting properties.

Therapeutic dose: 3–4 cups of organic green tea per day.

Pycnogenol

Extracted from grape seeds or pine bark, pycnogenol contains proantho-cyanidins, antioxidants 50 times more powerful than vitamins C and E. Proanthocyanidins can also increase the strength of collagen by cross-linking the fibers in the connective tissue matrix.[78] This makes the collagen more resistant to free radical damage from the arthritic process.

Therapeutic dose: 50–300 mg.

Quercetin

A bright yellow pigment, quercetin has outstanding anti-inflammatory properties useful in treating arthritis. It has several known anti-inflammatory mechanisms: It inhibits uric acid production (beneficial for gout), regulates the release of proinflammatory chemicals, decreases leukotrienes (immune cells that cause inflammation), and inhibits inflammation through down-regulation of the NFkB pathway.[79] Quercetin is also useful in helping correct intestinal permeability (leaky gut syndrome) and allergies.

Food sources: Onions and green tea.
Supplements: Quercetin works best when combined with the enzyme bromelain.
Therapeutic dose: 200–500 mg.

Enzymes

Enzymes are an important component of the metabolism of all living organisms. Over 3,000 different enzymes are present in the human body, each with a distinct task. Enzymes form new tissue, including bone, cartilage, muscle, and nerve cells. They are important in the normal detoxification processes, helping the body rid itself of toxins and cellular debris. Enzymes are also largely responsible for digestion, breaking down food into nutrients for use in the body. There are three primary types of enzymes the body produces to digest foods: amylases digest starch, lipases digest fat, and proteases digest proteins.

Essential Fatty Acids for Arthritis Relief

Essential fatty acids (EFAs) are unsaturated fats required in the diet. EFAs are converted into prostaglandins, hormonelike substances that regulate many metabolic functions, particularly inflammatory processes. Prostaglandins can be either pro-inflammatory (causing inflammation) or anti-inflammatory (decreasing inflammation), depending on which fatty acids are readily available from the diet, as well as the presence of enzymes and nutrients needed for prostaglandin production. These nutrients include vitamins B_3, B_6, and C, magnesium, and zinc. There are two types of EFAs, omega-3 and omega-6. The body needs more omega-6 than omega-3. However, in the case of arthritis, omega-6 fatty acids can be converted into inflammation-causing agents when levels of arachidonic acid are too high.

The omega-3 fatty acids EPA (eicosapentaenoic acid) and DHA (docosahexaenoic acid) have been shown to be effective in reducing and controlling inflammation in a variety of conditions, including heart disease and RA.[80] If enough omega-3 fatty acids are present in the body, they compete with arachidonic acid in the cyclooxygenase and lipoxygenase pathways. This interferes with the production of proinflammatory prostaglandins and suppresses inflammatory initiators, including thromboxane A2, interleukin-1alpha, tumor necrosis factor alpha (TNF-alpha), and COX II.[81] Patients who are moving toward a more natural management of inflammation may use omega-3 supplements along with drug therapies. Studies have shown that the dose of NSAIDs used for pain management can be reduced if omega-3 supplements are used.[82]

Food sources: Flaxseeds, hemp seed, wild game, and free-swimming fatty fish such as mackerel, salmon, and sardines.

Therapeutic dose: 500-3,000 mg omega-3 from foods and supplements combined.

Precautions: Since fish may contain high levels of mercury and other heavy metals, some manufacturers offer products described as "molecularly distilled," which they claim are free of heavy metals.

 For information about the **importance of EFAs in reducing inflammation**, see chapter 12, The Arthritis Diet, pages 225–256.

Many people with arthritis are deficient in proteases, which digest proteins from food and proteins in foreign cells. Protease supplements can decrease inflammation, reduce swelling and tenderness, and aid digestion. To treat pain and inflammation, enzymes should be taken on an empty stomach. Take them on a full stomach, immediately after eating, to digest food and prevent food allergens and toxins from migrating from the colon to the bloodstream.

Bromelain

Bromelain is a proteolytic enzyme extracted from the stems and fruits of the pineapple plant. It is helpful in several inflammatory diseases, including arthritis and inflammatory bowel disease.[83] Bromelain helps break down fibrin, which causes swelling by accumulating in inflamed areas and blocking off blood and lymph fluid. It also inhibits platelet aggregation and adherence of antigens to cell surfaces, which supports its widely observed antiallergic function. Anti-inflammatory effects may also be linked to bromelain's ability to alter leukocyte migration and activation. Bromelain interferes with the production of prostaglandins and other substances that contribute to the inflammatory cascade, including eicosanoids, cyclooxygenases, and lipoxygenases.[84]

Bromelain Juice Recipe

Bromelain juice is an excellent and delicious way to get high amounts of bromelain. Juice an organic nonirradiated pineapple along with half an organic lemon, and a 1/2-inch piece of fresh ginger root.

 Prostaglandins, hormonelike, complex fatty acids, affect smooth muscle function, inflammatory processes, and constriction and dilation of blood vessels. Essential fatty acids in the diet (omega-3s and omega-6s) provide the raw material for prostaglandin production; once ingested, these essential fatty acids can be converted to prostaglandins by nearly any cell in the body. Prostaglandins derived from omega-6s prostaglandins can have either proinflammatory or anti-inflammatory properties, while most prostaglandins converted from omega-3 sources help reduce pain and inflammation. For proper body function, an appropriate balance of both types of prostaglandins must be maintained.

For anti-inflammatory effects, bromelain should be taken on an empty stomach (taken with food, it helps improve digestion). For consistent therapeutic value, supplements containing specific amounts of bromelain should be used.

Therapeutic dose: 500–2,000 mg (2,400 mcu strength), three times daily. People who are allergic to bee stings, olive tree pollen, pineapple, grass pollen, and other allergens may also be sensitive to bromelain. As a digestive aid, bromelain is usually used in combination with ox bile and hydrochloric acid.

Papaya

Papayas contain the digestive enzyme papain, which aids in the digestion of protein. Papain helps to break down circulating immune complexes, which aggravate arthritis and inflammation. Papain is included in many digestive enzyme combinations, often along with bromelain and hydrochloric acid.

Therapeutic dose: 250–500 mg.

Homeopathic Remedies

Homeopathic medicine, established in Germany in the late eighteenth century, is based on three principles: that like cures like (law of similars); that the more a remedy is diluted, the greater its potency (law of infinitesimal dose); and that an illness is specific to the individual (a holistic medical model). According to homeopathy's founder, Dr. Samuel Hahnemann, disease can be permanently and rapidly reversed by using a medicine that is capable of producing the most similar and complete symptoms of the disease in a healthy person. Each homeopathic medicine is proven, or tested, in healthy people, and their symptoms are recorded. When treating ill patients, a homeopathic practitioner matches the patient's symptoms with a remedy that produced similar symptoms in a healthy person. Treating like with like works effectively to reverse disease because the homeopathic remedy works on an energetic level (having been diluted to the point that no chemical components remain).

Dr. Hahnemann found that the more a substance is diluted and shaken, the higher its potency. Homeopathic remedies are prepared in a series of dilution steps using water and succussing (vigorous shaking). Potency levels are designated with X and C. The X means that the homeopathic remedy has been serially diluted on a 1:10 scale (1 part substance to 9 parts water), and the C means the remedy has been diluted on a 1:100 scale (1 part substance to 99 parts water). A number value is placed before the scale designator to identify how many dilutions the remedy has undergone. A remedy designated 6X has undergone six dilutions at 1 part substance to 9 parts water; a remedy that is designated 12X has undergone 12 dilutions and is stronger than the 6X remedy. Common potencies available over the counter are 6X, 12X, 30X, 6C, 12C, and 30C.

Classical homeopathic remedies are prescribed for each patient based on their unique and distinguishing symptoms. This individualized prescription considers not only the person's physical symptoms but also their mental and emotional states. This is vastly different from conventional medicine, wherein many people with a specific disease condition are prescribed exactly the same medications. In homeopathy, any number of homeopathic remedies could be prescribed for that condition, but a specific remedy is selected only after reviewing the person's individual symptoms.

Hydrochloric Acid for Improving Digestion

Many people with arthritis are deficient in digestive factors (hydrochloric acid and pancreatic enzymes) needed to adequately break down food so that cells can absorb important nutrients. When digestion is incomplete or inadequate, food molecules can be inappropriately absorbed into the bloodstream, contributing to the onset of arthritis and other diseases.

Inside the stomach, an acidic environment with a very low pH is needed to break down food. To maintain the optimal pH (around 2, which is very acidic), the stomach secretes hydrochloric acid (HCl). HCl levels tend to decline with age, leading to impaired digestion. Research has shown that insufficient HCl is common in people suffering from RA.[85]

In order to determine HCl levels, physicians use the Heidelberg gastric analysis. After a 12-hour fast, the patient swallows a Heidelberg capsule, a device about the size of a vitamin that has a pH meter and radio transmitter inside. Once the capsule is swallowed, the patient drinks a solution of sodium bicarbonate, which stimulates the stomach to secrete HCl. The capsule measures and transmits the changing pH levels to a receiver placed over the patient's stomach, indicating whether or not the person is producing adequate HCl. The capsule can easily pass through the gastrointestinal tract for excretion.

A combination of physical symptoms can also indicate low levels of HCl or a deficiency in digestive and pancreatic enzymes. If you answer yes to at least three of the questions below, your body may not be producing enough digestive enzymes for optimal digestion.

After eating, do you suffer from any of these symptoms?

- Gas
- Bloating
- Abdominal discomfort
- Undigested food in your stool

The correct dose of HCl supplementation can often be determined by experimenting. Typically, start with 600 mg of HCl for a medium-size meal; if you feel a warm sensation in your stomach afterward, decrease the amount of HCl for meals of the same size in the future.

Building the Totality of Symptoms

The main symptom profile includes physical complaints, the effect of motion and temperature on pain, food cravings, and personality or emotional disposition. In homeopathy, the subjective quality of how a pain feels is extremely useful in identifying a remedy. When pursuing homeopathic treatment, pay attention to your pain and try to match it to the following categories.

- Sharp: Stabbing, cutting, stitching, piercing, pricking, splinterlike, stinging
- Shooting: Radiates from one location to another

- Stiff: Constricted or contracted
- Pressing: Squeezing, compressing, crushing, pinching
- Changeable: Wandering in any direction or hard to locate
- Burning: Cold or hot needles
- Lame: Dislocated, broken, sprained, or paralytic
- Other types of pain: Throbbing or pulsating, digging, twisting, drawing, pulling

Frequency and duration of symptoms are also important. Do they occur regularly, at a particular time, or in correlation with the weather? Do they come on strongly and persist for only a short time? In musculoskeletal diseases, physical signs are also part of the patient profile. The affected areas may be swollen and discolored (red, white, pale, waxy, or bruised), or hot or cold to the touch. Protrusions or bone deformities may be visible, especially on finger joints, as arthritis progresses. Although most Americans seldom consider that their emotional disposition affects their physical ailments, in homeopathy, these factors are as important as the location and duration of pain. Homeopathic doctors look for the following emotional patterns: restlessness, irritability, quick to overreact, or cries easily. Traits such as a strong desire for rest or remaining still, a constant need for motion or activity, desire to be outdoors, or fear of crowds all figure into the personality profile.

Common Homeopathic Remedies for Arthritis

Many different homeopathic remedies can be effective in treating arthritis, depending upon the type of arthritis, location of the pain, affinity for warmth or cold, and emotional state. Below, Ann Seipt, N.D., a homeopathic practitioner in Phoenix, Arizona, describes the most commonly prescribed remedies for arthritis and the symptom profile for which each is appropriate. If a remedy is well-suited for your condition, after taking it you'll experience immediate improvements or, in some cases, a healing crisis (a brief worsening of symptoms followed by improvement). If symptoms persist, however, it indicates an incorrect potency, dosage, or remedy, or perhaps deeper underlying problems. As with all medicinal substances, be cautious in self-prescribing homeopathic remedies and seek professional medical advice before beginning a course of homeopathic treatment.

Remedies for Inflammation

Apis mellifica: Symptoms of acute arthritis that come on rapidly; wandering joint pain that feels stiff and sore to any pressure; burning and stinging pains; stiffness and lameness in the shoulder blades; edema (swelling) in affected parts; sensation of joints being stretched tightly; red or shiny white coloration in affected parts; worsening of pain and swelling when the temperature is warm and improvement from application of cold water.

Bryonia alba: Symptoms of pale, tense, and swollen joints that come on slowly, continuously, or remittently; stitching and tearing pains aggravated by motion and relieved after rest; desire to remain still and quiet; extremely irritable disposition; white-coated tongue; dry mouth and lips; no thirst or, alternatively, great thirst; frequent constipation.

Dulcamara: Symptoms of rheumatism during sudden changes of weather from hot and dry to cold and damp; rheumatic complaints alternating with diarrhea; rheumatism following suppression of a skin eruption; pins-and-needles sensation in limbs.

Formica rufa: Symptoms of intense pain that come and go suddenly; red and swollen joints typically in the right side of the body; decreased swelling when pressure is applied to the joint.

Kali bichromium: Symptoms of gouty pains alternating with gastric complaints; rheumatism in spring and summer; pains that occur at the same time every year; pain in small spots that wander within a period of a few days or weeks; pricking pain or stiffness all over; joint symptoms alternating with diarrhea or nasal discharge.

Rhus toxicodendron: Symptoms of painful joints, ligaments, tendons, and skin; joints red, shiny, and swollen; stiffness and lameness of the affected parts; tearing and burning pain, as if sprained; tendency to affect the left side of the body; stiffness compelling the person to move around but pain worsening from overexertion; pain relief through warmth or massage; worsens in damp, cold weather; cravings for cold milk.

Remedies for Degenerative Changes

Causticum: Symptoms of stiff and cracking joints, especially knees; contracted muscles and tendons in the fingers and palm of hand; contractions drawing the limbs out of shape and causing deformed joints; aching shoulders; paralysis of deltoid muscle (triangular muscle covering the shoulder joint); symptoms decreasing in damp weather and worsening in dry, cold weather; aversion to sweet foods and cravings for smoked meats.

Guaiacum: Symptoms of immovable stiffness of contracted parts; rheumatic pain worsening around heat and improving around cold; pain increasing with slight motion and the affected part feeling hot; nodosities (conspicuous protuberances) on the joints and contracted tendons, hamstrings, and left wrist; craving for apples and aversion to milk.

Ruta graveolens: Symptoms of pain in the back or coccyx (lower end of spinal column) as if bruised; pain with an affinity for tendons and bones of the feet causing the patient to walk lightly; all body parts feeling bruised, especially the right wrist and both feet; pain worsening around heat; thirst for ice-cold water.

Remedies for Arthritis in Small Joints

Actaea spicata: Symptoms of swelling and severe pain in the joints of the feet, hands, wrists, and ankles; stiffness increasing after rest; weakness in the hands; swelling of the small joints during or after walking.

Colchicum: Symptoms of acute arthritis or gout of small joints; a white spot remaining on the skin after being pressed by a finger; sudden onset or increase of tearing or stitching pain, especially in the fingers; pain traveling from left to right; dark red, swollen joints; enlarged gouty joint nodosities; dark urine with white sediment; thick nasal discharge; irritable disposition; sensitive to noise, light, or odors.

Ledum palustre: Symptoms of arthritis starting in the feet and moving upward, especially in small joints; soreness in the feet and soles; swelling of body parts that feel cold to the touch; tearing pain in joints with accompanying weakness; pain changing place quickly with little or no swelling; pain improving with cold water or cold applications; pain worse at night when getting warm in bed; sensitive to wine; arthritic nodosities developing in later stages. This remedy is specific for Lyme disease.

Phosphorus: Symptoms of arthritic wrists and finger joints; pains that feel as if sprained or cut; pain usually occurring on the left side; back feeling as if it's broken; stiffness of knees and the feet; stiffness in the morning; symptoms worsening with cold applications and improving with warm applications; prominent stiffness, especially in the neck, back, and shoulders, or when rising from a sitting position.

Rhododendron: Symptoms of arthritic nodes on smaller joints like the fingers, neck, and heel; pain worsening before a storm or from cold weather, but lessening once a storm begins; pain increasing with rest and subsiding with motion; improved sleep when legs are crossed.

Remedies for Arthritis in the Neck and Back

Cimicifuga racemosa: Symptoms of fibromyalgia, arthritis, and rheumatism, accompanied by great pain; rheumatism alternating with depression; wandering pains that feel like an electric shock; frequent pains in the neck that cause stiffness; heat and swelling occurring in affected parts; menses exacerbating fibromyalgia; menstrual and uterine problems.

Ferrum phosphoricum: Symptoms of several joints affected at the same time; stinging and tearing pains that cause constant motion; pain improving from slow motion; face turning red with only minimal exertion.

Remedies for Arthritis in the Lower Back and Extremities

Berberis vulgaris: Symptoms of shooting, tearing, or burning pains radiating in low back muscles and knees; pain changing rapidly within minutes or hours; sticking pain near the kidneys; lameness after walking a short distance; kidney stones or gallstones.

Kali carbonicum: Symptoms of tearing pain in the small joints; sharp stitching pain in lumbar region that shoots into the buttocks or thighs; back pain; deformed joints; irritable with pain; sensitive to drafts or easily chilled.

Lac caninum: Symptoms of rheumatism that migrate and alternate from one side of the body to the other, or from one site to another.

Pulsatilla: Symptoms of red, hot, and swelling knees and feet; erratic pains that shift rapidly from joint to joint, or one-sided pains; drawing, tearing, and shifting pains; pain worsening at twilight or in a warm, stuffy room; craving fresh air and gentle exercise or motion; crying easily.

Ranunculus bulbosa: Symptoms of pain in the nerves and muscles in the back and upper arms and between the ribs; pains tending to occur on the left side; pain worsening in a cold and damp place or when the temperature changes from warm to cold; pain worsening with motion; possibly associated with herpes zoster (shingles); sensitive to wine.

fourteen

Exercises and Physical Therapies

While daily exercise and physical activity are important components of any healthy lifestyle, they are an absolute necessity for people with arthritis. Regular exercise improves energy levels, provides nourishment for muscles and connective tissues, and helps maintain a healthy weight. When muscles are toned and fit, they can adequately support joints. Muscle fitness also helps reduce pain and stiffness and helps halt the progression of arthritis.

An ideal exercise program for arthritis should target flexibility, strength, circulation of blood and lymph fluid, and relaxation. We recommend working with a qualified health-care practitioner or physical therapist to develop a daily routine to suit your specific type of arthritis and physical limitations. Start off slowly, with home or office stretches, then add aerobic exercises. Isometric exercises (resistance training) and aquatic exercises build muscle and increase flexibility without placing excessive strain on the joints. Tai chi, yoga, and other meditative exercises achieve the same goals while also focusing an anxious and scattered mind.

If exercise causes pain that persists for more than an hour, you're overexercising, which can stress your joints and cartilage and lead to subsequent damage or deterioration. High-impact aerobic exercises such as jogging aren't recommended for patients with arthritis in their knees, hips, or ankles. The type of exercise you choose, along with frequency and duration, should be tailored to your weight, age, sex, cartilage health, and many other factors. Consult with a health-care practitioner to design a program that will suit your individual profile.

Daily exercise should be complemented with massage, acupressure, or other physical therapies that promote relaxation and improve the circulation of blood and lymphatic fluid. You may want to incorporate therapeutic baths and other water treatments into your daily routine as well. Water has a therapeutic effect and can help improve circulation, detoxify the body, and initiate healing of internal organs. In this chapter, we discuss some of the most widely available physical therapies so that you and your health-care professional can determine which would be most beneficial for you.

Exercises

People with arthritis should ease into an exercise program and never try to do too much too quickly. Gentle stretches are an excellent way to gain flexibility and begin exercising joints and muscles. Other exercise therapies, including isometric and aquatic exercises, tai chi, qigong, and yoga, provide an effective workout without putting excessive strain on the body. They are also effective for relieving stress and focusing the mind.

Stretches for Home and Work

This program is designed to help reduce muscle tension and stress in the neck, shoulders, and back, with stretching routines to be done at work and at home.[1] It should be undertaken in conjunction with a sound exercise and nutrition program. See pages 298–302 for instructions and illustrations for this program.

 You should feel tightness but never pain while doing these exercises. If you experience any pain, stop and check with your doctor.

Isometric Exercises

In arthritis, muscles stay abnormally contracted for long periods, causing a buildup of waste products in the muscle tissues and even a shortening of the muscle. This can starve portions of the cartilage (or disks in spinal arthritis), leading to degeneration and OA. The goal of an isometric exercise is to relax a muscle so that it will stretch to its normal length and move more freely, eliminating wastes and feeding cartilage more efficiently. An isometric exercise applies resistance (or force) to a contracted (stiffened) muscle in order to improve motion and flexibility. The basic premise is that a muscle is easier to stretch after it has been contracted for at least 10 to 15 seconds. In an isometric contraction, the muscle is opposed by an immovable force (a wall, for example); after holding the contraction, the muscle is relaxed and will then stretch with more ease.

Aquatic Exercise

Water exercises make the muscles work harder because of the water's increased resistance, but the body's buoyancy diminishes shock and trauma to bones and joints. Swimming is one of the best water exercises and can be used as an aerobic exercise if continued for 20 minutes or more. Try different strokes to exercise different muscles and joints. Using flotation devises like kickboards and water wings can give more support to the body. If the lower half of your body needs special attention, walking in water is also highly recommended; the faster you walk, the greater the resistance the muscles encounter and the better the workout. There are also water aerobics classes available at most gyms and health clubs that have a pool.

Tai Chi

Tai chi is a unique Chinese system of slow, continuous, flowing movements that create a sense of tranquility, vitality, and calmness. Tai chi is

A Simple Isometric Exercise

If you experience pain when you straighten an elbow, the following isometric exercise may help.

1. Straighten out the arm to the point where you begin to feel discomfort and hold it there.

2. Grab the wrist of that hand with your other hand, hold it firmly in place, and then, for a count of 10 seconds, continue to try to straighten the elbow, applying gentle force in the opposite direction with the arm that is holding it.

3. Release your hold on the wrist. Relax the painful arm and attempt to straighten it further. When you release the opposing force, you'll find that your painful elbow moves more easily.

You can model exercises for other joints on this one. Doing such exercises several times a day, for about 10 seconds for each stiff joint, should increase mobility of the joint and decrease pain in about a week. If pain persists or increases in intensity after a day or two, stop doing the exercise and consult your health-care practitioner. Flexibility can be further increased by first rubbing an analgesic salve on the joint or using a hot pack before stretching.

Daily Office Routine

If you spend eight hours or more sitting at a desk or standing behind a counter, your joints and muscles are not receiving the proper amount of motion necessary for healthy flexibility. Be sure to take a break from your normal working position to walk around and stretch your muscles, thereby helping to circulate nutrients to muscles and other tissues. Or take a walk during your lunch break to reduce stress and avoid afternoon weariness. The stretches described below can be done at your desk throughout the day with only minimal disruption of your work schedule. Take a 10-minute break to do these exercises; repeat the entire routine two to three times a day. Work into each stretch slowly and hold it steadily for 15 to 30 seconds; try to avoid a bouncing motion, as this stresses the joints. Do two to three repetitions of each position and remember to take deep, relaxing breaths during each stretch.

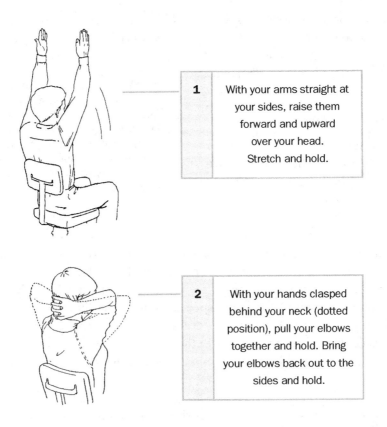

1 With your arms straight at your sides, raise them forward and upward over your head. Stretch and hold.

2 With your hands clasped behind your neck (dotted position), pull your elbows together and hold. Bring your elbows back out to the sides and hold.

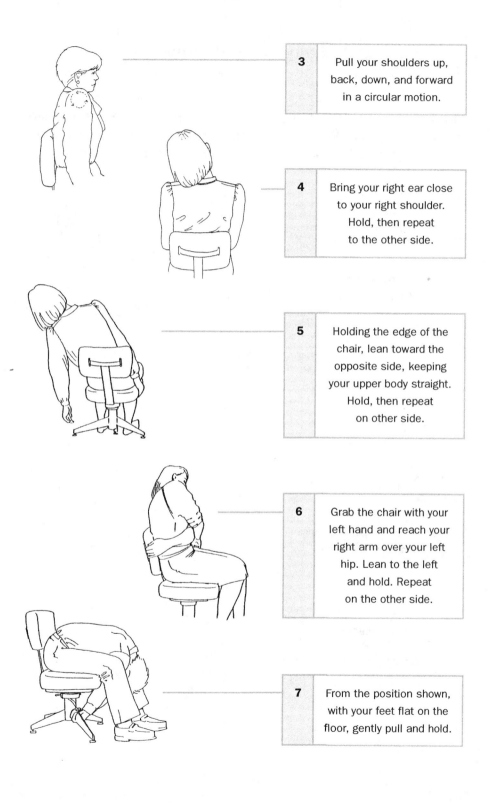

3 Pull your shoulders up, back, down, and forward in a circular motion.

4 Bring your right ear close to your right shoulder. Hold, then repeat to the other side.

5 Holding the edge of the chair, lean toward the opposite side, keeping your upper body straight. Hold, then repeat on other side.

6 Grab the chair with your left hand and reach your right arm over your left hip. Lean to the left and hold. Repeat on the other side.

7 From the position shown, with your feet flat on the floor, gently pull and hold.

Daily Home Routine

The stretches described below can be done in the morning after waking or before going to bed at night. Do the entire routine and repeat particular stretches that cater to areas of your body that are tight or sore. Before beginning the routine, warm up your muscles with a brisk walk or a soak in a warm tub for 10 to 20 minutes.

Back

Lie flat on the floor. Pull one knee to your chest and raise your head to the knee. Hold the stretch, then switch legs and repeat.

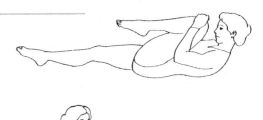

Upper body

Sit in a chair. From the position shown, with arms extended, twist your body and head. Hold the stretch, then repeat on the other side.

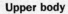

Hamstrings

From the position shown, use a belt or towel to pull your upper body gently forward. Hold the stretch, then switch legs and repeat.

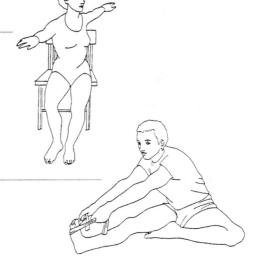

Shoulders

Put one elbow behind your head. Gently pull your elbow toward the center of your back. Hold the stretch, then switch arms and repeat.

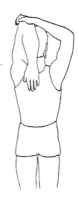

Exercises for Specific Parts of the Body

These exercises target the head, neck, shoulders, and upper back. For many people, stress and tension tend to build up in these areas, causing muscle contractions and pain. Do these exercises two to three times per day to stretch contracted muscles and strengthen weakened joints. When doing these stretches, concentrate on breathing to provide a deeper, more relaxed stretch.

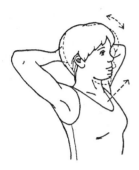

Base of head and neck

1. With your chest up, tuck your chin down and in, rocking your head on your neck.
Don't bend your neck or bob your head.
Don't hold your breath while nodding.

2. Turn your head to left and repeat step 1, then repeat on the right.

Neck, shoulders, and upper back

1. This is the starting and ending position. (The exercise can be done sitting or standing.)

2. While exhaling, turn your head slightly and use your left hand to pull your head and neck down in a diagonal direction, then release the pressure from your hand.

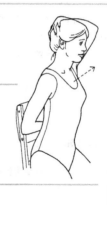

3. When your head reaches the end point in step 2, maintain the pressure from your hand and rotate your head away from your arm about 40 degrees. Repeat this rotation several times before returning to the starting position. Repeat several times on this side, then do the other side.

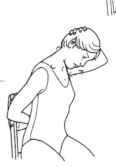

Shoulders and middle back

These exercises target the shoulders and middle back. For many people, stress and tension tend to build up in these areas, causing muscle contractions and pain. Do these exercises two to three times per day to stretch contracted muscles and strengthen weakened joints. When doing these stretches, concentrate on breathing to provide a deeper, more relaxed stretch.

Upper back

With your chin in and arms straight, raise your upper back toward the ceiling and inhale. Relax, exhale, and lower your spine, letting your shoulder blades come close to each other.

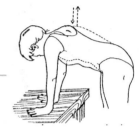

Upper chest and shoulders

With your hands at the level shown, exhale and lean in toward the corner, keeping your chest up. Interlock your fingers behind your back and raise your arms as high as possible while exhaling. Keep your chest up and your chin in.

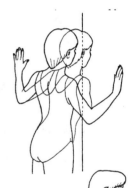

Shoulders and middle back

Interlock your fingers behind your back and raise your arms as high as possible while exhaling. Keep your chest up and your chin in.

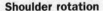

Shoulder rotation

Hold a length of stretchy rubber tubing with your hands about shoulder width apart. Move hands apart while exhaling and pinching your shoulder blades together slightly. Keep your chest up and keep your elbows bent at a 90-degree angle and close to your sides.

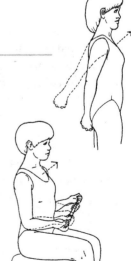

a perfect exercise for those with arthritis because it involves little impact (no bouncing motions). It is gentle and yet effective in stretching muscles, loosening and lubricating the joints, and promoting blood circulation. Traditional Chinese medicine (TCM) holds that tai chi stimulates and nourishes the body's internal organs by circulating qi, while also facilitating emotional and mental well-being and teaching the mind how to control the body.[2] The art of tai chi can be practiced by almost anyone, and movements can be modified for those with arthritis. We suggest you begin your practice with a structured class, which will teach you the fundamentals for exercises that you can eventually practice at home.

Qigong

Similar to tai chi, qigong (also referred to as chi kung) is an ancient exercise that stimulates and balances the flow of qi along acupuncture meridians (energy pathways). Qigong cultivates inner strength, calms the mind, and restores the body to its natural state of health. Although less artistic and dynamic than tai chi, qigong is much easier to learn and can be done by the severely disabled as well as the healthy. Qigong practice can range from simple calisthenics-type movements with breath coordination to complex exercises that direct brain wave frequencies, deep relaxation, and breathing to improve strength and flexibility and reverse damage caused by prior injuries and disease.

Qigong can be especially helpful to arthritis patients because it initiates relaxation, moderates pain and depression, and regulates the immune system. It also enhances flow of lymphatic fluids, which improves the body's ability to detoxify and deliver vital, replenishing nutrients to target tissues. Qigong can also balance the function of hormone-producing glands, which mediate pain and mood. After six months of qigong, several patients maintained that the stiffness and pain in their hands had lessened and the deformed knuckles characteristic of arthritis were starting to return to normal.[3]

Yoga

Yoga is one of the most ancient systems of self-healing practiced today. It teaches a basic principle of mind-body unity and maintains that if the mind is chronically restless and agitated, the health of the body will be compromised. Similarly, if the body is in poor health, mental strength and clarity will be adversely affected. The art of yoga can bring about harmony and oneness of mind, body, and spirit.

Classical yoga is divided into eight branches that give guidance as to

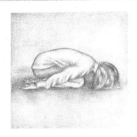
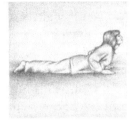
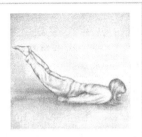

Yoga postures or asanas: child's posture, cobra, and locust.

the proper diet, hygiene, detoxification regimes, and physical and psychological practices to help the individual integrate their personal, psychological, and spiritual awareness. The most well-known and popular of the yogic branches is hatha yoga, which teaches certain asanas (postures) and breathing techniques to create profound changes in the body and mind. The two types of asana, therapeutic and meditative, are designed to improve health and physical well-being and were originally prescribed for those with neck, back, and joint pain.

Yoga can benefit most illnesses if done on a regular basis. One goal of yoga is to harness and stimulate the flow of prana, or life energy (similar to qi in the Chinese system). The blockage of prana, whether due to improper diet, lifestyle stressors, or imbalance in one's physical, emotional, or spiritual health, can lead to illness. Breathing techniques and the duration for which certain postures are held remove barriers to the flow of prana and can improve oxygen intake by as much as seven times in a single, normal breath.

In addition to improving circulation of blood, lymph, and prana, yoga corrects hormone imbalances by regulating chakras (the energy centers that correspond to hormone-producing glands). The lymphatic system (SEE QUICK DEFINITION) doesn't have a pump of its own; instead, it depends on movement

The **lymphatic system** consists of lymph fluid and the structures (vessels, ducts, and nodes) involved in transporting it from tissues to the bloodstream. Lymph fluid occupies the space between the body's cells and contains plasma proteins, foreign particles, and cellular wastes. Lymph nodes are clusters of immune tissue that work as filters or "inspection stations" for detecting and removing foreign and potentially harmful substances in the lymph fluid. While the body has over 500 lymph nodes, they are mostly clustered in the neck, armpits, chest, groin, and abdomen. The lymphatic system is the body's master drain, collecting and filtering the lymph fluid and conveying it to the bloodstream, thereby clearing waste products and cellular debris from the tissues.

of the body to transport fluid in and out of tissues. When a person is inactive or if motion is imbalanced, the lymphatic fluid can become stagnant and create disease. Through yoga's stretches and postures, lymphatic fluid is pumped throughout the body, removing toxins and waste products from cells and delivering fresh nutrients. The health of all cartilage is dependent on this very process.

The safest and most reliable way to use yoga therapeutically is to follow a balanced program of postures to achieve an overall normalizing and health-inducing effect. It's best for beginners to start with a simple program of basic postures. A structured course can teach the fundamental breathing techniques and postures, which you can later practice on your own. Books and videos are also good resources for beginners.

Physical Therapies

A number of physical therapies can be effective in treating all types of arthritis, particularly hydrotherapy, massage, and energy medicine. The most effective forms of hydrotherapy include contrast hydrotherapy, hyperthermic hydrotherapy, hot packs, ice packs, heat compresses, and baths, showers, and whirlpools. Of the many types of bodywork that are helpful, we'll discuss massage, Rolfing, osseous manipulation, Oriental body therapies, and reflexology. Energy medicine primarily refers to microcurrent therapy and magnet therapy.

Hydrotherapy

Hydrotherapy is the use of water, ice, steam, and hot and cold temperatures to maintain and restore health. Treatments include full body immersion, steam baths, saunas, and the application of hot and cold compresses. Therapeutically, hot water soothes and relaxes the body, muscles, and connective tissues. Applications of hot water produce a response that stimulates the immune system and causes white blood cells to clean up toxins and assist in eliminating wastes. Organs are affected through the reflex action of the surface nerves located in the skin.

Cold water, on the other hand, discourages inflammation by means of vasoconstriction (narrowing the blood vessels) and making the blood vessels less permeable. Cold water also tones muscular weakness. When applications of hot and cold water are alternated (known as contrast hydrotherapy), their therapeutic benefits are combined. Contrast therapy stimulates the endocrine system, liver, skin, and lymphatic system. It also improves circulation of fresh blood (containing oxygen, nutrients, and hormones) to the tissues and removal of waste products (such as inflammatory molecules and carbon dioxide).

Contrast hydrotherapy and hyperthermic hydrotherapy should only be pursued under the supervision of a trained health-care practitioner. However, the other techniques we'll describe, many of which are used in spas or clinics, can be performed in the comfort of your own home with little equipment or expense. Hot and cold compresses and packs are particularly effective for applying heat or cold to specific parts of the body to relieve muscle spasms, produce local hyperthermia (fever), and help relieve pain.

Contrast Hydrotherapy. No other therapy can initiate a sense of relaxation, well-being, and relief from spasms and pain as well as whole-body contrast hydrotherapy. The treatment begins with a 10- to 15-minute session in a whirlpool, Finnish sauna, or Russian steam cabinet. After the patient's body has warmed, the practitioner sprays cool water on him or her, starting on the back of the legs and working up the back along the spine, trunk, and head. The cool spray lasts for about 30 seconds. This process is repeated on the front side of the patient for another 30 seconds. The patient immediately returns to the source of heat for three to four minutes. After returning to the heat, they should feel a pleasant tingling sensation caused by the dilation of blood vessels. The application of alternating cold and hot is repeated two more times, ending in a shorter cool application.

CAUTION Low blood pressure upon standing rapidly may occur during contrast hydrotherapy. Patients taking hypertension medication should proceed with caution. Although it rarely happens, patients have fainted from this therapy. Follow all contrast hydrotherapy by drinking 8 ounces of mixed vegetable juice.

Contrast applications to arthritic joints and tight muscles are the most effective therapy for increasing blood flow through an area. This aids in removing wastes (which cause pain and inflammation) from joints and connective tissues and helps bring nutrients and oxygen into the area.[4] It also increases the functional activity of the organs; for example, a cool spray of water over the small of the back where the kidneys and adrenal glands are located increases the function of these organs. Again, contrast hydrotherapy must be supervised by a trained health-care practitioner.

Hyperthermic Hydrotherapy. Hyperthermic hydrotherapy deliberately induces fever in a patient who is unable to mount a natural fever response. Fever is helpful for the body; it's an intelligent physical response to an internal imbalance or invader and stimulates the immune system by increasing the production of antibodies and white blood cells. Hyperthermia is used in arthritis for detoxification of fat-stored chemicals and drug residues, stimulation of the lymphatic system, or treatment of infections. This treatment can be quite intense and must be provided by a trained practitioner.

 For more about **detoxifying fat-stored chemicals and other toxins**, see chapter 4, General Detoxification, pages 66–87.

The entire hyperthermia procedure takes about 75 to 90 minutes and includes immersion of the entire body in hot water, followed by a sweating period and then a tepid shower. Before beginning the treatment, the patient should empty their bladder. The practitioner records the patient's temperature, pulse, and blood pressure, then the patient drinks a cup of tea (peppermint, yarrow, elder, ginger, cayenne, or boneset) and climbs into the whirlpool. The temperature of the water should be 104 to 106°F throughout the treatment. The patient is immersed in the water to raise their body temperature; by immersing more body surface area, their temperature will increase more rapidly. A washcloth dipped in ice water is used as a cold compress for the patient's head and brow; liberal use of the compress is advised (if using a sauna, a cup of water will periodically be poured over the body). Oral temperature and pulse are taken every 5 to 10 minutes. Once the patient's temperature reaches 103°F, they are helped out of the water and escorted to a bed to begin the second phase of the treatment, the diaphoretic, or sweating, period.

The patient is wrapped in sheets and covered with five to seven layers of wool blankets. Under the blankets, the patient will begin to sweat profusely. We have found that sweating occurs even in people who report a difficult time perspiring. It is important to create a relaxed atmosphere during treatment; soothing or meditative music can be used to induce sleep or a sense of calm. This phase of the treatment usually lasts

 Hyperthermia treatment should be conducted only by a qualified health-care practitioner trained in hydrotherapy. Do not attempt this alone or without proper training.

for an hour, by which time the patient's temperature has dropped to 99°F. A tepid shower will return the body temperature to normal. Vegetable juice or water with trace minerals can be sipped after the shower. The patient should return home and rest, as this treatment can be exhausting.

Baths and Showers. Bathtubs and showers provide the easiest and cheapest form of home hydrotherapy. Baths and showers are both mentally and

Mineral Baths

Some of the most therapeutic baths come directly from the earth. For instance, seawater contains a similar balance of minerals to that found in human blood. Soaking in the ocean or a bath of dissolved sea salts (use Celtic or Dead Sea salts, which are prepared through evaporation of seawater) can help balance the body's mineral ratios, which is especially helpful for those with mineral deficiencies.[5] Because seawater so closely resembles human blood, these minerals can be readily absorbed by the skin in a form that cells can use.

Natural springs are also a source of concentrated minerals such as sodium, calcium, magnesium, and sulfur. Sulfur is especially helpful for rheumatic and arthritic complaints. A vital component of cartilage and synovial fluid, sulfur levels are lower than normal in the joints of many people with arthritis. Bathing in sulfur-rich water may support cartilage formation and pain relief.

Another earth-based therapy is immersion in mineral-rich mud. Originally used in the healing spas of Europe, fango is a combination of mineral-rich clay, anti-inflammatory herbs, and paraffin wax especially useful for arthritis. Fango clay is heated to approximately 116°F and applied as a localized heat pack on problem joints and muscles. The clay molds to the body like a cast and the healing minerals (such as sulfur) and powerful botanicals are absorbed by the skin. Blood flow and metabolic activity increase as capillaries enlarge and pores open, releasing waste products. Other muds, such as green argillite mud, can be used in place of fango.[6]

physically soothing. They help relieve general aches and pains and can also ease internal congestion and digestive problems. Hot baths and showers stimulate the immune system and induce detoxification through perspiration. Cold baths and showers tone muscles and reduce inflammation. Alternating between hot and cold (similar to the procedure used in contrast hydrotherapy) can also be used to increase circulation of blood and lymphatic fluid. We advise warming the body with a hot shower (at a tolerable temperature) for five minutes, then changing the temperature of the water to warm for two minutes, and finally to cold for one to two minutes. Repeat the cycle three times, always ending with cold water.

Whirlpool Baths. We prescribe whirlpool baths for all of our arthritis patients. Whirlpools can rehabilitate injured muscles and joints and alleviate the stresses and strains of everyday life. Although most gyms and clinics have whirlpools, many people with arthritis have found that installing one in their home is affordable and easy. The cost of installing a whirlpool into your home for medical purposes may even be tax deductible. To qualify as tax deductible, these expenses must be prescribed in writing by a physician or licensed health-care practitioner "for the mitigation, treatment, or prevention of disease or for the purpose of affecting any structure or function of the body." Save receipts and check with your tax advisor to see if your whirlpool expenses qualify.

In a whirlpool or bathtub, you can prepare the following bath for relief of aches and pains: Dissolve 5 pounds (or more) of Epsom salts or Dead Sea salts and 10 drops of lavender essential oil in a bath of hot water. Soak for 10 to 15 minutes, using a cold compress to keep your forehead and head cool. Follow the bath with a cold shower. Perform this soak four times per week if you're in severe pain or twice a week for less debilitating conditions. Epsom salts and Dead Sea salts are available at grocery or health food stores, drugstores, or through the Internet.

 CAUTION Always use the buddy system when using a hot bath or whirlpool for an extended period. Consult with a physician before using a new therapy, especially if you're pregnant, on prescription medications, or have any cardiovascular, thyroid, lung, or diabetic conditions. Use caution when entering and exiting any potentially slippery area. Get out of a hot bath slowly and carefully; be ready to put your head lower than your heart if you feel faint or dizzy. Direct hydrotherapy over the kidneys (if a person has kidney stones) or the liver (if a person has gallstones) can cause the stones to move, creating a medical emergency. Constantly monitor the skin if using cold or hot applications for thermal effects.

Hot Packs. Use a commercial hot pack or hot water bottle; if these are not available, use towels that have been soaked in hot water (the water should be hot but not unbearable). Prepare hot packs to 120°F. Place two or three layers of toweling over the area to be treated, then place the hot pack on the toweling and cover with an insulating layer of towels. Leave the pack in place for 5 to 20 minutes; the pack may need to be reheated if it cools too much. Follow with a 30-second cold application. Localized redness and perspiration will occur, indicating circulation of oxygen and nutrients to the area. A number of herbs, oils, and minerals may be used in this procedure for enhanced therapeutic benefits: Chamomile soothes skin, opens pores, eliminates blackheads, aids digestive problems, and promotes sleep. Ginger relaxes sore muscles, improves circulation, and tones the skin. Oat straw relieves sore feet, ingrown toenails, and blisters, and sage stimulates the sweat glands. Prepare the herbs as you would for tea. Or add tinctures or oils directly to a small basin of hot water. Soak a towel in the basin, wring it out, and apply it directly to the skin; cover with an insulating layer.

Precautions: Always test a small area of skin for sensitivity to heat or herbs. In general, hot packs using towels wrung from hot tap water are the safest; carefully monitor the skin to avoid burning.

Ice Packs. Helpful in reducing swelling, inflammation, pain, or congestion, ice packs are easy to prepare and inexpensive. Prepare an ice pack

Aromatherapy Can Help Arthritis Sufferers

Aromatherapy uses the essential oils of plants for medicinal purposes. Through steam distillation or cold-pressing, the volatile constituents of the plant's oil are extracted from its flowers, leaves, branches, or roots. Essential oils contain beneficial vitamins, minerals, enzymes, and hormones that are easily absorbed into the body's tissues. The benefits of essential oils can be obtained through inhalation or external application. Diffusers are devices that disperse tiny particles of essential oils into the air; inhaling these oils can affect the portion of the brain that controls heart rate, blood pressure, breathing, memory, stress, and hormone balance. Diffused oils are particularly helpful for decreasing muscle tension and increasing relaxation.

For people with arthritis, aromatherapy can reduce inflammation and pain in aching and stiff joints. Aromatherapy can also address other factors involved in arthritis; for example, calming and dispelling anxiety. It can also address infections or other underlying causes of the disease. The following are particularly helpful for arthritis.

- Cedarwood: Promotes elimination through mucous membranes and acts as an antiseptic and sedative
- Wintergreen, menthol, and camphor: Anti-inflammatory and cooling (apply topically to inflamed joints)
- Clove, cinnamon, and thyme: Anti-inflammatory and warming (use with arthritis that's worse in cold, damp weather)

- Lemon: Increases urine flow and acts as an antiseptic
- Rose: Stimulates liver and stomach functions and acts as an antidepressant
- Tea tree: Enhances skin function and can be used as an antifungal and antibiotic

Include essential oils in baths, saunas, soaks, and showers to increase their therapeutic value. Essential oils can also be added directly to warm compresses wrapped on a joint to soothe pain. Since the oils are readily absorbed through the skin, direct topical application of oils is extremely beneficial. However, true essential oils can be very strong and may irritate sensitive skin, so it's usually better to dilute a few drops of essential oil in a carrier oil, such as almond or sesame oil.

When purchasing essential oils, watch for labels that state "pure botanical perfume" or "pure fragrance essence." This is a sure indication that the oils are not true essential oils but rather have synthetic chemicals added. Completely pure oil is marked "100% pure essential oil."

Chemical components of essential oils are readily altered by exposure to sun or heat; always keep essential oils in dark containers away from damp, moist, or warm places. Essential oils are also sensitive to oxidation when exposed to the air, so keep bottles tightly sealed. When properly stored, they should remain fresh for one year.

by freezing water in a waxed paper cup. Once it's completely frozen, remove it from the freezer and peel away a portion of the paper cup. Hold onto the remaining paper cup and rub the exposed portion of the ice over joints, muscles, or other painful areas. Use for 20 minutes or less, then rest for five minutes before applying the ice again; repeat two to three times.

Precautions: Take frequent breaks so as to not damage the skin. Applying ice for longer than 20 minutes at a time can cause blood vessels to dilate, creating more inflammation.

Heat Compresses. To use a heat compress, start with a cold compress and allow it to be heated by the body. Heat compresses are recommended for edema, inflammation, and redness in joints or an injured area. The compress encourages blood flow and increased metabolic activity in the area. Soak a cotton cloth in ice water, then wring it out and apply it to the area to be treated. Cover the cotton cloth with a piece of wool cloth, wrap plastic around the entire area, and secure it in place. Leave the wrap in place for several hours; after the cool sensation wears off, the body will warm the compress. This is an excellent application to leave on overnight or when napping.

Bodywork

Hands-on therapies such as massage, deep tissue manipulation, movement awareness, and energy balancing are used to improve the structure and functioning of the human body. Bodywork in all its forms helps to reduce pain, soothe injured muscles, stimulate blood and lymphatic circulation, and promote deep relaxation.

Massage. Massage is used for general well-being, stress reduction, resolution of embedded emotions or psychological problems, recovery from sports injuries or muscle soreness, or as an adjunct therapy for medical conditions. Massage is one of the most important therapies for the treatment of arthritis and fibromyalgia. People with arthritis often experience prolonged muscle tension, which interferes with the elimination of chemical wastes in the muscles and surrounding tissues. Poor

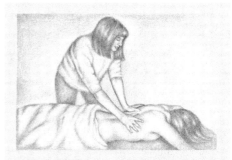

The Therapeutic Effects of Massage

Studies indicate that massage provides many health benefits.

- Sedates the nervous system and promotes voluntary muscle relaxation
- Relieves certain types of pain
- Provides effective treatment of chronic inflammatory conditions by increasing lymphatic circulation
- Improves circulation through the capillaries, veins, and arteries, and increases blood flow through the muscles
- Triggers reflex actions in the body to stimulate organs
- Promotes recovery from fatigue

circulation in muscle tissues can cause nerve and muscle pain, which may spread to other areas of the body. Nerves that supply the muscles also supply the supporting structures of the joint.

Pains that seem to emanate from the joints may actually be coming from trigger points, focal areas where wastes have accumulated in the muscles. Massage helps break up muscular waste deposits and stimulates circulation to troubled regions in the body. Deep pressure on trigger points stretches tissues and loosens shortened muscles to restore muscular balance and proper functioning. Most importantly, certain types of pain can be relieved by massage, as the rhythmic motions sedate the nervous system and promote voluntary muscle relaxation. We recommend that patients with arthritis receive massages at least two to three times per week in the early treatment stages of treatment, then once a week for several months, and ultimately twice a month for maintenance. Remember, massage therapies should be designed to fit individual profiles, including physical needs and economic limitations.

Rolfing. Rolfing, also referred to as structural integration, is a unique system of soft-tissue manipulation designed to restore flexibility and improve muscle function and body motion. Developed by biochemist Ida P. Rolf, Ph.D., Rolfing repositions the head, thorax, pelvis, and legs so that they are correctly aligned with gravity's force. According to Dr. Rolf, if the body is struggling against gravity to maintain imbalanced postures (while standing, walking, or sitting), the muscles become more contracted over time and eventually the fascial tissues (sheets of connective tissues that envelop muscles, tissues, and organs) begin to break down.[7] This stress causes the fascial tissues to lose their elasticity and become solid, rigid, or sticky, restricting movement of muscles and joints. OA can eventually set in as joints are abnormally compressed and the protective coating between bones deteriorates. Dr. Rolf also observed that physical dysfunction caused the onset of further chronic illness, fatigue, and emotional and psychological problems.

Dr. Rolf reasoned that by manually manipulating and stretching the fascial tissues, she could change the posture and biomechanics of the patient's movement. By applying pressure with the fingers, knuckles, or elbows, the practitioner reorganizes the fascial tissues so that the body's segments regain balance. Educational classes (called Rolfing Movement Education) help the person develop more balanced posture and movement. Our OA patients who had Rolfing sessions experienced improvement in everyday motions. They reported feeling less strain when walking, doing housework, or standing. X-rays of their affected joints revealed a decrease in the erosion of cartilage and bone surrounding the joint. We have also found that chiropractic adjustments to the spine or other joints remain in alignment longer if the patient completes the standard course of initial Rolfing treatments—a specifically designed and organized series of 10 sessions. Rolfing's combination of bodywork, education, and reinforcement of proper posture helps bones stay in alignment after they are manipulated.

Osseous Manipulation. Osseous manipulation is the repositioning of bones, including the bones of the spinal column, cranium, and other moveable joints. Chiropractors, as well as naturopathic doctors and qualified osteopathic physicians, are trained and licensed to practice this type of therapy. Chiropractic is concerned with the relationship of the spinal column and the musculoskeletal structures of the body to the nervous system. The nervous system holds the key to the body's incredible potential to heal itself because it controls the functions of all other systems of the body.

The spinal column acts as a switchboard for the nervous system, and when slight misalignments of the spine (called subluxations) interfere, the transmissions of the nervous system can be altered, as when an electrical wire has been crimped. This not only causes localized pain in the spine, it can also interfere with neurological information being transmitted to the major organs and cause dysfunction or disease. By adjusting the spine to remove subluxations, normal nerve function can be restored. Manipulation can help arthritis (particularly OA in the spine) by restoring proper movement and positioning of the joints. Balanced movement

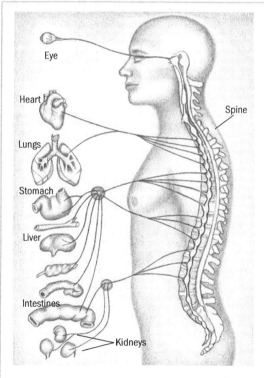

The spinal vertebrae and related organ systems.

prevents wear-and-tear damage to joints, ligaments, and cartilage. Frequent osseous manipulations help decrease the accumulation of scar tissue after injury, thus preventing later osteoarthritic changes in the joints. Chiropractic adjustments, combined with proper nutrition, can improve and in some cases reverse OA.[8]

Oriental Bodywork. The Oriental body therapies, such as acupuncture or acupressure, work to balance the flow of qi (vital life energy) through energy meridians. These meridians run throughout the body and are associated with different organs, and if there's a block in the energy meridian, it will be expressed as health problems in the organs associated with the blocked meridian. Blocked qi can be released by applying pressure to specific points along the energy meridians. Acupuncture uses needles, while acupressure (such as shiatsu and Jin Shin Do) uses rubbing, kneading, or other types of pressure from the fingers and hands.

Shiatsu, which means "finger pressure" in Japanese, was originally developed from ancient Chinese acupressure techniques. Shiatsu uses a sequence of firm rhythmic pressure applied to specific points for 3 to 10 seconds. Like acupuncture, it's designed to awaken, calm, and harmonize the meridians. Shiatsu affects not only the acupressure points, but the entire mind and body, making it one of the most effective forms of bodywork for arthritis. Jin Shin Do, another Japanese bodywork technique, is based on the original Jin Shin Jyutsu founded by Jiro Murai. Master Murai based his system on moving qi through the meridians by using certain combinations of acupressure points in a special sequence. Pressure is held for a minute or more until the practitioner can feel the flow of blood and qi through the point. Opening and releasing sequences move the qi in the proper direction.

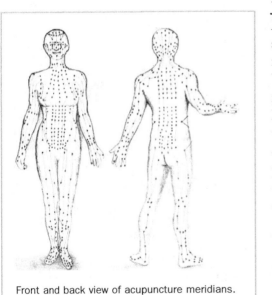
Front and back view of acupuncture meridians.

Reflexology. Reflexology is the application of pressure to areas of the feet, hands, and earlobes to influence and heal internal organs. Precise pressure releases block-

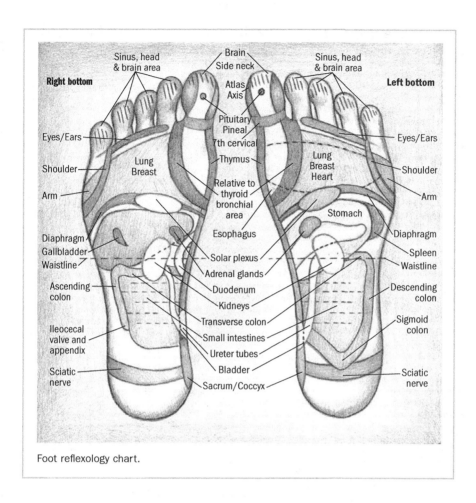

Foot reflexology chart.

ages that inhibit energy flow and cause pain and disease. This pressure is thought to affect internal organs and glands by stimulating reflex points of the body. Typically, practitioners use their thumbs to press on the various areas of the feet that correspond to specific organs or other structural components of the body. Reflexology can benefit those with arthritis by helping detoxify organs such as the kidneys and liver and stimulating sluggish glands, like the thyroid and adrenals.

We use reflexology as an integral part of our physical therapies, as exemplified in the case of Sarah, 53, who came to our office complaining of a frozen shoulder. She'd had difficulty moving her shoulder for the last three years. First, we soaked her feet in warm water with lavender oil for 3 minutes. After examining the shoulder reflexology points on Sarah's feet, we found that they were quite tender. We applied pressure to each

Daily Exercise and Physical Medicine Protocol for Arthritis

- Mornings: Do the daily home routine of stretches (see page 300). If it fits into your schedule, consider enrolling in a morning yoga or water aerobics class that meets two to three times a week.

- Afternoons: Do isometric exercises or the daily office routine (see pages 298–299). Take a brief walk after lunch.

- Early evenings: If you work, consider taking evening yoga or water aerobics classes.

- Before bedtime: Use some form of hydrotherapy, such as a bath, shower, whirlpool, or sauna. Repeat your morning stretching routine.

- Weekends: Try to devote more time to stretching, exercise, and meditation. A 1-mile walk, tai chi or qigong classes, and isometric exercises can be distributed throughout the weekend.

- Two to three times a week: See a licensed professional for massage, reflexology, and chiropractic therapies. Your health-care professional can design a weekly schedule with the types and frequency of treatments tailored to your unique situation.

foot for 30 minutes, focusing specifically on her shoulder reflex points. She didn't realize how beneficial the treatment had been until she put on her coat to leave. To her surprise, she easily lifted her arm into the sleeve of her coat—a motion that had been troublesome for years. On Sarah's next visit, she brought her husband so that they could both learn the basic techniques of reflexology to use on each other. Reflexology is safe and can be practiced by anyone; however, treatment by a professional reflexologist is more effective.

Energy Medicine

Energy medicine uses therapies that employ an energy field (electrical, magnetic, sonic, acoustic, or subtle) to treat health conditions by detecting and correcting imbalances in the body's own energy fields. Microcurrent treatment and magnet therapy are two forms of energy medicine that can be helpful for arthritis.

Microcurrent Treatment. Microcurrent treatment devices generate infinitesimally low levels of electrical current in a form compatible with the body's own biocurrents occurring in healthy tissues. Used to heal muscle-related back injuries or reduce muscle pain, these almost subsensory signals are applied to damaged muscles to recharge the cellular "battery," which in turn leads to healing. Pain relief comes from decreases in swelling and spasms and increases in muscle flexibility. Microcurrent is one application within the larger treatment field, electrotherapy, which uses stronger electrical currents for pain reduction. Nearly all U.S. chiropractic offices, physical therapy clinics, and hospital rehabilitation departments employ some form of electrotherapy for pain control, such as ultrasound or the well-known TENS (transcutaneous electrical nerve stimulation).

TENS works by applying constant electrical stimulation to a painful

A Quick Overview of Magnet Basics

All magnets have two poles: positive (or S for south, usually marked in red) and negative (or N for north, usually marked in green). If you are using magnets for therapeutic purposes, be sure to only use magnets that are specifically designed for this purpose. Do not substitute refrigerator or commercial magnets. Negative magnetic energy normalizes and calms systems of the human body, while positive magnetic energy overstimulates or disrupts the biological system. For this reason, negative poles are most frequently directed toward the body. Do not apply positive magnetic poles directly to the body unless under medical supervision.

The most common types of magnets used in magnetic therapy are ceramic and neodymium (a rare-earth element) mixed with iron to increase the magnet's strength or the duration of magnetic charge. The most powerful (and expensive) magnets are neodymium, while ceramic magnets are less expensive but still keep their charge for many years. These types of magnetic materials are incorporated into various types of products available at health food stores or through mail-order catalogs. Ceramic and neodymium magnets are available as wrist and back supports, seat pads, strips worn inside shoes, and plastiform strips that attach to the skin via an elastic adhesive. Magnetic blankets and mattress pads for promoting sleep and reducing stress are also available, however, we recommend you limit the use of magnetic therapy to one to two hours per day. We do not recommend sleeping on a magnetic pad for a full night's sleep.

The strength of a magnet is measured in gauss units (which measure the intensity of magnetic flux). Every magnetic device has a manufacturer's gauss rating; however, the actual strength of the magnet at the skin surface is often much less than this number. For example, a 4,000-gauss magnet transmits about 1,200 gauss to the patient. Magnets placed in pillows or bed pads will render even lower amounts of field strength at the skin surface, because a magnet's strength quickly decreases with the distance from the subject. The strength of the magnet also depends on its size and thickness. Therapeutic magnets use from 200 gauss to 1,500 gauss (only a fraction of what an MRI machine emits), while a common refrigerator magnet emits 10 gauss.[9]

---

area of the body. By stimulating certain nerves, TENS reduces the neural transmission of pain and produces large amounts of endorphins (natural opiates that block the transmission of pain messages between the brain and the extremities). There are two types of nerve fibers in the arms, legs, and thorax: nerve fibers with a large diameter that tend to inhibit pain transmission and prevent pain, and nerve fibers with small diameters that tend to facilitate transmission of pain. The application of electrical stimulus to painful areas causes the large-diameter nerves (pain inhibitors) to override the small-diameter nerves (pain transmitters), resulting in reduced sensations of pain.

Magnet Therapy. Magnetic fields exist everywhere: emanating from the earth, from changes in the weather, and even from the human body. The

Maintain a Healthy Posture

The way you hold your body when sitting, sleeping, or standing can affect breathing, energy use, movement of muscles and joints, and circulation of blood and lymph fluid. Poor or imbalanced posture requires a lot of energy to maintain and interferes with circulation. It also contributes to muscle and joint tension, creating the foundation for the development or exacerbation of arthritic changes in the joints. Chiropractic and Rolfing (see pages 312–314) are two of the many alternative health therapies that correct poor posture and internal imbalance. Here are a few guidelines for correcting posture and reducing muscle tension.

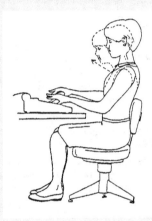

Sitting: When you sit properly, with your spine erect, pelvis centered, and the weight of your upper body supported by your pelvis, your body is actually at rest. Sit toward the front of your chair. Place your feet flat on the floor, parallel and hip-width apart, with your knees in line with your hips.[10] Sit erect, with your chest pointing slightly upward and your head and shoulders level. Don't slump or hold your head, neck, or shoulders forward. Choose a chair with an unyielding straight back and an adjustable seat. Don't look down at your work by moving your head, neck, and shoulders forward. Move only your head and keep the rest of your body still. Take deep breaths, soften your gaze, and release the tension in your jaw and mouth. When reading, place a pillow under your arms to alleviate stress on your neck, shoulders, and low back. Reading material should be at eye level.

use of magnetic devices to generate controlled magnetic fields has proven to be an effective diagnostic tool (magnetic resonance imaging, or MRI, is one example); it also provides beneficial therapies for rheumatoid disease, inflammation, cancer, circulatory problems, and other illnesses. Magnetic therapy can influence the flow of varying electrical currents (normally present in all organisms) that govern the nervous system and other biological systems. Controlled use of magnetic fields can improve arthritic conditions by increasing blood flow and providing more oxygen to the cells, relieving and even stopping pain, reducing inflammation and fluid retention, inhibiting microorganisms, and dissolving fat and calcium deposits.

Standing: Hold your chest slightly up and forward and keep your head and shoulders level. This posture may be strenuous at first, but continue practicing it without using excessive force. To relieve the stress on weight-bearing joints, stand with your knees bent or with one foot elevated (on a box or stool).

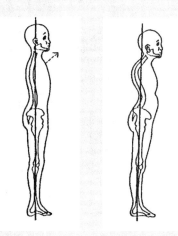

Sleeping: Sleep on your back or side, not on your stomach. Support your neck by using a specialized neck pillow (consult with a physical therapist about the correct position). When sleeping on your back, support your lower back by placing a pillow under your knees. When sleeping on your side, use a pillow under your upper arm and between your knees.

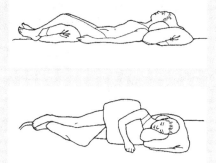

Using magnet to reduce swelling due to inflammation or fluid retention: Place the magnet directly on the swollen area for about an hour. After you feel a slight reduction in pain, move the magnet 2 to 3 inches toward the heart. Leave the magnet at the new location for an hour or until you experience further pain reduction. Negative magnetic energy has a pulling effect on fluids, actually drawing them away from the swollen area toward the heart, where excess fluids can be eliminated from the body. Removing these excess fluids also reduces pain.

Using magnet to dissolve calcium deposits: The body attempts to cushion injured joints by placing calcium around the injured area. These deposits

There are conflicting methods of naming the magnetic poles. To be effective, magnets need to be marked correctly, so be sure to use magnets marked according to the Davis-Rawls system (developed by Dr. Albert Roy Davis in 1936). Avoid touching the sides of thick, therapeutic magnets and never use magnets with holes in the middle. Keep magnets one to two feet away from your computer, audiotapes, videotapes, computer disks, credit cards, and the like. People with cancer, candida, or any infection—viral or bacterial—should avoid exposure to bipolar magnets. Don't use magnets on your chest if you have a pacemaker; a pregnant woman should not use magnets on her abdomen. Don't use magnetic beds for longer than 8 to 10 hours a day. For long-term results, use magnets at night and supplement during the day. It is best to use magnets under the guidance and supervision of a health-care professional.

can be broken down with the application of magnets, but doing so requires six weeks to six months of treatment, depending on magnet strength and the severity of the condition. Once the calcium deposits are removed, flexibility returns to the joints and further healing can take place.[11]

Sample Treatment Protocols for Arthritis

The following protocols are meant to serve as general guidelines for each type of arthritis. More specific and detailed information on diet, supplements, exercise, and other topics is provided in the appropriate chapters in this book. Evaluation by a qualified health-care practitioner is always recommended as a first step in the treatment of arthritis. Tests and other diagnostic tools can then be used to design an individual therapeutic program, monitor its effectiveness, and modify it as needed.

Osteoarthritis

Step One: Natural Pain Management

Since pain is a complex interaction of physical, perceptual, cognitive, emotional, environmental, and other factors, a great deal can be done to alleviate pain due to arthritis. In order to wean yourself off synthetic drugs, or to use far less toxic natural remedies, it is important to begin

 Allopathic medication cannot and should not be discontinued rapidly without medical supervision. Have your physician diagnose and correct as many of the underlying factors contributing to your condition as possible. Also note that vitamins, minerals, herbs, and other nutritional supplements often have potential interactions with pharmaceutical drugs. They may decrease the activity of the drug or increase the activity of the drug. Both situations may warrant a change in the amount of the prescription drug that should be used. Consult with your health-care provider before using any nutritional supplements if you are taking prescription drugs.

to use alternative therapies to dampen your pain and inflammation. It's often necessary to use conventional drugs along with natural therapies and supplements in the early stages of treatment, carefully shifting in favor of the nontoxic approach as time goes on (if possible). This is usually the first step in OA treatment.

1. For pain relief, take the following supplements daily.

- Adrenal cortex glandular extract: Dosage depends on brand and whether liquid or capsule. DHEA or pregnenolone can also be substituted, but use only under supervision; monitor via blood tests.
- Adrenal tonics, such as rehmannia and *Glycyrrhiza glabra* (monitor blood pressure and increase potassium), as well as appropriate tonic herbs (that is, standardized ashwaghandha or eleuthero) and nervine herbs (*Passiflora*, *Scutellaria*) to rebuild the adrenal function.
- Multivitamin-multimineral (without iron or copper if pain or inflammation is high).
- Vitamin E (mixed tocopherols with tocotrienols): 1,000–3,000 IU daily in divided doses with meals.
- Vitamin K_1 (phytonadione from plant sources): 20–40 mg.
- Selenium: 400–1,000 mcg daily in divided doses with meals.
- EPA/DHA (omega-3 essential fatty acids): 3–5 grams daily in divided doses.
- MSM (methylsulfonylmethane): 250 mg, four times daily.
- SAMe (S-adenosylmethionine): 500 mg, three times daily.
- DL-phenylalanine: 6 grams daily, in divided doses on an empty stomach, no later than 5 P.M. Double the dose in 3 weeks if no relief seen. **Warning**: Patients with phenylketenuria should not take this supplement.
- Proanthocyanidins (may be labeled PCOs or OPCs): 3 mg per pound body weight/per day in divided doses with meals.
- Lipoic acid: 250 mg daily in divided doses.
- *Glycyrrhiza glabra* (licorice) solid extract 6:1: ¼ teaspoon, three to four times daily. Use this dosage only if your blood pressure and potassium levels are being monitored by a physician or practitioner trained in botanical medicine.
- Proteolytic enzymes with bromelain: Several tablets between meals.

2. Use a high-quality standardized oral botanical anti-inflammatory and analgesic formula and a topical botanical analgesic simultaneously. We recommend the following herbs for the oral formula, in singles and/or a combination of products. All of these are not necessarily needed at once.

- Standardized *Salix alba* or *Salix* spp. (white willow stem bark: minimum of 240 mg salicin daily.
- *Boswellia serrata* (boswellia): 400 mg of boswellic acids daily.
- *Tanacetum parthenium* (feverfew) 6:1: 4 mg parthenolides daily.
- *Corydalis ambigua* 5:1: 1,500 mg daily.
- Kava: Use a solvent-free water extraction of active kavalactones from *Piper methysticum* to reduce strain on liver.
- *Zingiber officinale* (ginger root) 5:1: 1,000 mg daily.
- *Angelica* spp. (*du huo*) 4:1: 800–1,000 mg daily.
- *Cimicifuga racemosa* (black cohosh).
- *Piscidia erythrina* (Jamaican dogwood) 5:1.
- *Uncaria tomentosa* (cat's claw) 5:1.
- *Harpagophytum procumbens* (devil's claw).
- *Guaicum officinale* (lignum vitae root).
- *Dipsacus japonicus* (teasel root): 6 grams daily as a standardized, freeze-dried decoction.
- *Valeriana officinalis* (valerian) 8:1.
- Bromelain from pineapple (2,400 MCU/gram): 1,000 mg daily on an empty stomach.
- *Curcuma longa* (turmeric) extract (standardized to contain 97% curcumin): 150 mg augmented with piperine from black pepper, four times daily on an empty stomach.
- Chinese patent formulas: Yan Hu Suo Zhi Tong Pian, Du Zhong Hu Gu Wan, Yun Nan Feng Shi Ling, and Feng Shi Xiao Tong Wan.

3. Topical botanical formulas, in the form of salve, cream, gel, or liniment, should be massaged into the inflamed joint, muscle, or ligament at least four times daily. These formulas should include combinations of the following botanicals: menthol (*Mentha* spp.), camphor (*Cinnamomum camphora*), frankincense, myrrh, boswellia, cloves, allspice, prepared aconite, ginger, cinnamon, wintergreen

(methyl salicylate), capsicum, arnica, rue, *Erythrina variegata*, and *Dipsacus japonicus*. **Note:** You may have to avoid these phenolic, strong-smelling topical medicines if you're actively taking a homeopathic remedy, as they may cancel out or interfere with the effects of the remedy.

Homeopathic salves can greatly relieve muscle and joint pains but must be applied frequently. The following ingredients are commonly used in homeopathic pain preparations, as both oral and topical applications (they are usually found at 3X to 6X potencies): *Arnica montana, Rhus toxicodendron, Bryonia alba, Ruta graveolens, Aconitum napellus, Chamomilla, Belladonna, Symphytum officinale, Bellis perennis, Calendula officinalis, Cuprum, Echinacea angustifolia, Echinacea* spp., *Hamamelis virginiana, Hypericum perforatum, Millefolium, Hepar sulphuris calcareum, Colocynthis, Guaiacum, Ledum palustre, Colchicum, Dulcamara, Magnesium Phosphoricum, Ferrum phosphoricum, Causticum, Rhododendron, Mercurius solubilis*, and many others.

4. Follow the arthritis diet. After pharmaceutical medications are discontinued, follow the fasting procedure outlined in this book (see "Fasting" in chapter 4, pages 79–87). Continue to take your natural pain supplements during your fast. You can expect pain to begin to diminish around the fourth day. **Precautions:** Some allopathic medicine can cause severe damage to the gastrointestinal system when taken on an empty stomach. Since fasting necessitates the restriction of all solid food, it cannot be accomplished while using NSAIDs, prednisone, and other drugs, which must be taken with food.

5. Use contrast hydrotherapy several times daily to assist in pain relief.

6. Ice massage: See "Ice Packs" in chapter 14, pages 309–311, for instructions on how to do ice massage.

7. Use acupuncture and electrical stimulation (such as TENS) to increase endogenous endorphins.

8. Use mind-body therapies for pain, such as stress management techniques, meditation, hypnosis, relaxation, guided imagery, biofeedback, and cognitive therapy.

9. Get regular physical medicine from a naturopath, chiropractor, osteopath, or physiatrist, such as soft tissue and osseous manipulation, gait and postural analysis, or orthotic treatment. See a physical therapist, massage therapist, Rolfer, Feldenkrais proactitioner, or Alexander practitioner for postural integration and trigger point evaluation or regular treatment. (Other physical medicine techniques

for pain include ultrasound, moist heat, strain-counterstrain stretching, interferential therapy, diathermy, and needle-free trigger point release.)

10. Stretching and strengthening are critical for providing support to weakened or damaged joints.

Step Two: Detoxification

Undergo standard tests, especially diagnostic imaging of the joints. See a health-care practitioner to determine your digestive capacity, food allergies,

 Use the appropriate homeopathic remedies for pain, based on individual signs and symptoms. For more on **selecting homeopathic remedies for pain relief**, see chapter 13, Supplements for Arthritis, pp. 257–294. For more on **massage and other physical therapies**, see chapter 14, Exercises and Physical Therapies, pp. 295–320. For **mind-body therapies**, see chapter 11, Mind-Body Approaches to Arthritis, pp. 200–224. For more information on **TENS and other physical therapies**, see chapter 14, Exercises and Physical Therapies, pages 295–320.

intestinal permeability, adrenal and thyroid status, and colonic microflora. Follow therapies discussed in this book to correct imbalances. Use lymphatic drainage remedies, fasting, and other detoxification procedures to detoxify the body four times per year.

Step Three: Cartilage Rebuilding

The following program of supplements and nutritional support helps rebuild cartilage.

- Glucosamine: 1,500–3,000 mg daily in divided doses on an empty stomach.
- Collagen-building amino acids, vitamins, and related amino sugars (L-glycine, L-glutamine, L-proline, vitamin C to bowel tolerance, N-acetylglucosamine (NAG), N-acetylcysteine): Several grams of each daily on an empty stomach.
- Chondroitin polysulfates (maximum 8%–10% absorption).
- Sea cucumber extract: 50 mg daily.
- Hydrolyzed organic cartilage (bovine, deer antler, shark): 1,000–4,000 mg daily depending on the product used. Check label dosage.
- Cetyl myristoleate: 30 mg daily.
- Undenatured type II collagen from chicken sternum cartilage: 200–500 mg daily.
- Hyaluronic acid: 5 mg daily

 If you have severe OA and have 85% or more cartilage destruction, consult with an orthopedic physician who is knowledgeable on the use of injectable hyaluronic acid preparations.

- *Crataegus* spp. (hawthorn) solid extract 6:1: ¼ teaspoon, three to four times daily
- Bioflavonoids: Consume several cups daily of blueberries, blackberries, black cherries, acerola cherries, or hawthorn berries. (You can puree any of these fruits, or a combination of them, and mix with organic gelatin. Drink as is, or refrigerate until firm to make joint-healthy snack.)
- Multiple bioflavonoid complex supplement (containing grape seed polyphenols, green tea, hawthorn berry, mixed citrus bioflavonoids, acerola cherries, gotu kola extracts, amla (Indian gooseberries), and/or quercetin).

Step Four: Stabilization

1. Consult with a physician trained in physical medicine, manipulation, and restoration of proper biomechanics to restore normal range of motion of your joints, attain muscular balance, correct posture or flat feet, correct ergonomic issues, strengthen weak muscles, and stretch short muscles.

2. Get 45 minutes of exercise four times per week. Especially useful are yoga, tai chi, and aquatic exercises. Perform regular stretching and muscle strengthening.

3. Maintain all of the above therapies in steps 1 through 4 until you're 90% pain free for one month. When you're no longer in pain, decrease dosages or discontinue all herbs for pain and DL-phenylalanine but continue taking all other supplements. Continue with physical medicine therapies but adjust them to your individual needs and schedule.

4. Attain a desirable weight for your height and an optimum percentage of body fat, as obesity worsens OA.

5. Seek advice from your alternative health-care practitioner to individualize your program as you become increasingly well.

6 . If your joints are so damaged that you don't achieve sufficient relief through this program, nontoxic injection therapy into the synovium with homeopathic remedies, growth factors, or stem cells may be warranted before joint replacements are performed.

Autoimmune Arthritis

This protocol is effective for RA, ankylosing spondylitis, systemic lupus erythematosus, juvenile RA, and other autoimmune problems.

Step One: Natural Pain Management

Since pain is a complex interaction of physical, perceptual, cognitive, emotional, environmental, and other factors, a great deal can be done to alleviate pain due to arthritis. In order to wean yourself off synthetic drugs, it is important to begin to use alternative therapies to dampen the amount of pain and inflammation. It's often necessary to use conventional drugs along with natural therapies and supplements in the early stages of treatment, carefully shifting in favor of the nontoxic approach as time goes on (if possible).

1. For pain relief, take the following supplements daily.

   - Adrenal cortex glandular extract: Dosage depends on brand and whether liquid or capsule. DHEA or pregnenolone can be substituted, but use only under supervision and monitor via blood tests.

   - Adrenal tonics such as rehmannia and *Glycyrrhiza glabra* (monitor blood pressure and increase potassium), as well as appropriate tonic herbs (that is, standardized ashwaghandha or eleuthero) and nervine herbs (*Scutellaria*) to rebuild the adrenal function.

   - Multivitamin-multimineral (without iron or copper if pain or inflammation is high).

   - Vitamin E (mixed tocopherols with tocotrienols): 1,000–3,000 IU daily in divided doses with meals.

   - Vitamin K_1 (phytonadione from plant sources): 20–40 mg.

   - Selenium: 400–1,000 mcg daily in divided doses with meals.

 CAUTION Allopathic medication cannot and should not be discontinued rapidly without medical supervision. Have your physician diagnose and correct as many of the underlying factors contributing to your condition as possible. Also note that vitamins, minerals, herbs, and other nutritional supplements often have potential interactions with pharmaceutical drugs. They may decrease the activity of the drug or increase the activity of the drug. Both situations may warrant a change in the amount of the prescription drug that should be used. Consult with your health-care provider before using any nutritional supplements if you are taking prescription drugs.

- EPA/DHA (omega-3 essential fatty acids): 3–5 grams daily in divided doses.
- MSM (methylsulfonylmethane): 250 mg, four times daily.
- SAMe (S-adenosylmethionine): 500 mg, three times daily.
- DL-phenylalanine: 4–6 grams daily, in divided doses on an empty stomach, no later than 5 P.M. Double the dose in three weeks if no relief seen. **Warning:** Patients with phenylketenuria should not take this supplement.
- Proanthocyanidins (may be labeled PCOs or OPCs): 3 mg per pound body weight/per day in divided doses with meals.
- Lipoic acid: 250 mg daily in divided doses.
- *Glycyrrhiza glabra* (licorice) solid extract 6:1: ¼ teaspoon, three to four times daily. Use at this dose only if your blood pressure and potassium levels are being monitored by a physician or practitioner trained in botanical medicine.
- Proteolytic enzymes: Several tablets between meals.

2. Use a high-quality standardized oral botanical anti-inflammatory and analgesic formula and a topical botanical analgesic simultaneously. We recommend the following herbs for the oral formula, in singles and/or a combination of products. All of these are not necessarily needed at once.

- Standardized *Salix alba* or *Salix* spp. (white willow stem bark): minimum of 240 mg salicin daily.
- *Boswellia serrata* (boswellia): 400 mg of boswellic acids daily.
- *Tanacetum parthenium* (feverfew) 6:1: 4 mg parthenolides daily.
- *Corydalis ambigua* 5:1: 1,500 mg daily.
- Kava: Use a solvent-free water extraction of active kavalactones from *Piper methysticum* to reduce strain on liver.
- *Zingiber officinale* (ginger root) 5:1: 1,000 mg daily.
- *Angelica* spp. (*du huo*) 4:1: 800–1,000 mg daily.
- *Cimicifuga racemosa* (black cohosh).
- *Piscidia erythrina* (Jamaican dogwood) 5:1.
- *Uncaria tomentosa* (cat's claw) 5:1.
- *Harpagophytum procumbens* (devil's claw).
- *Guaicum officinale* (lignum vitae root).

- *Dipsacus japonicus* (root): 6 grams daily as a standardized, freeze-dried decoction.
- *Valeriana officinalis* (valerian) 8:1.
- Bromelain from pineapple (2,400 GDU/gram): 1,000 mg daily on an empty stomach.
- *Curcuma longa* (turmeric) extract (standardized to contain 97% curcumin): 150 mg augmented with piperine from black pepper, four times daily on an empty stomach.
- Chinese patent formulas: Yan Hu Suo Zhi Tong Pian, Du Zhong Hu Gu Wan, Yun Nan Feng Shi Ling, and Feng Shi Xiao Tong Wan.

3. Topical botanical formulas, in the form of salve, cream, gel, or liniment, should be massaged into the inflamed joint, muscle, or ligament at least four times daily. These formulas should include combinations of the following botanicals: menthol (*Mentha* spp.), camphor (*Cinnamomum camphora*), frankincense, myrrh, boswellia, cloves, allspice, prepared aconite, ginger, cinnamon, wintergreen (methyl salicylate), capsicum, arnica, rue, *Erythrina variegata*, and *Dipsacus japonicus*. **Note:** You may have to avoid these phenolic, strong-smelling topical medicines if you're actively taking a homeopathic remedy, as they may cancel out or interfere with the effects of the remedy.

   Homeopathic salves can greatly relieve muscle and joint pains but must be applied frequently. The following ingredients are commonly used in homeopathic pain preparations, as both oral and topical applications (they are usually found 3X to 6X potencies): *Arnica montana, Rhus toxicodendron, Bryonia alba, Ruta graveolens, Aconitum napellus, Chamomilla, Belladonna, Symphytum officinale, Bellis perennis, Calendula officinalis, Cuprum, Echinacea angustifolia, Echinacea* spp., *Hamamelis virginiana, Hypericum perforatum, Millefolium, Hepar sulphuris calcareum, Colocynthis, Guaiacum, Ledum palustre, Colchicum, Dulcamara, Magnesium Phosphoricum, Ferrum phosphoricum, Causticum, Rhododendron, Mercurius solubilis*, and many others.

4. Follow the arthritis diet. After pharmaceutical medications are discontinued, follow the fasting procedure outlined in this book (see "Fasting" in chapter 4, pages 79–87). Continue to take your natural pain supplements during your fast. You can expect pain to begin to diminish around the fourth day. **Precautions:** Some allopathic medicine can cause severe damage to the gastrointestinal system when

taken on an empty stomach. Since fasting necessitates the restriction of all solid food, it cannot be accomplished while using NSAIDs, prednisone, and other drugs, which must be taken with food.

5. Use contrast hydrotherapy several times daily to assist in pain relief.

6. Ice massage: See "Ice Packs" in chapter 14, pages 309–311, for instructions on how to do ice massage.

7. Use acupuncture and electrical stimulation (such as TENS) to increase endogenous endorphins.

8. Use mind-body therapies for pain, such as stress management techniques, meditation, hypnosis, relaxation, guided imagery, biofeedback, and cognitive therapy.

9. Get regular physical medicine from a naturopath, chiropractor, osteopath, physiatrist, or conventional doctor, such as soft tissue and osseous manipulation, gait and postural analysis, or orthotic treatment. See a physical therapist, massage therapist, Rolfer, Feldenkrais proactitioner, or Alexander practitioner for postural integration and trigger point evaluation or regular treatment. (Other physical medicine techniques for pain include ultrasound, moist heat, strain-counterstrain stretching, interferential therapy, diathermy, and needle-free trigger point release.)

 Use the appropriate homeopathic remedies for pain, based on individual signs and symptoms. For more on **selecting homeopathic remedies and other supplements for pain relief**, see chapter 13, Supplements for Arthritis, pp. 257–294.

10. Stretching and strengthening are critical for providing support to weakened or damaged joints.

Step Two: Detoxification

Undergo standard tests, especially diagnostic imaging of the joints. See a health-care practitioner to determine your digestive capacity, food allergies, intestinal permeability, adrenal and thyroid status, and colonic microflora. Follow therapies discussed in this book to correct imbalances. Use lymphatic drainage remedies, fasting, and other detoxification procedures to detoxify the body four times per year.

Step Three: Cartilage Rebuilding

The following program of supplements and nutritional support helps rebuild cartilage.

- Glucosamine: 1,500–3,000 mg daily in divided doses on an empty stomach.
- Collagen-building amino acids, vitamins, and related amino sugars (L-glycine, L-glutamine, L-proline, vitamin C to bowel tolerance, N-acetylglucosamine (NAG), N-acetylcysteine): Several grams of each daily on an empty stomach.
- Chondroitin polysulfates (maximum 8%–10% absorption).
- Sea cucumber extract: 50 mg daily.
- Hydrolyzed organic cartilage (bovine, deer antler, shark): 1,000–4,000 mg daily depending on the product used. Check label dosage.
- Cetyl myristoleate: 30 mg daily.
- Undenatured type II collagen from chicken sternum cartilage: 200–500 mg daily.
- Hyaluronic acid: 5 mg daily
- *Crataegus* spp. (hawthorn) solid extract 6:1: 1/4 teaspoon, 3–4 times daily
- Bioflavonoids: Consume several cups daily of blueberries, black-berries, black cherries, acerola cherries, or hawthorn berries. (You can puree any of these fruits, or a combination of them, and mix with organic gelatin. Drink as is, or refrigerate until firm to make joint-healthy snack.)
- Multiple bioflavonoid complex supplement (containing grape seed polyphenols, green tea, hawthorn berry, mixed citrus bioflavonoids, acerola cherries, gotu kola extracts, amla (Indian gooseberries), and/or quercetin).

Step Four: Desensitizing Autoimmunity

1. Have your physician prepare an oral auto-sanguis nosode (take 15 drops, three times daily between meals). Use injectable auto-sanguis therapy from your doctor.
2. Consider urine therapy.
3. Consider one or several of the following herbs and supplements:
   - *Hemidesmus indicus* 1:2: 1 teaspoon, three to four times daily.
   - MSM (methylsulfonylmethane): 3,000 mg daily in divided doses.
   - *Ganoderma* supercritical CO_2 extract: 12 ml daily 1:2 fluid extract (or 2–6 grams daily of the raw herb).

- Rehmannia: 2–6 grams daily of raw herb or 12 ml daily 1:2 fluid extract.
- Standardized nettle leaf: 1 gram daily.
- DHEA (or its precursor pregnenolone): Use per your physician's instructions of physician and based on lab tests; doses vary.
- EPA/DHA (omega-3 essential fatty acids): 3–5 grams daily in divided doses.
- *Glycyrrhiza glabra* (licorice) solid extract 6:1: 1/4 teaspoon, three times daily. Include several grams of potassium with that dose to avoid water retention.
- *Stephania tetrandra*: 2–10 grams daily of raw herb or 12 ml daily 1:2 fluid extract.
- Smilax solid extract: 1/2 teaspoon, two times daily.
- *Tripterygium wilfordii* : 15–30 ml of the tincture in divided doses. Or use Leigongteng Pian: 1–2 tablets two to three times daily. Use this herb only if you're unresponsive to other therapies and only under the supervision of a health-care practitioner trained in traditional Chinese medicine.

Step Five: Stabilization

1. Consult with a physician trained in physical medicine, manipulation, and restoration of proper biomechanics to restore normal range of motion of your joints, attain muscular balance, correct posture or flat feet, correct ergonomic issues, strengthen weak muscles, and stretch short muscles.

2. Get 45 minutes of exercise four times per week. Especially useful are yoga, tai chi, and aquatic exercises. Perform regular stretching and muscle strengthening.

3. Maintain all of the above therapies in steps 1 through 4 until you're 90% pain free for one month. When you're no longer in pain, discontinue all herbs for pain and DL-phenylalanine but continue taking all other supplements. Continue with physical medicine therapies but adjust them to your individual needs and schedule.

4. Attain a desirable weight for your height and an optimum percentage of body fat, as obesity worsens all forms of arthritis.

5. Seek advice from your alternative health-care practitioner to individualize your program as you become increasingly well.

6. If your joints are so damaged that you don't achieve sufficient relief through this program, nontoxic injection therapy into the synovium with homeopathic remedies, growth factors, or stem cells may be warranted before joint replacements are performed.

Gout

1. Take the following supplements daily.

   - Multivitamin-multimineral (low potency, with no more than 100 mg of vitamin C).
   - Folic acid: 10 mg daily during an acute gout attack.
   - Omega-3 oils: 3 tablespoons.
   - Bioflavonoids: Take a high-potency bioflavonoid supplement at least 5,000 mg two times daily.
   - Quercetin: 600 mg, three times daily. Combine quercetin with bromelain for an increased anti-inflammatory effect.
   - Reduce your intake of vitamin C and niacin (vitamin B_3), and stop taking these supplements completely during an acute gout attack, as they increase blood acidity levels and precipitate uric acid crystallization. Continue with low-level supplementation (levels typically found in a high-quality multivitamin) when the acute attack is over.

2. Follow the arthritis diet and drink lots of fresh vegetable juices during gout attacks.

3. Eat ½ pound of fresh organic cherries, blueberries, and hawthorn berries daily. These fruits contain flavonoid components that block the enzyme that increases uric acid. No uric acid buildup means no

 CAUTION Allopathic medication cannot and should not be discontinued rapidly without medical supervision. Have your physician diagnose and correct as many of the underlying factors contributing to your condition as possible. Also note that vitamins, minerals, herbs, and other nutritional supplements often have potential interactions with pharmaceutical drugs. They may decrease the activity of the drug or increase the activity of the drug. Both situations may warrant a change in the amount of the prescription drug that should be used. Consult with your health-care provider before using any nutritional supplements if you are taking prescription drugs.

gout attack. Use potent concentration of flavonoids to support the joints.

4. Avoid eating the following purine-rich foods: Most beans (including soy products) and all animal products (including meats—especially liver and other organ meats, sausages and other processed meats, anchovies, crab, and shrimp—milk, and eggs).

5. Drink 2 to 3 quarts of filtered water daily to help keep the urine diluted and to flush out uric acid crystals.

6. Stop all consumption of alcohol, especially beer. Alcohol increases purine production in the body and makes the blood more acidic. This starts the crystallization process.

7. Lose weight, as obesity is positively correlated with gout. Make a commitment to remaining on the arthritis diet and not falling back into unhealthy eating practices, which induce gout in those who are susceptible to it.

8. Have a health-care practitioner determine your digestive capacity, intestinal permeability, and whether you have a healthy balance of colon microflora. Follow the therapies detailed in this book to correct imbalances in these areas.

9. Use contrast hydrotherapy several times daily to induce a pumping action and flush the afflicted joints with blood and lymphatic fluid, thereby removing uric acid crystals. Continue hydrotherapy indefinitely (once or twice daily) even when not in an acute phase of gout.

10. For pain and inflammation, follow the advice offered in the other arthritis protocols in this appendix.

11. Cleanse your tissues of toxins and uric acid on a regular basis using the detoxification methods outlined in chapters 4 and 5.

12. Get checked for heavy metal toxicity (especially lead) and follow the advice of your alternative health-care practitioner for detoxification.

Psoriatic Arthritis

1. Take the following supplements daily.
   - Copper-free multivitamin-multimineral supplement.
   - Vitamin E: 800 IU.
   - Selenium: 200–600 mcg.
   - Zinc: 50–100 mg. Also use zinc ointment on skin lesions.

- EPA/DHA omega-3 oils: 3 tablespoons.
- Flaxseed oil: 1 tablespoon, five times a day.
- Glutathione: 200 mg.
- Bromelain: 2,000 mg.
- Sulfur, in the form of MSM: 2–3 grams daily.
- Folic acid: 5–10 mg daily.
- Pancreatic enzymes to support digestion: two to three, or as needed, with meals.
- Bitter tincture: ½ teaspoon in water 30 minutes before meals.
- N-acetylcysteine: 2 grams daily.

2. Pursue a fasting program consisting of an initial preparation period of juices and "green" drinks, followed by a supervised fast, and ending with a repetition of juices and green drinks.

3. Concentrate your detoxification therapy on colon cleansing and liver support. Detoxify copper and correct ratios of copper to zinc, copper to selenium, and copper to sulfur. Use detoxification herbs and protocols specific for the liver and colon (see chapter 5, pages 93–102). Detox toxic metals if warranted.

4. Have a health-care practitioner determine your digestive capacity, intestinal permeability, and whether you have a healthy balance of colon microflora. Follow the therapies detailed in this book to correct imbalances in these areas. Consume enough fiber daily to maintain colon health.

5. Massage sesame oil into your skin prior to a daily shower.

6. Get plenty of sunshine and go swimming in the ocean. Folkloric traditional medicine recommends this old time remedy, and our patients have confirmed its effectiveness. Avoid overexposure to the sun by limiting time to 20 minutes.

7. Use massage therapy, deep tissue work, neuromuscular therapy, or other physical therapies to facilitate lymphatic drainage of toxins. Use ultrasound over afflicted joints two to three times per week to provide relief. Provide optimum nutrition to the joints.

8. Use stress-management techniques, such as guided imagery, flotation therapy, biofeedback, visualization, and other mind-body therapies.

9. Eat a well-balanced vegan diet (no animal products, including eggs and dairy products, and especially no meat or shellfish) with plenty

of organic nuts, legumes, grains, fruits, and vegetables. Some wild cold-water fish is acceptable. However, avoid all beets, radishes, onions, lentils, spinach, and nightshades (tomatoes, peppers, eggplant, and potatoes), as they aggravate psoriasis.

10. To reduce psoriasis outbreaks, take plant-based antimicrobial herbs to reduce the pathogenic bacterial overgrowth in the colon. Detoxify the body and support the liver and adrenal glands as well as anti-inflammatory systems, and heal leaky gut syndrome (see chapter 8, page 140). Also, include the herbs *Coleus forskohlii*, *Momordica charantia* (Bitter melon), and *Smilax* spp. (sarsaparilla), which are used to help stop the skin lesions from enlarging. Use standardized or solid extracts when available.

11. Apply fresh parsley juice or essential oil of bergamot mixed into an almond oil base to psoriatic lesions before sunbathing to reduce the severity of lesions. But avoid excessive exposure, as these remedies may increase photosensitivity. For pain, utilize the suggestions listed under the other types of arthritis, both orally and topically as needed.

Infectious Arthritis and Lyme Disease

Step One: Natural Pain Management

Since pain is a complex interaction of physical, perceptual, cognitive, emotional, environmental, and other factors, a great deal can be done to alleviate pain due to arthritis. In order to wean yourself off synthetic drugs, it is important to begin to use alternative therapies to dampen the amount of pain and inflammation. It's often necessary to use conventional drugs along with natural therapies and supplements in the early stages of treatment, carefully shifting in favor of the nontoxic approach

 CAUTION Allopathic medication cannot and should not be discontinued rapidly without medical supervision. Have your physician diagnose and correct as many of the underlying factors contributing to your condition as possible. Also note that vitamins, minerals, herbs, and other nutritional supplements often have potential interactions with pharmaceutical drugs. They may decrease the activity of the drug or increase the activity of the drug. Both situations may warrant a change in the amount of the prescription drug that should be used. Consult with your health-care provider before using any nutritional supplements if you are taking prescription drugs.

as time goes on (if possible). This is usually the first step in infectious arthritis treatment.

1. For pain relief, take the following supplements daily.

   - Adrenal cortex glandular extract: Dosage depends on brand and whether liquid or capsule. DHEA or pregnenolone should be used only under supervision and monitored via blood tests.

   - Adrenal tonics, such as rehmannia and *Glycyrrhiza glabra* (monitor blood pressure and increase potassium), as well as appropriate tonic herbs (that is, standardized ashwaghandha or eleuthero) and nervine herbs (*Passiflora, Scutellaria*) to rebuild the adrenal function.

   - Multivitamin-multimineral (without iron or copper if pain or inflammation is high).

   - Vitamin E (mixed tocopherols with tocotrienols): 1,000–3,000 IU daily in divided doses with meals.

   - Vitamin K_1 (phytonadione from plant sources): 20–40 mg.

   - Selenium: 400–1,000 mcg daily in divided doses with meals.

   - "EPA/DHA (omega-3 essential fatty acids): 3–5 grams daily in divided doses.

   - MSM (methylsulfonylmethane): 250 mg, four times daily.

   - SAMe (S-adenosylmethionine): 500 mg, three times daily.

   - DL-phenylalanine: 4–6 grams daily, in divided doses on an empty stomach, no later than 5 P.M. Double the dose in three weeks if no relief seen. **Warning:** Patients with phenylketenuria should not take this supplement.

   - Proanthocyanidins (may be labeled PCOs or OPCs): 3 mg per pound body weight/per day in divided doses with meals.

   - Lipoic acid: 250 mg daily in divided doses.

   - *Glycyrrhiza glabra* solid extract 6:1: 1/4 teaspoon, three to four times daily. Use at this dose only if your blood pressure and potassium levels are being monitored by a physician or practitioner trained in botanical medicine.

   - Proteolytic enzymes: Several tablets between meals.

2. Use a high-quality standardized oral botanical anti-inflammatory and analgesic formula and a topical botanical analgesic simultaneously. We recommend the following herbs for the oral formula, in singles

and/or a combination of products. All of these are not necessarily needed at once.

- Standardized *Salix alba* or *Salix* /spp. (white willow stem bark) (delivering a minimum of 240 mg salicin daily)
- *Boswellia serrata* (boswellia): 400 mg of boswellic acids daily.
- *Tanacetum parthenium* (feverfew) 6:1: 4 mg parthenolides daily.
- *Corydalis ambigua* 5:1: 1,500 mg daily.
- Kava: Use a solvent-free water extraction of active kavalactones from *Piper methysticum* to reduce strain on liver.
- *Zingiber officinale* (ginger root) 5:1: 1,000 mg daily.
- *Angelica* spp. (*du huo*) 4:1: 800–1,000 mg daily.
- *Cimicifuga racemosa* (black cohosh).
- *Piscidia erythrina* (Jamaican dogwood) 5:1.
- *Uncaria tomentosa* (cat's claw) 5:1.
- *Harpagophytum procumbens* (devil's claw).
- *Guaicum officinale* (lignum vitae root).
- *Dipsacus japonicus* (root): 6 grams daily as a standardized, freeze-dried decoction.
- *Valeriana officinalis* (valerian) 8:1.
- Bromelain from pineapple (2,400 GDU/gram): 1,000 mg daily on an empty stomach.
- *Curcuma longa* (turmeric) extract (standardized to contain 97% curcumin): 150 mg augmented with piperine from black pepper, four times daily on an empty stomach.
- Chinese patent formulas: Yan Hu Suo Zhi Tong Pian, Du Zhong Hu Gu Wan, Yun Nan Feng Shi Ling, and Feng Shi Xiao Tong Wan.

3. Topical botanical formulas, in the form of salve, cream, gel, or liniment, should be massaged into the inflamed joint, muscle, or ligament at least four times daily. These formulas should include combinations of the following botanicals: menthol (*Mentha* spp.), camphor (*Cinnamomum camphora*), frankincense, myrrh, boswellia, cloves, allspice, prepared aconite, ginger, cinnamon, wintergreen (methyl salicylate), capsicum, arnica, rue, *Erythrina variegata*, and *Dipsacus japonicus*. **Note:** You may have to avoid these phenolic, strong-smelling

topical medicines if you're actively taking a homeopathic remedy, as they may cancel out or interfere with the effects of the remedy.

Homeopathic salves can greatly relieve muscle and joint pains but must be applied frequently. The following ingredients are commonly used in homeopathic pain preparations, as both oral and topical applications (they are usually found at 3X to 6X potencies): *Arnica montana, Rhus toxicodendron, Bryonia alba, Ruta graveolens, Aconitum napellus, Chamomilla, Belladonna, Symphytum officinale, Bellis perennis, Calendula officinalis, Cuprum, Echinacea angustifolia, Echinacea* spp., *Hamamelis virginiana, Hypericum perforatum, Millefolium, Hepar sulphuris calcareum, Colocynthis, Guaiacum, Ledum palustre, Colchicum, Dulcamara, Magnesium Phosphoricum, Ferrum phosphoricum, Causticum, Rhododendron, Mercurius solubilis,* and many others.

4. Follow the arthritis diet. After pharmaceutical medications are discontinued, follow the fasting procedure outlined in this book (see "Fasting" in chapter 4, pages 79–87). Continue to take your natural pain supplements during your fast. Your pain should begin to diminish around the fourth day. **Precautions:** Some allopathic medicine can cause severe damage to the gastrointestinal system when taken on an empty stomach. Since fasting necessitates the restriction of all solid food, it cannot be accomplished while using NSAIDs, prednisone, and other drugs, which must be taken with food.

5. Use contrast hydrotherapy several times daily to assist in pain relief.

6. Ice massage: See "Ice Packs" in chapter 14, pages 309–311, for instructions on how to do ice massage.

7. Use acupuncture and electrical stimulation (such as TENS) to increase endogenous endorphins.

 For more information on **TENS and other physical therapies**, see chapter 14, Exercises and Physical Therapies, pages 295–320.

8. Use mind-body therapies for pain, such as stress management techniques, meditation, hypnosis, relaxation, guided imagery, biofeedback, and cognitive therapy.

9. Get regular physical medicine from a naturopath, chiropractor, osteopath, physiatrist, or conventional doctor, such as soft tissue and osseous manipulation, gait and postural analysis, or orthotic treatment. See a physical therapist, massage therapist, Rolfer, Feldenkrais practitioner, or Alexander practitioner for postural integration and trigger point evaluation or regular treatment. (Other physical medicine techniques for pain include ultrasound, moist heat,

strain-counterstrain stretching, interferential therapy, diathermy, and needle-free trigger point release.)

10. Stretching and strengthening are critical for providing support to weakened or damaged joints.

Step Two: Detoxification

1. See your alternative health-care practitioner to undergo testing of your hair, urine, or stool to document heavy metal toxicity, which often causes immunosuppression and hampers mounting an efficient offensive against the Lyme spirochete. Follow their advice for removal of any heavy metal burden. Also consult a health-care practitioner to determine your digestive capacity, food allergies, intestinal permeability, adrenal and thyroid status, and colonic microflora. Follow therapies discussed in this book to correct imbalances. Use lymphatic drainage remedies, fasting, and other detoxification procedures to detoxify the body four times per year.

2. For dysbiosis and infectious arthritis, a stool analysis will direct the physician to the proper therapies. In general, use plant-based antimicrobials.

3. Get two to three colonic hydrotherapy treatments per week for 12 weeks. For the first 8 weeks, use antimicrobial herbs and demulcents in the water. For the last 4 weeks, use lactobacillus and bifidobacterium cultures as an implant. Repeat the stool test to measure results. Repeat the intensive therapy if still positive, or continue with two treatments per month on a maintenance basis if your bowel flora is normalized.

4 . For botanical detoxification of all organs and to support the liver and anti-inflammatory systems use cleansing and tonic herbs, such as dandelion, milk thistle, and other detoxification strategies listed in chapter 5 (page 88). Treat intestinal permeability (see chapter 8, page 149).

5 . Use hyperthermic hydrotherapy: Have a naturopathic physician or other practitioner administer hyperthermia treatments three times per week, making sure to raise the body temperature to a minimum of 103°F for one hour. This will help kill the spirochetes associated with Lyme disease; beware of die-off reactions (the Jarisch-Herxheimer reaction) the day after treatment.

6. Use homeopathic Lyme nosode: 15 drops between meals, four times daily. Under the supervision of a homeopathic practitioner, take

Ledum 200C (1 dose daily for one week), which often arrests the case immediately and halts arthralgia, or have your practitioner prepare a nosode out of your blood or urine.

7. Use *Smilax, Glycyrrhiza, Lonicera, Dipsacus, Taraxacum, Dictamnus,* and *Portulaca*) in freeze-dried tea form (available in many Chinese apothecaries): 6 grams of each. One glass, sipped throughout the day.

8. Use cat's claw: 600 mg, three times daily.

Step Three: Cartilage Rebuilding

The following program of supplements and nutritional support helps rebuild cartilage.

- Glucosamine: 1,500–3,000 mg daily in divided doses on an empty stomach.
- Collagen-building amino acids, vitamins, and related amino sugars (L-glycine, L-glutamine, L-proline, vitamin C to bowel tolerance, N-acetylglucosamine (NAG), N-acetylcysteine): Several grams of each daily on an empty stomach.
- Chondroitin polysulfates (maximum 8%–10% absorption).
- Hydrolyzed organic cartilage (bovine, deer antler, shark), 1,000–4,000 mg daily, depending on the product used. Check label dosage.
- Cetyl myristoleate: 30 mg daily.
- Undenatured type II collagen from chicken sternum cartilage: 2–5 mg daily.
- Hyaluronic acid: 5 mg daily.
- *Crataegus* spp. (hawthorn) solid extract 6:1: 1/4 teaspoon, three to four times daily.
- Bioflavonoids: Consume several cups daily of blueberries, blackberries, black cherries, acerola cherries, or hawthorn berries. (You can puree any of these fruits, or a combination of them, and mix with organic gelatin. Drink as is, or refrigerate until firm to make joint-healthy snack.)
- Multiple bioflavonoid complex supplement (containing grape seed polyphenols, green tea, hawthorn

 For more information on hydrotherapy, see chapter 14, Exercises and Physical Therapies, pages 295–320. For more on tests used for diagnosing the underlying causes of arthritis, see chapter 3, Diagnosing Arthritis, pages 39–65.

berry, mixed citrus bioflavonoids, acerola cherries, gotu kola extracts, amla [Indian gooseberries], and/or quercetin).

Step Four: Stabilization

1. Consult with a physician trained in physical medicine, manipulation, and restoration of proper biomechanics to restore normal range of motion of your joints, attain muscular balance, correct posture or flat feet, correct ergonomic issues, strengthen weak muscles, and stretch short muscles.

2. Get 45 minutes of exercise four times per week. Especially useful are yoga, tai chi, and aquatic exercises. Perform regular stretching and muscle strengthening.

3. Maintain all of the above therapies in steps 1 through 4 until you're 90% pain free for one month. When you're no longer in pain, discontinue all herbs for pain and DL-phenylalanine, but continue taking all other supplements. Continue with physical medicine therapies, but adjust them to your individual needs and schedule.

4. Attain a desirable weight for your height and an optimum percentage of body fat, as obesity worsens all arthritis.

5. Seek advice from your alternative health-care practitioner to individualize your program as you become increasingly well.

6. If your joints are so damaged that you don't achieve sufficient relief through this program, nontoxic injection therapy into the synovium with homeopathic remedies, growth factors, or stem cells may be warranted before joint replacements are performed.

7. Don't consume hot, pungent, spicy, and sour foods. Avoid vinegar and all pickled foods, alcohol, and salt. Limit garlic to a minimum. Avoid all oils except for olive, fish, coconut, flaxseed, hemp seed, and walnut oils. Emphasize cooling spices and herbs, such as cilantro, parsley, dill, mint, fennel coriander, and turmeric.

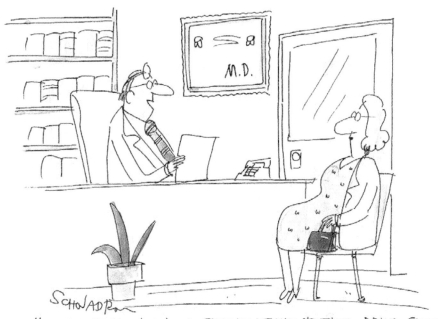

"I'M SENDING YOU TO A SPECIALIST WHO TREATS DRUG-SIDE EFFECTS FROM DRUG SIDE EFFECTS."

Resources

Herbs and Nutritional Supplements

Integrative Therapeutics, 9 Monroe Parkway, Suite 250, Lake Oswego, OR 97035; tel: 800-931-1709; fax: 800-380-8189; www.integrativeinc .com.

Lin Sister Herb Shop, 4 Bowery Street, New York, NY 10013; tel: 212-962-5417; email: linsisterherb@aol.com. Sells traditional Chinese medicine herbs and formulas.

Metagenics, 971 Calle Negocio, San Clemente, CA 92673; tel: 800-692-9400; fax: 714-366-0818; www.metagenics.com. (Available to professionals only.)

Nature's Answer, 75 Commerce Drive, Hauppauge, NY 11788; tel: 800-439-2324 or 631-231-7492; fax: 516-231-8391; www.naturesanswer.com.

Nutricology/Allergy Research Group, P.O. Box 55907, Hayward, CA 94544; tel: 510-487-8526 or 800-782-4274; fax: 510-487-8682; www.nutricology.com.

Pure Encapsulations, 490 Boston Post Road, Sudbury, MA 01776; tel: 800-753-2277 or 508-443-1999; fax: 888-783-2277; www.purecaps. com.

Scientific Botanicals, P.O. Box 31131, Seattle, WA 98103; tel: 206-527-5521; fax: 206-526-7948. (Available to professionals only.)

Source Naturals, Threshold Enterprises, 23 Janis Way, Scotts Valley, CA 95066; tel: 800-777-5677 or 831-438-1144; www.sourcenaturalscatalog .com.

Thorne Research, P.O. Box 25, Dover, ID 83825; tel: 800-228-1966 or 208-263-1337; fax: 208-265-2488; www.thorne.com.

Homeopathics

Boiron, 6 Campus Boulevard, Building A, Newtown Square, PA 19073;
tel: 800-264-7661 or 610-325-7464; www.boiron.ca.

Heel/BHI, 11600 Cochiti Road Southeast, Albuquerque, NM 87123;
tel: 800-621-7644 or 505-293-3843; www.heel.com.

HVS Labs, 3427 Exchange Avenue, Naples, FL 34104; tel: 800-521-7722;
www.hvslabs.com.

Nutritional Specialties Professional Health Products, P.O. Box 5897, Pittsburgh,
PA 15209; tel: 800-245-1313; fax: 412-821-0520; www.phpltd .com.

Aromatherapy

Amrita Aromatherapy, P.O. Box 2178, Fairfield, IA 52556; tel: 800-410-9651 or
515-472-9136; www.amrita.net.

Clinics

Eugene Zampieron, N.D., M.H. (A.H.G), 413 Grassy Hill, Woodbury, CT
06798; tel: 203-263-2970; email: DrZ@DrZnaturally.com; www.DrZnaturally
.com.

The American Institute for Cognitive Therapy, 136 E. 57th Street, Suite 1101,
New York, NY 10022; tel: 212-308-2440; www.cognitivetherapy nyc.com.

Bastyr University; www.bastyr.edu

Institute for Traditional Medicine and Preventive Health Care, 2017 Southeast
Hawthorne, Portland, OR 97215; tel: 800-544-7504 or 503-233-4907; fax: 503-
233-1012; www.itmonline.org.

National Center for Homeopathy, 801 North Fairfax Street, Suite 306,
Alexandria, VA 22314; tel: 703-548-7790; www.homeopathic.org.

National College of Naturopathic Medicine; www.ncnm.edu.

Neuro-Linguistic Programming University/Dynamic Learning Center, P.O. Box
1112, Ben Lomond, CA 95005; tel: 408-336-3457; fax: 408-336-5854; www.nlpu
.com.

William Rea, M.D., Environmental Health Center, 8345 Walnut Hill Lane, Suite
220, Dallas, TX 75231; tel: 214-368-4132; fax: 214-691-8432; www.ehcd.com.

Ann Seipt, N.D., 3003 North Central, Suite 103-117, Phoenix, AZ 85012;
tel: 602-274-1340; fax: 602-604-9655.

Virender Sodhi, M.D., N.D., 2115 112th Avenue NE, Bellevue, WA 98004;
tel: 425-453-8022; fax: 425-451-2670; http://ayurvedicscience.com.

Southwest College of Naturopathic Medicine; www.scnm.edu.

University of Bridgeport Naturopathic Medical Center, 60 Lafayette Avenue, Bridgeport, CT 06604; tel: 203-576-4349.

Kim Vanderlinden, N.D., D.T.C.M., West Coast Clinic of Integrated Medicine, 601 W. Broadway, Suite 204, Vancouver, BC, Canada V5Z 4C2; tel: 604-873-0046.

Peter Zilahy, D.C., 35 Candee Hill Road, Watertown, CT 06795; tel: 860-274-9641.

Laboratories

Diagnos-Tech, 6620 South 192nd Place, J-104, Kent, WA 98032;tel: 800-878-3787 or 425-251-0596; fax: 425-251-0637; www.diagnostechs.com. Offers adrenal stress index test.

Great Smokies Diagnostic Laboratory, 63 Zillicoa Street, Asheville, NC 28801; tel: 704-253-0621 or 800-522-4762; fax: 704-252-9303; www .gsdl.com. Offers comprehensive digestive stool analysis, functional liver detoxification profile, and oxidative stress profile.

Herbal Focus, P.O. Box 15178, Seattle, WA 98115-0178; tel: 206-524-1722; email: HerbalFocus@ktsweb.com. Offers herbal crystallization analysis (available to practitioners only).

Immuno Laboratories, 1620 West Oakland Park Boulevard, Fort Lauderdale, FL 33311; tel: 800-231-9197 or 954-486-4500; fax: 954-739-8583; www.immunolabs .com. Offers IgG ELISA test.

MetaMetrix Medical Laboratory, 5000 Peachtree Boulevard, Suite 110, Norcross, GA 30071; tel: 800-221-4640 or 770-446-5483; fax: 770-441-2237; www.meta metrix.com. Offers cell membrane lipid profile and toxic metal screening.

SpectraCell, 515 Post Oak Boulevard, Suite 830, Houston, TX 77027; tel: 713-621-3101 or 800-227-5227; www.spectracell.com. Offers functional intracellular analysis.

Hair Analysis

American College for Advancement in Medicine, 23121 Verdugo Drive, Suite 204, Laguna Hills, CA 92653; tel: 800-532-3688 or 714-583-7666; www.acam.org. Offers EDTA lead versenate 24-hour urine collection test.

Analytical Research Labs, 2225 West Alice Avenue, Phoenix, AZ 85069-7964; tel: 602-995-1580; fax: 602-371-8873; www.arltma.com.

Doctor's Data, 3755 Illinois Avenue, St. Charles, IL 60174-2420.

Organic and Nontoxic Products

American Water Council, tel: 866-278-2634; www.aquamd.com. Provides water testing services.

Chef Elieth Ameni Harris, Nature's Feast Catering, 37 Geraldine Circle, Trumbull, CT 06611; tel: 203-261-6256; www.integrativewellnessllc.com. Offers personal and phone consultations on diet.

Consumer Health Research, P.O. Box 1884, Bandon, OR 97411; tel: 800-282-9274 or 609-645-1110; fax: 609-645-8881; www.vegiwash.com. Makers of VegiWash.

EarthSafe, National Research & Chemical Company, 15600 New Century Drive, Gardena, CA 90248; tel: 310-515-1700; fax: 310-527-9963; www.earthsafe.net.

Environmental Detoxification Consultants, 413 Grassy Hill Road, Woodbury, CT 06798; tel/fax: 203-263-2970; www.drznaturally.com.

The Fresh Air Company, 1181 North Hollywood Drive, Reedley, CA 93654; tel: 800-860-4244 or 209-638-7908; fax: 619-723-0603; www.freshairmachine.com. Specialists in air filtration.

Northeast Organic Farmers Association (NOFA), 411 Sheldon Road, Barre, MA 01005; tel: 978-355-2853; www.nofamass.org.

Organic Consumers Association, 6771 South Silver Hill Drive, Finland, MN 55603; tel: 218-353-7454; fax: 218-353-7652; www.organicconsumers.org.

Seventh Generation, One Mill Street, Box A-26, Burlington, VT 05401; tel: 800-456-1191 or 802-658-3773; fax: 802-658-1771; www.seventhgeneration .com. Offers environmentally friendly cleaning products.

Walnut Acres Organic Farms, Walnut Acres Road, Penns Creek, PA 17862; tel: 800-433-3998 or 570-837-0601; www.walnutacres.com. Offers a wide selection of organically grown foods.

Electronic Testing and Treatment Devices

Aum Himalaya Sanjeevini Essences Pvt. Ltd., Dr. Rupa Shah, MD, and Dr. Atul Shah, MD; www.aumhimalaya.com. Offers Electromagnetic Field Deflecting Devices and flower and gemstone essence remedies.

Electromagnetic Bio-Communications, Ráth Gy. u. 16. H-1122 Budapest, Hungary; tel/fax: +36-1-214-5591; www.Hippocampus-brt .com.

United States Psychotronic Association, P.O. Box 45, Elkhorn, WI 53121; tel: 262-742-4790; fax: 262-742-3670; www.psychotronics.org.

Exercise and Bodywork

American Chiropractic Association, 1701 Clarendon Boulevard, Arlington, VA 22209; tel: 703-276-8800; www.amerchiro.org.

American Massage Therapy Association, 820 Davis Street, Suite 100, Evanston, IL 60201; tel: 312-761-2682; www.amtamassage.org.

International Institute of Reflexology, P.O. Box 12462, St. Petersburg, FL 33733; tel: 813-343-4811; www.reflexology-usa.net.

International Rolf Institute, P.O. Box 1868, Boulder, CO 80306; tel: 303-449-5903; www.rolf.org.

Workshops

The authors, Ellen Kamhi, Ph.D., R.N., and Eugene Zampieron, N.D., M.H. (A.H.G.), conduct the *EcoTours for Cures* series of workshops internationally, focusing on the ethnobotany of wild edible and medicinal plants. For more information on any of the *EcoTours for Cures* workshops, call 800-829-0918 or check out these websites: www.naturalnurse.com; www.drz naturally.com; and www.ecotoursfor cures.com.

Endnotes

Chapter 1. Arthritis Can Be Reversed

1. Arthritis Foundation, *The Facts about Arthritis* (Atlanta, GA: Arthritis Foundation, 2003.) (Available from: Arthritis Foundation, 1330 West Peachtree Street, Atlanta, GA 30309; 404-872-7100; fax: 404-872-8694; website: www.arthritis.org/resources/gettingstarted/default.asp.)

2. Ibid.

3. Michael T. Murray, *Arthritis* (Rocklin, CA: Prima Publishing, 1994), 28.

4. Medical Economics, *The PDR Family Guide to Prescription Drugs*, 2nd ed. (Montvale, NJ: Medical Economics, 1994), 804–808.

5. P. M. Brooks et al., "NSAIDs and Osteoarthritis—Help or Hindrance?" *Journal of Rheumatology* 9 (1982): 3–5; P. J. Verschure and C. J. Van Noorden, "The Effects of Interleukin-1 on Articular Cartilage Destruction as Observed in Arthritic Diseases, and Its Therapeutic Control," *Clinical and Experimental Rheumatology* 8, no. 3 (1990): 303–313.

6. N. M. Newman et al., "Acetabular Bone Destruction Related to NSAIDs," *The Lancet* 2 (1985): 11–13; L. Soloman, "Drug Induced Arthropathy and Necrosis of the Femoral Head," *Journal of Bone and Joint Surgery* 55B (1973): 246–251; J. T. Dingle, "The Effects of NSAID on the Matrix of Human Articular Cartilages," *Zeitschrift fur Rheumatologie* 58, no. 3 (1999): 125–129.

7. B. F. McAdam et al., "Systemic Biosynthesis of Prostacyclin by Cyclo-oxygenase (COX)-2: The Human Pharmacology of a Selective Inhibitor of COX-2" *Proceedings of the National Academy of Sciences* 96, no. 1 (1999): 272–277; D. W. Gilroy et al., "Inducible Cyclooxygenase May Have Anti-Inflammatory Properties," *Nature Medicine* 5, no. 6 (1999): 698–701.

8. D. J. Graham et al., "Risk of Acute Myocardial Infarction and Sudden

Cardiac Death in Patients Treated with Cyclo-oxygenase 2 Selective and Non-selective Non-steroidal Anti-inflammatory Drugs: Nested Case-Control Study," *Lancet* 365, no. 9458 (2005): 475–481.

9. M. Battistella et al., "Risk of Upper Gastrointestinal Hemorrhage in Warfarin Users Treated with Nonselective NSAIDs or COX-2 Inhibitors," *Archives of Internal Medicine* 165, no. 2 (2005): 189–192.

10. American Heart Association website: www.americanheart.org/presenter .jhtml?identifier=3029633.

11. Adverse effects listed on Enbrel website: http://www.enbrel.com/global/ enbrel-important.jsp?ms=5.

Chapter 2. What Is Arthritis?

1. T. Dorner et al., "Rheumatoid Factor Revisited," *Current Opinion in Rheumatology* 16, no. 3 (2004): 246–253; A. J. Silman and J. E. Pearson, "Epidemiology and Genetics of Rheumatoid Arthritis," *Arthritis Research* 4, suppl. 3 (2002): S265–S272; D. Holderbaum et al., "Genetics and Osteoarthritis: Exposing the Iceberg," *Arthritis and Rheumatism* 42 (1999): 397–405.

2. David S. Pisetsky with Susan Flamholtz Trien, *Duke University Medical Center Book of Arthritis* (New York: Ballantine Books, 1995), 75–76.

3. I. Shrier, "Muscle Dysfunction versus Wear and Tear as a Cause of Exercise Related Osteoarthritis: An Epidemiological Update," *British Journal of Sports Medicine* 38, no. 5 (2004): 526–535; E. L. Rabin et al., eds., *Mechanics of Joint Degeneration: Practical Biomechanics for the Orthopedic Surgeon* (New York: John Wiley and Sons, 1979).

4. C. A. Hitchon CA and H. S. El-Gabalawy, "Oxidation in Rheumatoid Arthritis," *Arthritis Research and Therapy* 6, no. 6 (2004): 265–278.

5. E. Gomez-Barrena et al., "Sequential Changes of Parathyroid Hormone Related Protein (PTHrP) in Articular Cartilage during Progression of Inflammatory and Degenerative Arthritis," *Annals of the Rheumatic Diseases* 63, no. 8 (2004): 917–922.

6. R. H. Straub et al., "How Psychological Stress via Hormones and Nerve Fibers May Exacerbate Rheumatoid Arthritis," *Arthritis and Rheumatism* 52, no. 1 (2005): 16–26.

7. W. Miehle, "Vitamin E in Active Arthroses and Chronic Polyarthritis: What Is the Value of Alpha-tocopherol in Therapy?" *Fortschritte der Medizin* 115, no. 26 (1997): 39–42.

8. J. M. May and Z. C. Qu, "Transport and Intracellular Accumulation of Vitamin C in Endothelial Cells: Relevance to Collagen Synthesis," *Archives of Biochemistry and Biophysics* 434, no. 1 (2005): 178–186; G. Krystal et al., "Stimulation of DNA Synthesis by Ascorbate in Cultures of Articular Chondrocytes," *Arthritis and Rheumatism* 25 (1982): 318–325.

9. M. F. McCarty and A. L. Russell, "Niacinamide Therapy for Osteoarthritis: Does It Inhibit Nitric Oxide Synthase Induction by Interleukin 1 in Chondrocytes?" *Medical Hypotheses* 53, no. 4 (1999): 350–360.

10. R. E. Newnham, "Essentiality of Boron for Healthy Bones and Joints," *Environmental Health Perspectives* 102 suppl. 7 (1994): 83–85; R. L. Travers et al., "Boron and Arthritis: The results of a Double-Blind Pilot Study," *Journal of Nutrition in Medicine* 1 (1990): 127–132.

11. H. K. Choi, "Dietary Risk Factors for Rheumatic Diseases," *Current Opinion in Rheumatology* 17, no. 2 (2005): 141–146.

12. T. A. Mori and L. J. Beilin, "Omega-3 Fatty Acids and Inflammation," *Current Atherosclerosis Reports* 6, no. 6 (2004): 461–467.

13. S. Aratay et al., "The Effect of Individualized Diet Challenges Consisting of Allergenic Foods on TNF-alpha and IL-1beta Levels in Patients with Rheumatoid Arthritis," *Rheumatology (Oxford)* 43, no. 11 (2004): 1429–1433.

14. Arthritis Foundation, *Primer on Rheumatic Disease*, 8th ed. (Atlanta, GA: Arthritis Foundation, 1983), 39; J. P. Kulka et al., "Early Joint Lesions of Rheumatoid Arthritis," *Archives of Pathology* 59 (1955): 129–150; H. R. Schumacher, "Synovial Membrane and Fluid Morphological Alterations in Early Rheumatoid Arthritis: Microvascular Injury and Virus-Like Particles," *Annals of the New York Academy of Sciences* 256 (1975): 39–64.

15. N. Balandraud et al., "Epstein-Barr Virus and Rheumatoid Arthritis," *Autoimmunity Reviews* 3, no. 5 (2004): 362–367.

16. J. P. Katz and G. R. Lichtenstein, "Rheumatologic Manifestations of Gastrointestinal Diseases," *Gastroenterology Clinics of North America* 27, no. 3 (1998): 533–562, v; P. Picco et al., "Increased Gut Permeability in Juvenile Chronic Arthritides: A Multivariate Analysis of the Diagnostic Parameters," *Clinical and Experimental Rheumatology* 18, no. 6 (2000): 773–778.

17. R. S. Panesh et al., "Delayed Reactions to Food: Food Allergy in Rheumatic Disease," *Annals of Allergy* 56 (1986): 500–503; M. A. Van de Laar and J. K. Ander Korst, "Food Intolerance in Rheumatoid Arthritis: A Double-Blind Controlled Trial of the Clinical Effects of Elimination of Milk Allergens and Azo Dyes," *Annals of Rheumatological Disease* 51 (1992): 298–302; J. A. Hickland, "The Effect of Diet in Rheumatoid Arthritis," *Journal of Clinical Allergy* 10 (1980): 463–467; Gail Darlington et al., "Placebo-Controlled, Blind Study of Dietary Manipulation Therapy in Rheumatoid Arthritis," *The Lancet* 1, no. 8475 (1986): 236–238; F. MacCrae et al., "Diet and Arthritis," *Practitioner* 230 (1986): 359–361; H. M. Buchanan et al., "Is Diet Important in Rheumatoid Arthritis?" *British Journal of Rheumatology* 30 (1991): 125–134; Gail Darlington et al., "Clinical Review of Dietary Therapy for Rheumatoid Arthritis," *British Journal of Rheumatology* 32 (1993): 507–514.

18. K. Hadjigogos, "The Role of Free Radicals in the Pathogenesis of Rheumatoid Arthritis," *Panminerva Medica* 45, no. 1 (2003): 7–13; R. Bergholm et al., "Impaired Responsiveness to NO in Newly Diagnosed Patients with Rheumatoid Arthritis," *Arteriosclerosis, Thrombosis, and Vascular Biology* 22, no. 10 (2002): 1637–1641.

19. Richard Leviton, "Rheumatoid Arthritis and Multiple Sclerosis: The Cause May Be in the Blood," *Alternative Medicine Digest* 18 (1997): 64–68.

20. Hans-Henrich Reckeweg, *Homotoxicology: Illness and Healing Through Anti-Homotoxic Therapy* (Albuquerque, NM: Menaco Publishing, 1980).

21. G. E. Comstock et al., "Serum Concentrations of Alpha-Tocopherol, Beta Carotene, and Retinol Preceding the Diagnosis of Rheumatoid Arthritis and Systemic Lupus Erythematosus," *Annals of Rheumatic Disease* 56, no. 5 (1997): 323–325.

22. L. De Rycke et al., "Rheumatoid Factor and Anticitrullinated Protein Antibodies in Rheumatoid Arthritis: Diagnostic Value, Associations with Radio-logical Progression Rate, and Extra-Articular Manifestations," *Annals of the Rheumatic Diseases* 63, no. 12 (2004): 1587–1593.

23. H. K. Choi et al., "Alcohol Intake and Risk of Incident Gout in Men: A Study," *The Lancet* 363, no. 9417 (2004): 1277–1281.

24. Gail Darlington and Linda Gamlin, *Diet and Arthritis* (London: Vermilion, 1996), 247.

25. S. Jorstad et al., "Effects of Cascade Apheresis in Patients with Psoriasis and Psoriatic Arthropathy," *Blood Purification* 16, no. 1 (1998): 37–42.

26. M. Azzini et al., "Fatty Acids and Antioxidant Micronutrients in Psoriatic Arthritis," *The Journal of Rheumatology* 22, no. 1 (1995): 103–108.

27. Ibid.

28. M. M. Griffiths, "Arthritis Induced by Bacteria and Viruses" in B. Henderson et al., eds., *Mechanisms and Models in Rheumatoid Arthritis* (London: Academic Press, 1995), 411–430.

29. M. Segal et al., "Microbial Products Induce Autoimmune Disease by an IL-12 Dependent Pathway," *Journal of Immunology* 158 (1997): 5087–5090.

30. J. H. Schwab, "Bacterial Cell Wall Induced Arthritis: Models of Chronic Recurrent Polyarthritis and Reactivation of Monoarticular Arthritis" in B. Henderson et al., eds., *Mechanisms and Models in Rheumatoid Arthritis* (London: Academic Press, 1995), 431–446.

31. Centers for Disease Control (CDC) website: www.cdc.gov/ncidod/dvbid/lyme/index.htm.

Chapter 3. Diagnosing Arthritis

1. S. Margetic et al., "Soluble Transferrin Receptor and Transferrin Receptor–Ferritin Index in Iron Deficiency Anemia and Anemia in Rheumatoid Arthritis," *Clinical Chemistry and Laboratory Medicine* 43, no. 3 (2005): 326–331.

2. Robert Berkow, *The Merck Manual*, 14th ed. (Rahway, NJ: Merck, 1982), 1177.

3. R. Roubenoff et al., "Abnormal Homocysteine Metabolism in Rheumatoid Arthritis," *Arthritis and Rheumatism* 40, no. 4 (1997): 718–722.

4. W. Emlen et al., "Measurement of Serum Hyaluronic Acid with Rheumatoid Arthritis: Correlation with Disease Activity," *Journal of Rheumatology* 23, no. 6 (1996): 974–978.

5. Robert Berkow, *The Merck Manual*, 14th ed. (Rahway, NJ: Merck, 1982), 1223.

6. U. Wagner et al., "HLA Markers and Prediction of Clinical Course and Outcome in Rheumatoid Arthritis," *Arthritis and Rheumatology* 40, no. 2 (1997): 341–351.

7. E. Neumann et al., "Local Production of Complement Proteins in Rheumatoid Arthritis Synovium," *Arthritis and Rheumatism* 46, no. 4 (2002): 934–945; M. Hakala et al., "Application of Markers of Collagen Metabolism in Serum and Synovial Fluid for Assessment of Disease Process in Patients with Rheumatoid Arthritis," *Annals of Rheumatic Disease* 54, no. 11 (1995): 886–890.

8. F. De Keyser et al., "Bowel Inflammation and the Spondyloarthropathies," *Rheumatic Disease Clinics of North America* 24, no. 4 (1998): 785–813, ix–x.

9. D. L. Gordon et al., "*Plesiomonas shigelloides* septic arthritis complicating rheumatoid arthritis," *Australian and New Zealand Journal of Medicine* 13, no. 3 (1983): 275–276.

10. A. N. Ellepola and C. J. Morrison, "Laboratory diagnosis of invasive candidiasis," *The Journal of Microbiology* 43 (2005): 65–84.

11. U. Bengtsson et al., "Survey of Gastrointestinal Reactions to Foods in Adults in Relation to Atopy, Presence of Mucus in the Stools, Swelling of Joints and Arthralgia in Patients with Gastrointestinal Reactions to Foods," *Clinical and Experimental Allergy* 26, no. 12 (1996): 1387–1394; Gail Darlington and Linda Gamlin, *Diet and Arthritis* (London: Vermilion Press, 1996); M. A. Van de Laar et al., "Food Intolerance in Rheumatoid Arthritis II: Clinical and Histological Aspects," *Annals of Rheumatic Disease* 51, no. 3 (1992): 303–306.

12. W. Atkinson et al., "Food Elimination Based on IgG Antibodies in Irritable Bowel Syndrome: A Randomised Controlled Trial," *Gut* 53, no. 10 (2004): 1459–1464.

13. G. E. Comstock et al., "Serum Concentrations of Alpha Tocopherol, Beta Carotene, and Retinol Preceding the Diagnosis of Rheumatoid Arthritis and Systemic Lupus Erythmatosus," *Annals of Rheumatic Disease* 56, no. 5 (1997): 323–355.

14. Centers for Disease Control (CDC), Division of Parasitic Diseases website: www.cdc.gov/ncidod/dpd/aboutdpd/default.htm.

15. Patrick R. Murray, ed., *Manual of Clinical Microbiology* (Washington, DC: ASM Press, 1999).

16. D. V. Parke and A. Sapota, "Chemical Toxicity and Reactive Oxygen Species," *International Journal of Occupational Medicine and Environmental Health* 9, no. 4 (1996): 331–340.

17. F. Suska et al., "In Vivo Cytokine Secretion and NF-kappaB Activation around Titanium and Copper Implants," *Biomaterials* 26, no. 5 (2005): 519–527.

18. G. J. Brewer, "Neurologically Presenting Wilson's Disease: Epidemiology, Pathophysiology and Treatment," *CNS Drugs* 19, no. 3 (2005): 185–192.

19. L. Knobeloch et al., "Fish Consumption, Advisory Awareness, and Hair Mercury Levels among Women of Childbearing Age," *Environmental Research* 97, no. 2 (2005): 220–227.

Chapter 4. General Detoxification

1. William J. Rea, *Chemical Sensitivity*, vol. 4 (Boca Raton, FL: CRC Lewis, 1997), 2434.

2. Environmental Working Group, Body Burden Study: www.ewg.org/issues/siteindex/issues.php?issueid=5004#report'%20or%20content_type='project.

3. Food and Drug Administration website: www.fda.gov/fdac/features/2003/503_fats.html.

4. R. J. Laumbach and H. M. Kipen, "Bioaerosols and Sick Building Syndrome: Particles, Inflammation, and Allergy," *Current Opinion in Allergy and Clinical Immunology* 5, no. 2 (2005): 135–139.

5. D. P. Wyon, "The effects of indoor air quality on performance and productivity," *Indoor Air* 14 suppl. 7 (2004): 92–101.

6. B. Thriene et al., "Man-Made Mineral Fiber Boards in Buildings: Health Risks Caused by Quality Deficiencies," *Toxicology Letters* 88, no. 1–3 (1996): 299–303.

7. B. McFadden, "Phenotypic Variation in Xenobiotic Metabolism and Adverse Environmental Response: Focus on Sulfur-Dependent Detoxification Pathways," *Toxicology* 111, no. 1–3 (1996): 43–65; B. Crotty "Ulcerative Colitis and Xenobiotic Metabolism" *The Lancet* 343, no. 8888 (1994): 35–38.

8. William Lee Cowden, "Is Your Shower Toxic? Some Pollution Solutions," *Alternative Medicine* 29 (1999): 69; Joseph Mercola, comments on Mercola.com: www.mercola.com/2004/sep/4/heavy_metals_water.htm.

9. M. E. Crespo-Lopez et al., "Mercury and Neurotoxicity," *Revista de Neurologia* 40, no. 7 (2005): 441; World Health Organization, *Environmental Health Criteria for Inorganic Mercury* (Geneva, Switzerland: World Health Organization, 1991), 118.

10. C. M. Galhardi et al., "Toxicity of Copper Intake: Lipid Profile, Oxidative Stress and Susceptibility to Renal Dysfunction," *Food and Chemical Toxicology* 42, no. 12 (2004): 2053–2060.

11. X. Y. Cheng and Z. H. Li, "Spectrophotometric Determination of Copper in the Hair of the Patients with Rheumatoid Arthritis," *Hunan Yi Ke Da Xue Xue Bao* 25, no. 2 (2000): 117–118.

12. H. Xu et al., "Exposure to Trichloroethylene and Its Metabolites Causes Impairment of Sperm Fertilizing Ability in Mice," *Toxicological Sciences* 82, no. 2 (2004): 590–597.

13. Bill Wolverton, *How to Grow Fresh Air: 50 Houseplants That Purify Your Home or Office* (New York, New York: Penguin, 1997).

14. K. Iwashige et al., "Calorie Restricted Diet and Urinary Pentosidine in Patients with Rheumatoid Arthritis," *Journal of Physiologocal Anthropology and Applied Human Science* 23, no. 1 (2004): 19–24; A. Michalsen et al., "Short-Term Therapeutic Fasting in the Treatment of Chronic Pain and Fatigue Syndromes: Well-Being and Side Effects with and without Mineral Supplements," *Forschende Komplementarmedizin und Klassische Naturheilkunde* 9, no. 4 (2002): 221–227; J. Palmblad et al., "Antirheumatic Effects of Fasting," *Rheumatic Disease Clinics of*

North America 17, no. 2 (1991): 351–352; J. Kjeldsen-Kragh et al., "Controlled Trial of Fasting and One-Year Vegetarian Diet in Rheumatoid Arthritis," *The Lancet* 338, no. 8772 (1991): 899–902; J. Kjeldsen-Kragh et al., "Vegetarian Diet after Fasting for Patients with Rheumatoid Arthritis—Status: Two Years after Introduction of the Diet," *Clinical Rheumatology* 13, no. 3 (1994): 475–482.

15. I. Hafstrom et al., "Effects of Fasting on Disease Activity, Neutrophil Function, Fatty Acid Composition, and Leukotriene Biosynthesis in Patients with Rheumatoid Arthritis," *Arthritis and Rheumatology* 31, no. 5 (1988): 585–592.

16. L. C. Wu et al., "Antioxidant and Antiproliferative Activities of Spirulina and Chlorella Water Extracts," *Journal of Agricultural and Food Chemistry* 53, no. 10 (2005): 4207–4212.

Chapter 5. Detoxifying Specific Organs

1. R. S. Barsoum, "Parasitic Infections in Organ Transplantation," *Experimental and Clinical Transplantation* 2, no. 2 (2004): 258–267.

2. J. B. Kaneene and R. Miller, "Problems Associated with Drug Residues in Beef from Feeds and Therapy," *Revue Science et Technique* 16, no. 2 (1997): 694–708.

3. Edmond Bordeaux Szekeley, *Essene Gospel of Peace* (London: International Biogenic Society, 1937), 16.

4. John Harvey Kellogg, "Should the Colon Be Sacrificed or May It Be Reformed?" *Journal of the American Medicine Association* 68, no. 26 (1917): 1957–1959.

5. D. Pizzetti et al., "Colonic Hydrotherapy for Obstructed Defecation," *Colorectal Disease* 7, no. 1 (2005): 107–108.

6. Dean J. Tuma and Carol A. Casey, "Dangerous Byproducts of Alcohol Breakdown: Focus on Adducts," National Institute on Alcohol Abuse and Alcoholism website: www.niaaa.nih.gov/publications/arh27-4/285-290-text. htm.

7. C. E. Ruhl and J. E. Everhart, "Coffee and Caffeine Consumption Reduce the Risk of Elevated Serum Alanine Aminotransferase Activity in the United States," *Gastroenterology* 128, no. 1 (2005): 24–32; L. K. T. Lam et al., "Isolation and Identification of Kahweol Palmitate and Cafestol Palmitate as Active Constituents of Green Coffee Beans That Enhance Glutathione-S-Transferase Activity in the Mouse," *Cancer Research* 42, no. 4 (1982): 1193–1198.

8. Michael Tierra, *The Way of Herbs* (Santa Fe, NM: Lotus Press, 1988), 263.

9. N. H. Shear et al., "Acetaminophen-Induced Toxicity to Human Epidermoid Cell Line A431 and Hepatoblastoma Cell Line Hep G2, in Vitro, Is Diminished by Silymarin," *Skin Pharmacology* 8, no. 6 (1995): 279–291.

10. Kerry Bone, "Picrorrhiza: Important Modulator of Immune Function," *Townsend Letter for Doctors and Patients* 1995: 88–94, website: www. herbalgram.org/herbclip/review.asp?i=41604.

11. Eugene Zampieron and Ellen Kamhi, *The Natural Medicine Chest* (New York: M. Evans, 1999), 65–67.

12. D. Chen D et al., "Inhibition of Human Liver Catechol-O-Methyltrans-

ferase by Tea Catechins and Their Metabolites: Structure-Activity Relationship and Molecular-Modeling Studies," *Biochemhemical Pharmacology* 69, no. 10 (2005): 1523–1531.

13. Eugene Zampieron, clinical observations (1986–2005).

14. A. Bhattacharya et al., "Body Acceleration Distribution and O₂ Uptake in Humans during Running and Jumping," *Journal of Applied Physiology* 49, no. 5 (1980): 881–887; Joan Bartlett et al., "Rebounding on a Mini-Trampoline: Implications for Physical Fitness and Coronary Risk Factors," *Journal of Cardiopulmonary Rehabilitation* 10 (1990): 401–408.

15. David L. Hoffmann, *The Herb User's Guide* (Wellingborough, Northhamptonshire, England: Thorsens, 1987), 141.

16. H. S. Wolf et al., "Detection of Polycyclic Aromatic Hydrocarbons in Skin Oil Obtained from Roofing Workers," *Chemosphere* 11 (1982): 595.

17. N. Kap-Soon et al., "Protein Biomarkers in the Plasma of Workers Occupationally Exposed to Polycyclic Aromatic Hydrocarbons," *Proteomics* 4, no. 11 (2004): 3505–3513.

18. D. W. Schnare et al., "Body Burden Reductions of PCBs, PBBs, and Chlorinated Pesticides in Human Subjects," *Ambio* 13 (1984): 5–6.

19. William J. Rea, *Chemical Sensitivity*, vol. 4 (Boca Raton, FL: CRC Lewis, 1997), 2463.

Chapter 6. Eradicating Bacteria and Yeast

1. A. Sullivan et al., "Effect of Antimicrobial Agents on the Ecological Balance of Human Microflora," *Lancet Infectious Diseases* 1, no. 2 (2001): 101–114.

2. A. Sekikawa et al., "Possible Role of REG I {alpha} Protein in Ulcerative Colitis and Colitic Cancer," *Gut* 54, no. 10: 1437–1444.

3. A. K. So et al., "Arthritis Is Linked to Local and Systemic Activation of Coagulation and Fibrinolysis Pathways," *J Thrombosis and Haemostasis* 1, no. 12 (2003): 2510–2515.

4. A. Scholin et al., "CRP and IL-6 Concentrations Are Associated with Poor Glycemic Control Despite Preserved Beta-Cell function during the First Year after Diagnosis of Type 1 Diabetes," *Diabetes/Metabolism Research and Reviews* 20, no. 3 (2004): 205–210.

5. A. Lombardo et al., "Inflammation as a Possible Link between Coronary and Carotid Plaque Instability," *Circulation* 2004 109, no. 25 (2004): 3158–3163.

6. Alan Ebringer et al., "Cross Reactivity between *Klebsiella aerogenes* Species and B27 Lymphocyte Antigens as an Etiological Factor in Ankylosing Spondylitis" in Jean Dausset and Arne Svejgaard, eds., *HLA and Disease* (Copenhagen: Williams & Wilkins, 1977), 27.

7. Alan Ebringer et al., "Ankylosing Spondylitis HLA-B27 and Klebsiella 11: Cross Reactivity Studies with Human Tissue Typing Sera," *British Journal of Experimental Pathology* 61 (1980): 92–96.

8. I. I. Maslova et al., "Antibodies to *Yersinia enterocolitica* and *Proteus mirabilis* in Blood Sera of Rheumatoid Arthritis Patients," *Zhurnal mikrobiologii, epidemi-*

ologii, i immunobiologii no. 4 (2004): 71–72; Alan Ebringer et al., "Rheumatoid Arthritis and *Proteus*: A Possible Aetiological Association," *Rheumatology International* 9, no. 3–5 (1989): 223–228.

9. A. S. Ramirez et al., "Relationship between Rheumatoid Arthritis and *Mycoplasma pneumoniae*: A Case-Control Study," *Rheumatology (Oxford)* 44, no. 7 (2005): 912–914.

10. W. Krause et al., "Fungaemia and Funguria after Oral Administration of *Candida albicans*," *The Lancet* 1, no. 7595 (1969): 598–599.

11. G. Pizzo et al., "Biotypes and Randomly Amplified Polymorphic DNA (RAPD) Profiles of Subgingival *Candida albicans* Isolates in HIV Infection," *The New Microbiologica* 28, no. 1 (2005): 75–82.

12. D. M. Gardiner et al., "The Epipolythiodioxopiperazine (ETP) Class of Fungal Toxins: Distribution, Mode of Action, Functions and Biosynthesis," *Microbiology* 151, no. 4 (2005): 1021–1032.

13. L. Brennan et al., "Gliotoxins Disrupt Alanine Metabolism and Glutathione Production in C6 Glioma Cells: A 13C NMR Spectroscopic Study," *Neurochemistry International* 45, no. 8 (2004): 1155–1165.

14. M. L. Freile et al., "Antimicrobial Activity of Aqueous Extracts and of Berberine Isolated from *Berberis heterophylla*," *Fitoterapia* 74, no. 7–8 (2003): 702–705.

15. Gudmundur Bergsson et al., "In Vitro Killing of *Candida albicans* by Fatty Acids and Monoglycerides," *Antimicrobial Agents and Chemotherapy* 45, no. 11 (2001): 3209–3212.

16. S. Delgado et al., "Antibiotic Susceptibility of *Lactobacillus* and *Bifidobacterium* Species from the Human Gastrointestinal Tract," *Current Microbiology* 50, no. 4 (2005): 202–207; Michael T. Murray, "Probiotics: Acidophilus, Bifidobacter, and FOS," *American Journal of Natural Medicine* 3, no. 4 (1996): 11–14; Elizabeth Lipski, *Digestive Wellness* (New Canaan, CT: Keats, 1996); John A. Catanzaro and Lisa Green, "Microbial Ecology and Dysbiosis in Human Medicine," *Alternative Medicine Review* 2, no. 3 (1997): 202–209; John A. Catanzaro and Lisa Green, "Microbial Ecology and Probiotics in Human Health (Part II)," *Alternative Medicine Review* 2, no. 4 (1997): 296–305; P. S. Moshchich et al., "Prevention of Dysbacteriosis in the Early Neonatal Period Using a Pure Culture of Acidophilic Bacteria," *Pediatriia* no. 3 (1989): 25–30; S. J. Bhatia et al., "*Lactobacillus acidophilus* Inhibits Growth of *Campylobacter pylori* in Vitro," *Journal of Clinical Microbiology* 27, no. 10 (1989): 2328–2330.

17. I. M. Bakri and C. W. Douglas, "Inhibitory Effect of Garlic Extract on Oral Bacteria," *Archives of Oral Biology* 50, no. 7 (2005): 645–651; Paul Bergner, *The Healing Power of Garlic* (Rocklin, CA: Prima Publishing, 1995), 98–100.

18. R. Bruck et al., "Allicin, the Active Component of Garlic, Prevents Immune-Mediated, Concanavalin A-induced Hepatic Injury in Mice," *Liver International* 25, no. 3 (2005): 613–621; Heinrich P. Koch and Larry D. Lawson, *Garlic: The Science and Therapeutic Application of Allium sativum L. and Related Species* (Baltimore, MD: Williams & Wilkins, 1996), 168–172.

19. N. Talpur et al., "Medicinal Herbal Oils: Antifungal Effects of the Edible Oil of Oregano," *Journal of the American College of Nutrition* 19, no. 5 (2000): 689;

Y. S. You et al., "Antimicrobial activity of some medical herbs and spices against *Streptococcus mutans*," *Korean Journal of Applied Microbiology and Bioengineering* 21, no. 2 (1993): 187–191; J. C. Stiles et al., "The Inhibition of *Candida albacans* by Oregano," *Journal of Applied Nutrition* 47, no. 4 (1995): 96–102.

20. J. A. Vazquez et al., "In Vitro Susceptibilities of *Candida* and *Aspergillus* Species to *Melaleuca alternafolia* (Tea Tree) Oil," *Revista Iberoamericana de Micologia* 17, no. 2 (2000): 60–63.

21. C. F. Carson and T. V. Riley, "Antimicrobial Activity of the Major Components of the Essential Oil of *Melaleuca alternifolia*," *Journal of Applied Bacteriology* 78, no. 3 (1995): 264–269.

Chapter 7. Eliminating Parasites

1. M. C. Hlavsa et al., "Giardiasis Surveillance—United States, 1998–2002," *Morbidity and Mortality Weekly Report* United States Centers for Disease Control, Surveillence Summary 54, no. 1 (2005): 9–16.

2. H. Auer and H. Aspock, "Nosology and Epidemiology of Human Toxocarosis: The Recent Situation in Austria," *Wiener Klinische Wochenschrift* 116 suppl. 4 (2004): 7–18.

3. A. Cali et al., "An Analysis of the Microsporidian Genus *Brachiola*, with Comparisons of Human and Insect Isolates of *Brachiola algerae*," *Journal of Eukaryotic Microbiology* 51, no. 6 (2004): 678–685.

4. A. Sing et al., "Reactive Arthritis Associated with Prolonged Cryptosporidial Infection," *Journal of Infection* 47, no. 2 (2003): 181–184.

5. P. E.. McGill, "Geographically Specific Infections and Arthritis, Including Rheumatic Syndromes Associated with Certain Fungi and Parasites, *Brucella* Species and *Mycobacterium leprae*," *Best Practice and Research. Clinical Rheumatology* 17, no. 2 (2003): 289–307.

6. L. H. Ghotekar et al., "Reactive Arthritis, Psoriasiform Lesions and Protein Loosing Enteropathy Secondary to Strongyloidiasis," *Journal of the Association of Physicians of India* 51 (2003): 395–396.

7. J. M. Shields and B. H. Olson, "*Cyclospora cayetanensis*: A Review of an Emerging Parasitic Coccidian," *International Journal for Parasitology* 33, no. 4 (2003): 371–391.

8. Patrick R. Murray, ed., *Manual of Clinical Microbiology* (Washington, DC: ASM Press, 1999).

9. G. Cancrini and A. Iori, "Traditional and Innovative Diagnostic Tools: When and Why They Should Be Applied," *Parassitologia* 46, no. 1–2 (2004): 173–176.

10. H. X. Wang and T. B. Ng, "Isolation of Cucurmoschin, a Novel Antifungal Peptide Abundant in Arginine, Glutamate and Glycine Residues from Black Pumpkin Seeds," *Peptides* 24, no. 7 (2003): 969–972.

11. S. R. Davis, "An Overview of the Antifungal Properties of Allicin and Its Breakdown Products: The Possibility of a Safe and Effective Antifungal Prophylactic," *Mycoses* 48, no. 2 (2005): 95–100.

12. B. A. Iwalokun et al., "In Vitro Antimicrobial Properties of Aqueous

Garlic Extract against Multidrug-Resistant Bacteria and *Candida* Species from Nigeria," *Journal of Medicinal Food* 7, no. 3 (2004): 327–333.

13. B. Y. Hwang et al., "Antimicrobial Constituents from Goldenseal (the Rhizomes of *Hydrastis canadensis*) against Selected Oral Pathogens," *Planta Medica* 69, no. 7 (2003): 623–627.

14. S. Gupte, "Use of Berberine in the Treatment of Giardiasis," *American Journal of Diseases of Children* 129 (1975): 866.

15. A. D. Azaz et al., "Composition and the in Vitro Antimicrobial Activities of the Essential Oils of Some *Thymus* Species," *Zeitschrift fur Naturforschung C* 59, no. 1–2 (2004): 75–80.

16. D. Kalemba and A. Kunicka, "Antibacterial and Antifungal Properties of Essential Oils," *Current Medicinal Chemistry* 10, no. 10 (2003): 813–829.

17. Z. Cvetnic and S. Vladimir-Knezevic, "Antimicrobial Activity of Grapefruit Seed and Pulp Ethanolic Extract," *Acta Pharmaceutica* 54, no. 3 (2004): 243–250.

18. R. A. Giove Nakazawa, "Traditional Medicine in the Treatment of Enteroparasitosis," *Revista de Gastroenterologia del Peru* 16, no. 3 (1996): 197–202.

19. N. Beloin et al., "Ethnomedicinal Uses of Momordicacharantia (Cucurbitaceae) in Togo and Relation to Its Phytochemistry and Biological Activity," *Journal of Ethnopharmacology* 96, no. 1–2 (2005): 49–55.

Chapter 8. Alleviating Leaky Gut Syndrome

1. A. Barton et al., "Increased Prevalence of Sicca Complex and Fibromyalgia in Patients with Irritable Bowel Syndrome," *American Journal of Gastroenterology* 94, no. 7 (1999): 1898–1901.

2. T. Y. Ma et al., "Mechanism of TNF-α Modulation of Caco-2 Intestinal Epithelial Tight Junction Barrier: Role of Myosin Light-Chain Kinase Protein Expression," *American Journal of Physiology. Gastrointestinal and Liver Physiology* 288, no. 3 (2005): G422–G430.

3. P. Picco et al., "Increased Gut Permeability in Juvenile Chronic Arthritides: A Multivariate Analysis of the Diagnostic Parameters," *Clinical and Experimental Rheumatology* 18, no. 6 (2000): 773–778.

4. P. J. Fortun and C. J. Hawkey, "Nonsteroidal Antiinflammatory Drugs and the Small Intestine," *Current Opininion in Gastroenterology* 21, no. 2 (2005): 169–175.

5. R. K. Rao et al., "Recent Advances in Alcoholic Liver Disease I. Role of Intestinal Permeability and Endotoxemia in Alcoholic Liver Disease," *American Journal of Physiology. Gastrointestinal and Liver Physiology* 286, no. 6 (2004): G881–884.

6. E. Husebye, "The Pathogenesis of Gastrointestinal Bacterial Overgrowth," *Chemotherapy* 51 suppl. 1 (2005): 1–22; R. Wiest and G. Garcia-Tsao, "Bacterial Translocation (BT) in Cirrhosis," *Hepatology* 41, no. 3 (2005): 422–433.

7. P. Nava et al., "The Rotavirus Surface Protein VP8 Modulates the Gate and Fence Function of Tight Junctions in Epithelial Cells," *Journal of Cell Science* 117, no. 23 (2004): 5509–5519.

8. K. Iwashige et al., "Calorie Restricted Diet and Urinary Pentosidine in Patients with Rheumatoid Arthritis," *Journal of Physiological Anthropology and Applied Human Science* 23, no. 1 (2004): 19–24; L. G. Darlington et al., "Diets for Rheumatoid Arthritis," *The Lancet* 333 (1991): 1209; H. Lithell et al., "A Fasting and Vegetarian Diet Treatment Trial on Chronic Inflammatory Disorders," *Acta Dermato-Venereologica* 63 (1983): 397–403; L. Skoldstam et al., "Impaired Con A Suppressive Cell Activity in Patients with Rheumatoid Arthritis Shows Normalization during Fasting," *Scandinavian Journal of Rheumatology* 12:4 (1983): 369–373; T. Sundqvist et al., "Influence of Fasting on Intestinal Permeability and Disease Activity in Patients with Rheumatoid Arthritis Showing Normalization during Fasting," *Scandinavian Journal of Rheumatology* 11 (1982): 33–38.

9. A. M. Uden et al., "Neutrophil Function and Clinical Performances after Total Fasting in Patients with Rheumatoid Arthritis," *Annals of Rheumatic Disease* 42 (1983): 45–51; J. Palmblad et al., "Acute Energy Deprivation in Man: Effect on Serum Immunoglobulins Antibody Response Complement Factors Three and Four, Acute Phased Reactants and Interferon Producing Capacity of Blood Lymphocytes," *Clinical Experimental Immunology* 30 (1977): 55.

10. R. Saller et al., "Dyspeptic Pain and Phytotherapy: A Review of Traditional and Modern Herbal Drugs," *Forschende Komplementarmedtarmedizin und Klassische Naturheilkdkunde* 8, no. 5 (2001): 263–273.

11. David Hoffman, *The Herb User's Guide* (Northamptonshire, England: Thorsens Publishers, 1987), 55.

12. John Lust, *The Herb Book* (New York: Bantam Books, 1974), 270.

13. T. Otamiri and C. Tagesson, "*Ginkgo biloba* Extract Prevents Mucosal Damage Associated with Small-Intestinal Ischaemia," *Scandanavian Journal of Gastroenterology* 24, no. 6 (1989): 666–670.

14. Z. A. Khan et al., "Inhibition of Oxalate Nephrolithiasis with *Ammi visnaga* (AI-Khillah)," *International Urology and Nephrology* 33, no. 4 (2001): 605–607.

15. S. Park et al., "Preventive Effect of the Flavonoid, Wogonin, against Ethanol-Induced Gastric Mucosal Damage in Rats," *Digestive Diseases and Sciences* 49, no. 3 (2004): 384–394.

16. O. H. Kang et al., "Inhibition of Interleukin-8 Production in the Human Colonic Epithelial Cell Line HT-29 by 18 Beta-glycyrrhetinic Acid," *International Journal of Molecular Medicine* 15, no. 6 (2005): 981–985.

17. S. H. van Uum, "Liquorice and hypertension," *The Netherlands Journal of Medicine* 63, no. 4 (2005): 119–120.

18. C. A. Calliste et al., "Free Radical Scavenging Activities Measured by Electron Spin Resonance Spectroscopy and B16 Cell Antiproliferative Behaviors of Seven Plants," *Journal of Agricultural and Food Chemistry* 49, no. 7 (2001): 3321–3327.

19. H. Sakai and M. Misawa, "Effect of Sodium Azulene Sulfonate on Capsaicin-Induced Pharyngitis in Rats," *Basic and Clinical Pharmacology and Toxicology* 96, no. 1 (2005): 54–59.

20. B. Y. Hwang et al., "Antimicrobial Constituents from Goldenseal (the

Rhizomes of *Hydrastis canadensis*) against Selected Oral Pathogens," *Planta Medica* 69, no. 7 (2003): 623–627.

21. M. Comalada et al., "In Vivo Quercitrin Anti-inflammatory Effect Involves Release of Quercetin, Which Inhibits Inflammation through Down-Regulation of the NF-kappaB Pathway," *European Journal of Immunology* 35, no. 2 (2005): 584–592.

22. R. A. Kozar et al., "Enteral Glutamine but Not Alanine Maintains Small Bowel Barrier Function after Ischemia/Reperfusion Injury in Rats," *Shock* 21, no. 5 (2004): 433–437; R. R. van der Hulst et al., "Glutamine and the Preservation of Gut Integrity," *The Lancet* 334 (1993): 1363–1365.

23. E. C. Clark et al., "Glutamine Deprivation Facilitates Tumour Necrosis Factor Induced Bacterial Translocation in Caco-2 Cells by Depletion of Enterocyte Fuel Substrate," *Gut* 52, no. 2 (2003): 224–230; H. Chun et al., "Effect of Anteral Glutamine on Intestinal Permeability and Bacterial Translocation after Abdominal Radiation Injury in Rats," *Journal of Gastroenterology* 32, no. 2 (1997): 189–195.

24. C. A. Hitchon and H. S. El-Gabalawy, "Oxidation in rheumatoid arthritis," *Arthritis Research and Therapy* 6, no. 6 (2004): 265–278.

25. A. Witschi et al., "The Systemic Availability or Oral Glutathione," *European Journal of Clinical Pharmacology* 43 (1992): 667–669.

26. M. J. Montisci et al., "Gastrointestinal Transit and Mucoadhesion of Colloidal Suspensions of *Lycopersicon esculentum L.* and *Lotus tetragonolobus* Lectin-PLA Microsphere Conjugates in Rats," *Pharmaceutical Research* 18, no. 6 (2001): 829–837.

27. S. Sierra et al., "Il-10 Expression Is Involved in the Regulation of the Immune Response by Omega-3 Fatty Acids," *Nutricion Hospitalaria* 19, no. 6 (2004): 376–382; T. Pischon et al., "Habitual Dietary Intake of n-3 and n-6 Fatty acids in relation to inflammatory markers among US men and women," *Circulation* 108, no. 2 (2003): 155–160.

28. E. A. Miles et al., "The Influence of Different Combinations of Gamma-linolenic, Stearidonic and Eicosapentaenoic Acids on the Fatty Acid Composition of Blood Lipids and Mononuclear Cells in Human Volunteers," *Prostaglandins, Leukotrienes, and Essential Fatty Acids* 70, no. 6 (2004): 529–538.

29. H. Sies et al., "Nutritional, Dietary and Postprandial Oxidative Stress," *The Journal of Nutrition* 135, no. 5 (2005): 969–972.

30. M. Montalto et al., "*Lactobacillus acidophilus* Protects Tight Junctions from Aspirin Damage in HT-29 Cells," *Digestion* 69, no. 4 (2004): 225–228.

Chapter 9. Allergies and Arthritis

1. S. Karatay et al., "The Effect of Individualized Diet Challenges Consisting of Allergenic Foods on TNF-alpha and IL-1beta Levels in Patients with Rheumatoid Arthritis," *Rheumatology (Oxford)* 43, no. 11 (2004): 1429–1433.

2. A. Berstad et al., "Food Hypersensitivity-Immunologic (Peripheral) or

Cognitive (Central) Sensitisation?" *Psychoneuroendocrinology* 30, no. 10 (2005): 983–989.

3. G. Sellge et al., "Development of an In Vitro System for the Study of Allergens and Allergen-Specific Immunoglobulin E and Immunoglobulin G: Fcepsilon Receptor I Supercross-Linking Is a Possible New Mechanism of Immunoglobulin G–Dependent Enhancement of Type I Allergic Reactions," *Clinical and Experimental Allergy* 35, no. 6 (2005): 774–781.

4. S. Aoki and T. Mitsui, "Histological Features of Rheumatoid Arthritis Patients Having Antibodies to Enterobacterial Common Antigens: Correlation of Antibody Levels with Semiquantitative Histologic Scores and Laboratory Markers," *Clinical and Experimental Rheumatology* 23, no. 1 (2005): 13–18.

5. S. Karatay et al., "The Effect of Individualized Diet Challenges Consisting of Allergenic Foods on TNF-alpha and IL-1beta Levels in Patients with Rheumatoid Arthritis," *Rheumatology (Oxford)* 43, no. 11 (2004): 1429–1433.

6. A. Bener et al., "Genetics and Environmental Risk Factors Associated with Asthma in Schoolchildren," *Allergie et Immunologie (Paris)* 37, no. 5 (2005): 163–168.

7. T. T. Macdonald and G. Monteleone, "Immunity, Inflammation, and Allergy in the Gut," *Science* 307, no. 5717 (2005): 1920–1925.

8. R. S. Pinals, "Arthritis Associated with Gluten-Sensitive Enteropathy," *Journal of Rheumatology* 13, no. 1 (1986): 201–204.

9. U. Lindqvist et al., "IgA Antibodies to Gliadin and Coeliac Disease in Psoriatic Arthritis," *Rheumatology (Oxford)* 41, no. 1 (2002): 31–37.

10. S. B. Matthews et al., "Systemic Lactose Intolerance: A New Perspective on an Old Problem," *Postgraduate Medical Journal* 81, no. 953 (2005): 167–173.

11. Norman F. Childers, *A Diet to Stop Arthritis* (Somerville, NJ: Somerset Press, 1991).

12. K. Engvall et al., "Sick Building Syndrome and Perceived Indoor Environment in Relation to Energy Saving by Reduced Ventilation Flow during Heating Season: A 1 Year Intervention Study in Dwellings," *Indoor Air* 15, no. 2 (2005): 120–126.

13. R. J. Laumbach and H. M. Kipen, "Bioaerosols and Sick Building Syndrome: Particles, Inflammation, and Allergy," *Current Opinion in Allergy and Clinical Immunology* 5, no. 2 (2005): 135–139.

Chapter 10. Desensitizing the Autoimmune Reaction

1. Joseph Pizzorno, *Total Wellness* (Rocklin, CA: Prima Publishing, 1996), 167–168.

2. Cell Mediated Immunity Information: http://users.rcn.com/jkimball.ma.ultranet/BiologyPages/C/CMI.html.

3. S. Norlin et al., "Nuclear Factor-κB Activity in β-Cells Is Required for Glucose-Stimulated Insulin Secretion," *Diabetes* 54, no. 1 (2005): 125–132.

4. M. Helenius et al., "Characterization of Aging-Associated Up-Regulation of Constitutive Nuclear Factor-kappa B Binding Activity," *Antioxidant and Redox Signaling* 3, no. 1 (2001): 147–156.

5. C. H. Leung et al., "Novel Mechanism of Inhibition of NF-κB DNA-Binding Activity by Diterpenoids Isolated from *Isodon rubescens*," *Molecular Pharmacology* 68, no. 2 (2005): 286–297.

6. D. Y. Chen et al., "Predominance of Th1 Cytokine in Peripheral Blood and Pathological Tissues of Patients with Active Untreated Adult Onset Still's Disease," *Annals of the Rheumatic Diseases* 63, no. 10 (2004): 1300–1306.

7. M. Westman et al., "Expression of Microsomal Prostaglandin E Synthase 1 in Rheumatoid Arthritis Synovium," *Arthritis and Rheumatism* 50, no. 6 (2004): 1774–1780.

8. Arthritis Foundation drug guide website: www.arthritis.org/conditions/DrugGuide/types.asp.

9. D. E. Trentham et al., "Effects of Oral Administration of Type II Collagen on Rheumatoid Arthritis," *Science* 261, no. 5129 (1993): 1727–1730.

10. P. J. Pussinen et al., "High Serum Antibody Levels to *Porphyromonas gingivalis* Predict Myocardial Infarction," *European Journal of Cardiovascular Prevention and Rehabilitation* 11, no. 5 (2004): 408–411.

11. R. H. Milston et al., "Short-Term Exposure of Chinook Salmon (*Oncorhynchus tshawytscha*) to o,p-DDE or DMSO during Early Life-History Stages Causes Long-Term Humoral Immunosuppression," *Environmental Health Perspective* 111, no. 13 (2003): 1601–1607.

12. S. H. Roth and J. Z. Shainhouse, "Efficacy and Safety of a Topical Diclofenac Solution (Pennsaid) in the Treatment of Primary Osteoarthritis of the Knee: A Randomized, Double-Blind, Vehicle-Controlled Clinical Trial," *Archives of Internal Medicine* 164, no. 18 (2004): 2017–2023.

13. Martha M. Christy, *Your Own Perfect Medicine* (Scottsdale, AZ: Future Medicine, 1994), 28.

14. C. W. M. Wilson and A. Lewis, "Autoimmune Bucal Urine Therapy (AIBUT) against Human Allergic Disease: A Physiologic Self-Defense Mechanism," *Medical Hypothesis* 12, (1983): 143.

15. M. R. Chevrier et al., "*Boswellia carterii* Extract Inhibits TH1 Cytokines and Promotes TH2 Cytokines In Vitro," *Clinical and Diagnostic Laboratory Immunology* 12, no. 5 (2005): 575–580.

16. S. Ahmed et al., "Green Tea Polyphenol Epigallocatechin-3-gallate (EGCG) Differentially Inhibits Interleukin-1 Beta-Induced Expression of Matrix Metalloproteinase-1 and -13 in Human Chondrocytes," *The Journal of Pharmacology and Experimental Therapeutics* 308, no. 2 (2004): 767–773.

17. S. Ahmed et al., "Green Tea Polyphenol Epigallocatechin-3-gallate Inhibits the IL-1 Beta-Induced Activity and Expression of Cyclooxygenase-2 and Nitric Oxide Synthase-2 in Human Chondrocytes," *Free Radical Biology and Medicine* 33, no. 8 (2002): 1097–1105.

18. M. N. Vankemmelbeke et al., "Selective Inhibition of ADAMTS-1, -4 and -5 by Catechin Gallate Esters," *European Journal of Biochemistry* 270, no. 11 (2003): 2394–2403.

19. Paul Schulick, *Ginger: Common Spice and Wonder Drug* (Brattleboro, VT: Herbal Free Press, 1994), 21.

20. R. D. Altman and K. C. Marcussen, "Effects of a ginger extract on knee pain in patients with osteoarthritis," *Arthritis and Rheumatism* 44, no. 11 (2001): 2531–2538.

21. I. Wigler et al., "The Effects of Zintona EC (a Ginger Extract) on Symptomatic Gonarthritis," *Osteoarthritis and Cartilage* 11, no. 11 (2003): 783–789.

22. B. B. Aggarwal and S. Shisodia, "Suppression of the Nuclear Factor-kappaB Activation Pathway by Spice-Derived Phytochemicals: Reasoning for Seasoning," *Annals of the New York Academy of Sciences* 1030 (2004): 434–441.

23. S. K. Biswas et al., "Curcumin Induces Glutathione Biosynthesis and Inhibits NF-kappaB Activation and Interleukin-8 Release in Alveolar Epithelial Cells: Mechanism of Free Radical Scavenging Activity," *Antioxidant and Redox Signaling* 7, no. 1–2 (2005): 32–41.

24. D. Chandra et al., "Anti-Inflammatory and Anti-Arthritic Activity of Volatile Oil of *Curcuma longa* (Haldi)," *Indian Journal of Medical Research* 60 (1972): 138–142.

25. Daniel J. McCarty et al., "Treatment of Pain due to Fibromyalgia with Topical Capsaicin: A Pilot," *Seminars in Arthritis and Rheumatism* 23, no. 6 suppl. 3 (1995): 41–47.

26. A. J. Nelson et al., "Capsaicin-Based Analgesic Balm Decreases Pressor Responses Evoked by Muscle Afferents," *Medicine and Science in Sports and Exercise* 36, no. 3 (2004): 444–450.

27. C. Randall et al., "Randomized Controlled Trial of Nettle Sting for Treatment of Base-of-Thumb Pain," *Journal of the Royal Society of Medicine* 93, no. 6 (2000): 305–309.

28. T. Teucher et al., "Cytokine Secretion in Whole Blood of Healthy Subjects Following Oral Administration of *Urtica dioica L.* Plant Extract," *Arzneimittelforschung* 46, no. 9 (1996): 906–910.

29. K. Riehemann et al., "Plant Extracts from Stinging Nettle (*Urtica dioica*), an Antirheumatic Remedy, Inhibit the Proinflammatory Transcription Factor NF-kappaB," *FEBS Letters* 442, no. 1 (1999): 89–94.

30. J. Broer and B. Behnke, "Immunosuppressant Effect of IDS 30, a Stinging Nettle Leaf Extract, on Myeloid Dendritic Cells In Vitro," *Journal of Rheumatology* 29, no. 4 (2002): 659–666.

31. X. Wang et al., "Immunosuppressive Sesquiterpenes from *Tripterygium wilfordii*," Chemical and Pharmaceutical Bulletin (Tokyo) 53, no. 6 (2000): 305–309.

32. A. R. Setty and L. H. Sigal, "Herbal Medications Commonly Used in the Practice of Rheumatology: Mechanisms of Action, Efficacy, and Side Effects," *Seminars in Arthritis and Rheumatism* 34, no. 6 (2005): 773–784.

33. J. Sylvester et al., "*Tripterygium wilfordii* Hook F Extract Suppresses Proinflammatory Cytokine-Induced Expression of Matrix Metalloproteinase Genes in Articular Chondrocytes by Inhibiting Activating Protein-1 and Nuclear Factor-kappaB Activities," *Molecular Pharmacology* 59, no. 5 (2001): 1196–1205.

34. Y. Deyong, "Clinical Observation of 144 Cases of Rheumatoid Arthritis

Treated with Glycoside of *Radix Tripterygium wilfordii,*" *Journal of Traditional Chinese Medicine* 3, no. 2 (1983): 125–129; S. Z. Qian et al., "Effects of *Tripterygium* on Male Fertility," *Advances in Contraception* 4, no. 4 (1988): 307–310.

35. M. S. Kotnis et al., "Renoprotective Effect of *Hemidesmus indicus,* a Herbal Drug Used in Gentamicin-Induced Renal Toxicity," *Nephrology (Carlton)* 9, no. 3 (2004): 142–152.

36. N. K. Mary et al., "In Vitro Antioxidant and Antithrombotic Activity of *Hemidesmus indicus* (L)," *Journal of Ethnopharmacology* 87, no. 2–3 (2003): 187–191.

37. Eugene Zampieron and Ellen Kamhi, *The Natural Medicine Chest,* (Oyster Bay, NY: Natural Alternatives Health, Education and Multimedia, 2000), 209–212.

38. Dan Bensky and Gamble Andrew, *Chinese Herbal Medicine Materia Medica* (Seattle,WA: Eastland Press, 1986), 144–145.

39. J. Xu et al., "Antiinflammatory Constituents from the Roots of *Smilax bockii* Warb," *Archives of Pharmacal Research* 28, no. 4 (2005): 395–399.

40. H. Sasaki et al., "Immunosuppressive Principles of *Rehmannia glutinosa* var. *hueichingensis,*" *Planta Medica* 55, no. 5 (1989): 458–462.

41. H. Kim et al., "Effect of *Rehmannia glutinosa* on Immediate Type Allergic Reaction," *International Journal of Immunopharmacology* 20, no. 4–5 (1998): 231–240.

42. T. Nakada et al., "Effect of Ninjin-youei-to on Th1/Th2 Type Cytokine Production in Different Mouse Strains," *The American Journal of Chininese Medicine* 30, no. 2–3 (2002): 215–223.

43. J. H. Lai, "Immunomodulatory Effects and Mechanisms of Plant Alkaloid Tetrandrine in Autoimmune Diseases," *Acta Pharmacologia Sinica* 23, no. 12 (2002): 1093–1101.

44. A. Niizawa et al., "Clinical and Immunomodulatory Effects of Fun-boi, an Herbal Medicine, on Collagen-Induced Arthritis In Vivo," *Clinical and Experimental Rheumatology* 21, no. 1 (2003): 57–62.

45. Him-che Yeung, *Handbook of Chinese Herbs: Chinese Materia Medica* (Rosemead, CA: Institute of Chinese Medicine, 1983), 306–307.

46. L. G. van der Hem et al., "Ling Zhi-8: Studies of a New Immunomodulating Agent," *Transplantation* 60, no. 5 (1995): 438–443.

47. Him-che Yeung, *Handbook of Chinese Herbs: Chinese Materia Medica.* (Rosemead, CA: Institute of Chinese Medicine, 1983), 346.

48. M. Dai et al., "Glucosides of *Chaenomeles speciosa* Remit Rat Adjuvant Arthritis by Inhibiting Synoviocyte Activities," *Acta Pharmacologia Sinica* 24, no. 11 (2003): 1161–1166.

Chapter 11. Mind-Body Approaches to Arthritis

1. M. Scofield, *Work Site Health Promotion* (Philadelphia: Hanley & Belfus, 1990), 459.

2. Timothy D. Schellhardt, "Company Memo to Stressed-Out Employees: 'Deal with It,'" *The Wall Street Journal* October 2, 1996.

3. J. L. Marx, "The Immune System 'Belongs to the Body,'" *Science* 277 (1985): 1190–1192.

4. Hans Selye, *Stress without Distress* (New York: New American Library, 1975); J. D. Beasley and J. Swift, *Kellogg Report: The Impact of Nutrition, Environment, and Lifestyle on the Health of Americans* (Annandale-on-Hudson, NY: Institute of Health Policy and Practice, The Bard College Center, 1989).

5. M. Marcenaro et al., "Rheumatoid Arthritis, Personality, Stress Response Style, and Coping with Illness: A Preliminary Survey," *Annals of the New York Academy of Sciences* 876 (1999): 419–425.

6. Arthur Guyton, *Textbook of Medical Physiology*, 7th ed. (Philadelphia, PA: W. B. Saunders, 1986), 910.

7. Redford B. William, "Hostility and the Heart" in Daniel Goleman and Joel Gurin, eds., *Mind Body Medicine* (Yonkers, NY: Consumer Reports Books, 1993), 66–67.

8. C. David Jenkins, "The Mind and the Body," *World Health* 47, no. 2 (1994): 6–7.

9. Louise L. Hay, *You Can Heal Your Life* (Santa Monica, CA: Hay House, 1984), 132.

10. Emrika Padus, *Using Emotions to Heal: The Happy Mind, Healthy Body Connection to Self Healing* (Emmaus, PA: Rodale Press, 1986), 7–8.

11. Dennis Jaffe, *Healing from Within* (New York: Simon & Schuster, 1980), 76, 135.

12. Louise L. Hay, *You Can Heal Your Life* (Santa Monica, CA: Hay House, 1984).

13. Brian Tracy, *The Psychology of Achievement* (Niles, IL: Nightingale-Conant Corporation, 1987), 4.

14. R. A. Chalmers et al., eds., *Scientific Research on Maharishi's Transcendental Meditation and TM-Sidih Program: Collected Papers*, vol. 2–4 (Vlodrop, Netherlands: Maharishi Vedic University Press, 1989).

15. R. K. Wallace et al., "Physiological Effects of Transcendental Meditation," *Science* 167, no. 926 (1970): 1751–1754; M. C. Dillbeck et al., "Physiological Differences between TM and Rest," *American Physiologist* 42 (1987): 879–881.

16. R. W. Cranson et al., "Transcendental Meditation and Improved Performance on Intelligence-Related Measures: A Longitudinal Study," *Personality and Individual Differences* 12, no. 10 (1991): 1105–1116.

17. D. H. Shapiro and R. N. Walsh, *Meditation: Classic and Contemporary Perspectives* (New York: Aldine, 1984).

18. Jon Kabat-Zinn, *Full Catastrophe Living: Using the Wisdom of Your Body and Mind to Face Stress, Pain and Illness* (New York: Delacorte Press, 1990).

19. Shad Helmsetter, *What to Say When You Talk to Yourself* (Scottsdale, AZ: Grindle Press/Audio, 1986).

20. R. Dilts and T. Hallbom, *Beliefs: Pathways to Health and Well-Being* (Portland, OR: Metamorphous Press, 1990), 1–2.

21. J. C. Parker et al., "Effects of Stress Management on Clinical Outcomes in Rheumatoid Arthritis," *Arthritis and Rheumatism* 38, no. 12 (1995): 1807–1818.

22. The Burton Goldberg Group, *Alternative Medicine: The Definitive Guide* (Tiburon, CA: Future Medicine Publishing, 1993), 77.

23. Leon Chaitow, *Amino Acids in Therapy: A Guide to the Therapeutic Application of Protein Constituents* (Wellingborough, Northhamptonshire, UK: Thorsens, 1985), 50–61.

24. N. Miller, "Learning of Visceral and Glandular Responses," *Science* 163, no. 866 (1969): 434–445, 627.

25. The Burton Goldberg Group, *Alternative Medicine: The Definitive Guide* (Tiburon, CA: Future Medicine Publishing, 1993), 245.

26. William Lowe Mundy, *Curing Allergy with Visual Imagery* (Shawnee Mission, KS: Munday & Associates, 1993), 45.

27. The Burton Goldberg Group, *Alternative Medicine: The Definitive Guide* (Tiburon, CA: Future Medicine Publishing, 1993), 244.

28. J. W. Turner and T. H. Fine, "Flotation/REST Used in the Treatment of Arthritis Pain" (paper presented at the Fourth Annual International Conference on REST, Washington, D.C., 1990); Roderick A. Borrie et al., "Flotation/ REST for the Management of Rheumatoid Arthritis" in *Proceedings of the Ninth Annual Conference on Interdisciplinary Health Care* (Stony Brook, NY: SAHP/SUNY, 1988), 277–282; T. H. Fine and J. W. Turner, Jr., "Flotation REST and Chronic Pain" (presented at the International Congress of Psychology, Acapulco, Mexico, 1984).

29. Peter Suedfeld et al., "Water Immersion and Flotation: From Stress Experiment to Stress Treatment," *Journal of Environmental Psychology* 3 (1983): 147–155.

30. T. H. Fine and J. W. Turner, Jr., "The Effect of Flotation/REST on EMG Biofeedback and Plasma Cortisol" in T. S. Fine and J. W. Turner, Jr., eds., *Proceedings of the First International Conference on REST and Self-Regulation* (Toledo, OH: IRIS, 1985), 148–155.

31. Based on clinical observations of Eugene R. Zampieron, N.D., A.H.G., Woodbury, CT, 1993–2005): 203, 263–2970, www.drznaturally.com

32. Based on clinical observations of Eugene R. Zampieron, N.D., A.H.G., Woodbury, CT, 1993–2005): 203, 263–2970, www.drznaturally.com

33. Larry Dossey, *Healing Words: The Power of Prayer and the Practice of Medicine* (San Francisco: HarperCollins, 1993), 268.

34. Marilyn Elias, "Attending Church Found Factor in Longer Life," *USA Today* August 8, 1999, 1A.

35. Harrington, A. Ed. *The Placebo Effect: An Interdisciplinary Exploration* (Cambridge, MA: Harvard Univ Press, 1997), 12–36.

36. G. Rein, "Effect of Conscious Intention on Human DNA." *International Forum on New Science*, (Denver, CO: Oct. 1996).

37. H. Walch, WB Jonas. "Placebo Research: The Evidence Base for Harnessing Self-healing Capacities." *Journal of Alternative and Complementary Medicine*, (2004;10 Suppl 1:S103–12).

38. L Colloca, F. Benedetti. *Placebos and Painkillers: Is Mind As Real As Matter?* Nature reviews. Neuroscience. (2005 Jul;6 (7):545–52).

39. R. B. Tisserand, *The Art of Aromatherapy* (Rochester, VT: Healing Arts Press, 1977).

40. G. H. Dodd, "Receptor Events in Perfumery" in S. van Toller and

G. H. Dodd, eds., *Perfumery: The Psychology and Biology of Fragrance* (London: Chapman and Hall, 1988).

41. J. Steele, "Brain Research and Essential Oils," *Aromatherapy Quarterly* 3 (1984): 5.

42. "Aromatherapy on the Wards: Lavender Beats Benzodiazepines," *International Journal of Aromatherapy* 1, no. 2 (1988): 1.

Chapter 12. The Arthritis Diet

1. Joseph Pizzorno, *Total Wellness* (Rocklin, CA: Prima Publishing, 1996), 264.

2. I. Hafstrom et al., "Effects of Fasting on Disease Activity, Neuotrophil Function, Fatty Acid Composition, and Leukotriene Biosynthesis in Patients with Rheumatoid Arthritis," *Arthritis and Rheumatology* 31, no. 5 (1988): 585–592.

3. J. Kjeldsen-Kragh et al., "Changes in Laboratory Variables in Rheumatoid Arthritis Patients during a Trial of Fasting and One-Year Vegetarian Diet," *Scandinavian Journal of Rheumatology* 24, no. 2 (1995): 85–93.

4. Sheldon Margen, *The Wellness Encyclopedia of Food and Nutrition* (New York: Rebus, 1992), 498; Udo Erasmus, *Fats That Heal, Fats That Kill* (Burnaby, British Columbia, Canada: Alive Books, 1993), 237.

5. L. G. Cleland et al., "Clinical and Biochemical Effects of Dietary Fish Oil Supplements in Rheumatoid Arthritis," *Journal of Rheumatology* 15, no. 10 (1988): 1471–1475.

6. J. M. Kremer et al., "Dietary Fish Oil and Olive Oil Supplementation in Patients with Rheumatoid Arthritis. Clinical and Immunologic Effects," *Arthritis and Rheumatology* 33, no. 6 (1990): 810–820.

7. Udo Erasmus, *Fats That Heal, Fats That Kill* (Burnaby, British Columbia, Canada: Alive Books, 1993), 264.

8. Personal communication with Vincent Buyck, Sr., Ph.D., National College of Complementary Medicine and Sciences, Washington, D.C.

9. J. A. Dudek and E. R. Elkins, Jr., "Effects of Cooking on the Fatty Acid Profiles of Selected Seafoods" in A. P. Simopopulos et al., eds., *Health Effects of Polyusaturated Fatty Acids in Seafoods* (New York: Academic Press, 1986), 431–450.

10. Ralph Golan, *Optimal Wellness* (New York: Ballantine Books, 1995), 50.

11. W. A. Newman Dorland, *American Illustrated Medical Dictionary* (Philadelphia: W. B. Saunders, 1946), 1122.

12. Udo Erasmus, *Fats That Heal, Fats That Kill* (Burnaby, British Columbia, Canada: Alive Books, 1993), 112.

13. M. Azzini et al., "Fatty Acids and Antioxidant Micronutrients in Psoriatic Arthritis," *Journal of Rheumatology* 22, no. 1 (1995): 103–108.

14. Julian Whitaker, "Article Title," *Health and Healing* 7, no. 11 (1997): 1–3.

Chapter 13. Supplements for Arthritis

1. H. K. Blomhoff, "Vitamin A Regulates Proliferation and Apoptosis of Human T- and B-cells," *Biochememical Society Transactions* 32, no. 6 (2004):

982–984; R. D. Semba, "Vitamin A, Immunity, and Infection," *Clinical Infectious Diseases* 19 (1994): 489–499.

2. H. Carlsen et al., "Molecular Imaging of the Transcription Factor NF-kappaB, a Primary Regulator of Stress Response," *Mutation Research* 551, no. 1–2 (2004): 199–211.

3. K. J. Rothman et al., "Teratogenecity of High Vitamin A Intake," *New England Journal of Medicine* 333 (1995): 1369–1373.

4. W. J. Blot et al., "Nutrition Intervention Trials in Linxian, China: Supplementation with Specific Vitamin/Mineral Combinations, Cancer Incidence, and Disease-Specific Mortality in the General Population," *Journal of the National Cancer Institute* 85 (1993): 1483–1491.

5. M. R. Namazi, "Nicotinamide: A Potential Addition to the Anti-psoriatic Weaponry," *The FASEB Journal: Official Publication of the Federation of American Societies for Experimental Biology* 17, no. 11 (2003): 1377–1379.

6. H. Wieneke et al., "Niacin—An Additive Therapeutic Approach for Optimizing Lipid Profile," *Medizinische Klinik (Munich)* 100, no. 4 (2005): 186–192.

7. E. C. Barton-Wright and W. A. Elliot, "The Pantothenic Acid Metabollism of Rheumatoid Arthritis," *The Lancet* 38 (1963): 862–863.

8. General Practitioner Research Group, "Calcium Pantothenate in Arthritic Conditions," *Practitioner* 224 (1980): 208–211.

9. A. R. Tovar et al., "Biochemical Deficiency of Pyridoxine Does Not Affect Interleukin-2 Production of Lymphocytes from Patients with Sjogren's Syndrome," *European Journal of Clinical Nutrition* 56, no. 11 (2002): 1087–1093.

10. A. M. Hvas et al., "Vitamin B_6 Level Is Associated with Symptoms of Depression," *Psychotherapy and Psychosomatics* 73, no. 6 (2004): 340–343.

11. A. Bendich and M. Cohen, Vitamin B_6 Safety Issues," *Annals of the New York Academy of Sciences* 585 (1990): 321–330.

12. T. E. McAlindon et al., "Do Antioxidant Micronutrients Protect against the Development and Progression of Knee Osteoarthritis?" *Arthritis and Rheumatism* 39 (1996): 648–656.

13. C. S. Johnston and B. Luo, "Comparison of the Absorption and Excretion of Three Commercially Available Sources of Vitamin C," *Journal of the American Dietetic Association* 94 (1994): 779–781.

14. F. P. Cantatore et al., "Osteocalcin Synthesis by Human Osteoblasts from Normal and Osteoarthritic Bone after Vitamin D_3 stimulation," *Clinical Rheumatology* 23, no. 6 (2004): 490–495.

15. F. Richy et al., "D-hormone Analog Alfacalcidol: An Update on Its Role in Post-menopausal Osteoporosis and Rheumatoid Arthritis Management," *Aging Clinical and Experimental Research* 17, no. 2 (2005): 133–142.

16. M. C. Morris et al., "Relation of the Tocopherol Forms to Incident Alzheimer Disease and to Cognitive Change," *American Journal of Clinical Nutrition* 81, no. 2 (2005): 508–514.

17. N. B. Roberts et al., "Serial Changes in Serum Vitamin K_1, Triglyceride, Cholesterol, Osteocalcin and 25-hydroxyvitamin D_3 in Patients after Hip

Replacement for Fractured Neck of Femur or Osteoarthritis," *European Journal of Clinical Investigation* 26, no. 1 (1996): 24–29.

18. M. I. Evans et al., "Impact of Folic Acid Fortification in the United States: Markedly Diminished High Maternal Serum Alpha-fetoprotein Values," *Obstetrics and Gynecology* 103, no. 3 (2004): 474–479.

19. A. Tiftikci et al., "Influence of Serum Folic Acid Levels on Plasma Homocysteine Concentrations in Patients with Rheumatoid Arthritis," *Rheumatology International* Epub ahead of print, January 12, 2005.

20. E. S. Stroes et al., "Folic Acid Reverts Dysfunction of Endothelial Nitric Oxide Synthase," *Circulation Research* 86, no. 11 (2000): 1129–1134.

21. R. L. Travers et al., "Boron and Arthritis: The Results of a Double-Blind Pilot Study," *Journal of Nutrition in Medicine* 1 (1990): 127–132.

22. S. L. Meacham et al., "Effect of Boron Supplementation on Blood and Urinary Calcium, Magnesium, and Phosphorus, Urinary Boron in Athletic and Sedentary Women," *American Journal of Clinical Nutrition* 61, no. 2 (1995): 341–345.

23. F. H. Nielsen, "Studies on the Relationship between Boron and Magnesium Which Possibly Affects the Formation and Maintenance of Bones," *Magnesium and Trace Elements* 9, no. 2 (1990): 61–69.

24. R. Recker, "Calcium Absorption and Achlorhydria," *New England Journal of Medicine* 313, no. 2 (1985): 70–73.

25. R. P. Heaney and C. M. Weaver, "Calcium Absorption from Kale," *American Journal of Clinical Nutrition* 51, no. 4 (1990): 656–657.

26. J. A. Harvey et al., "Superior Calcium Absorption from Calcium Citrate Than Calcium Carbonate Using External Forearm Counting," *Journal of the American College of Nutrition* 9, no. 6 (1990): 583–587.

27. O. M. Silverio Amancio et al., "Copper and Zinc Intake and Serum Levels in Patients with Juvenile Rheumatoid Arthritis," *European Journal of Clinical Nutrition* 57, no. 5 (2003): 706–712.

28. S. Margetic et al., "Soluble Transferrin Receptor and Transferrin Receptor–Ferritin Index in Iron Deficiency Anemia and Anemia in Rheumatoid Arthritis," *Clinical Chemistry and Laboratory Medicine* 43, no. 3 (2005): 326–331.

29. L. Mascitelli and F. Pezzetta, "High Iron Stores and Ischemic Heart Disease in Rheumatoid Arthritis and Systemic Lupus Erythematosus," *American Journal of Cardiology* 94, no. 7 (2004): 981; V. Gordeuk et al., "Iron Overload: Causes and Consequences," *Annual Review of Nutrition* 7 (1987): 485–508; P. Biemond et al., "Intra-articular Ferritin-Bound Iron in Rheumatoid Arthritis," *Arthritis and Rheumatism* 29 (1986): 1187–1193; J. T. Salonen et al., "High Stored Iron Levels Are Associated with Excess Risk of Myocardial Infarction in Eastern Finnish Men," *Circulation* 86 (1992): 803–811.

30. B. M. Altura, "Basic Biochemistry and Physiology of Magnesium: A Brief Review," *Magnesium and Trace Elements* 10 (1991): 167–171.

31. J. S. Lindberg et al., "Magnesium Bioavailability from Magnesium Citrate and Magnesium Oxide," *Journal of the American College of Nutrition* 9, no. 1 (1990): 48–55.

32. J. H. Yen et al., "Manganese Superoxide Dismutase Gene Polymorphisms in Psoriatic Arthritis," *Disease Markers* 19, no. 6 (2003–2004): 263–265.

33. S. Shilo et al., "Selenium Attenuates Expression of MnSOD and Uncoupling Protein 2 in J774.2 Macrophages: Molecular Mechanism for Its Cell-Death and Antiinflammatory Activity," *Antioxidants and Redox Signaling* 7, no. 1–2 (2005): 276–286.

34. O. Andersen and J. B. Nielsen, "Effects of Simultaneous Low-Level Dietary Supplementation with Inorganic and Organic Selenium on Whole-Body, Blood, and Organ Levels of Toxic Metals in Mice," *Environmental Health Perspectives* 102 suppl. 3 (1994): 321–324.

35. A. Prasad, "Clinical, Biochemical and Nutritional Spectrum of Zinc Deficiency in Human Subjects: An Update," *Nutrition Reviews* 41, no. 7 (1983): 197–208; T. E. Tuormaa, "Adverse Effect of Zinc Deficiency: A Review from the Literature," *Journal of Orthomolecular Medicine* 10 (1995): 149–162.

36. Y. Naveh et al., "Zinc Metabolism in Rheumatoid Arthritis: Plasma and Urinary Zinc and Relationship to Disease Activity," *Journal of Rheumatology* 24, no. 4 (1997): 643–646; J. R. Cerhan et al., "Antioxidant Micronutrients and Risk of Rheumatoid Arthritis in a Cohort of Older Women," *American Journal of Epidemiology* 157, no. 4 (2003): 345–354; P. C. Mattingly and A. G. Mowat, "Zinc Sulphate in Rheumatoid Arthritis," *Annals of the Rheumatic Diseases* 41, no. 5 (1982): 456–457.

37. T. E. McAlindon et al., "Glucosamine and Chondroitin for Treatment of Osteoarthritis: A Systematic Quality Assessment and Meta-analysis," *Journal of the American Medical Association* 283, no. 11 (2000): 1469–1475.

38. T. E. Towheed et al., "Glucosamine Therapy for Treating Osteoarthritis," *Cochrane Database Systematic Reviews* 2005 Apr 18;(2):CD002946.

39. N. Poolsup et al., "Glucosamine Long-Term Treatment and the Progression of Knee Osteoarthritis: Systematic Review of Randomized Controlled Trials," *The Annals of Pharmacotherapy* 39, no. 6 (2005): 1080–1087; J. Hua et al., "Preventive Actions of a High Dose of Glucosamine on Adjuvant Arthritis in Rats," *Inflammation Research* 54, no. 3 (2005): 127–132.

40. C. T. Leffler et al., "Glucosamine, Chondroitin, and Manganese Ascorbate for Degenerative Joint Disease of the Knee or Low Back: A Randomized, Double-Blind, Placebo-Controlled Pilot Study," *Military Medicine* 164, no. 2 (1999): 85–91.

41. M. M. Chou et al., "Effects of Chondroitin and Glucosamine Sulfate in a Dietary Bar Formulation on Inflammation, Interleukin-1beta, Matrix Metalloprotease-9, and Cartilage Damage in Arthritis," *Experimental Biology and Medicine* 230, no. 4 (2005): 255–262.

42. H. Matsuno et al., "Biochemical Effect of Intra-articular Injections of High Molecular Weight Hyaluronate in Rheumatoid Arthritis Patients," *Inflammation Research* 48, no. 3 (1999): 154–159.

43. R. J. Petrella, "Hyaluronic Acid for the Treatment of Knee Osteoarthritis: Long-Term Outcomes from a Naturalistic Primary Care Experience," *Americal Journal of Physical Medicine and Rehabilitation* 84, no. 4 (2005): 278–283; R.

Barbucci et al., "Hyaluronic Acid Hydrogel Added with Ibuprofen-Lysine for the Local Treatment of Chondral Lesions in the Knee: In Vitro and In Vivo Investigations," *Journal of Biomedical Materials Research* 75, no. 1 (2005): 42–48.

44. W. J. Kraemer et al., "Effect of a Cetylated Fatty Acid Topical Cream on Functional Mobility and Quality of Life of Patients with Osteoarthritis," *Journal of Rheumatology* 31, no. 4 (2004): 767–774.

45. W. I. Najm et al., "S-adenosyl Methionine (SAMe) versus Celecoxib for the Treatment of Osteoarthritis Symptoms: A Double-Blind Cross-Over Trial," *BMC Musculoskeletal Disorders* 5, no. 1 (2004): 6d.

46. S. H. Roth and J. Z. Shainhouse, "Efficacy and Safety of a Topical Diclofenac Solution (Pennsaid) in the Treatment of Primary Osteoarthritis of the Knee: A Randomized, Double-Blind, Vehicle-Controlled Clinical Trial," *Archives of Internal Medicine* 164, no. 18 (2004): 2017–2023.

47. E. Barrager et al., "A Multicentered, Open-Label Trial on the Safety and Efficacy of Methylsulfonylmethane in the Treatment of Seasonal Allergic Rhinitis," *Journal of Alternative and Complementary Medicine* 8, no. 2 (2002): 167–173.

48. G. M. Halpern, "Anti-inflammatory Effects of a Stabilized Lipid Extract of *Perna canaliculus* (Lyprinol)," *Allergie et Immunologie (Paris)* 32, no. 7 (2000): 272–278.

49. J. K. Grover and S. P. Yadav, "Pharmacological Actions and Potential Uses of *Momordica charantia*: A Review," *Journal of Ethnopharmacology* 93, no. 1 (2004): 123–132.

50. H. P. Ammon, "Boswellic Acids (Components of Frankincense) as the Active Principle in Treatment of Chronic Inflammatory Diseases," *Wiener Medizinische Wochenschrift* 152, no. 15–16 (2002): 373–378.

51. Leslie Taylor, *The Cat's Claw TOA / POA Controversy* November 15, 2002. www.rain-tree.com/toa-poa-article.htm.

52. J. E. Williams, "Review of antibicrobial and immunomoduality properties of plants of the Perruvian rainforest, with a particular emphasis on Una de Gato and Sangre de Grado," *Alternative Medicine Review* (2001): 567–79.

53. E. Mur et al., "Randomized Double Blind Trial of an Extract from the Pentacyclic Alkaloid-Chemotype of *Uncaria tomentosa* for the Treatment of Rheumatoid Arthritis," *Journal of Rheumatology* 29, no. 4 (2002): 656–658.

54. W. Keitel et al., "Capsicum Pain Plaster in Chronic Non-specific Low Back Pain," *Arzneimittel-Forschung* 51, no. 11 (2001): 896–903.

55. P. Navarro et al., "In Vivo Anti-inflammatory Activity of Saponins from *Bupleurum rotundifolium*," *Life Sciences* 68, no. 10 (2001): 1199–1206.

56. S. Hiai et al., "Stimulation of the Pituitary-Adrenocortical Axis by Saikosaponin of *Bupleuri radix*," *Chemical and Pharmaceutical Bulletin* 29, no. 2 (1981): 495–499.

57. E. J. Verspohl et al, "Antidiabetic Effect of *Cinnamomum cassia* and *Cinnamomum zeylanicum* In Vivo and In Vitro," *Phytotherapy Research* 19, no. 3 (2005): 203–206.

58. E. S. Johnson et al., "Efficacy of Feverfew as Prophylactic Treatment of Migraine," *British Medical Journal* 291, no. 6495 (1985): 569–573.

59. A. T. Smolinski and J. J. Pestka, "Comparative Effects of the Herbal Constituent Parthenolide (Feverfew) on Lipopolysaccharide-Induced Inflammatory Gene Expression in Murine Spleen and Liver," *Journal of Inflammation (London)* 2, no. 1 (2005): 6.

60. S. D. Jolad et al., "Fresh Organically Grown Ginger (*Zingiber officinale*): Composition and Effects on LPS-induced PGE Production," *Phytochemistry* 65, no. 13 (2004): 1937–1954.

61. B. B. Aggarwal and S. Shishodia, "Suppression of the Nuclear Factor-κB Activation Pathway by Spice-Derived Phytochemicals: Reasoning for Seasoning," *Annals of the New York Academy of Science* 1030 (2004): 434–441.

62. F. Kiuchi et al., "Inhibition of Prostaglandin and Leukotriene Biosynthesis by Gingerols and Diarylheptanoids," *Chemical and Pharmaceutical Bulletin* 40, no. 2 (1992): 387–391.

63. K. C. Srivastava and T. Mustafa, "Ginger (*Zingiber officinale*) in Rheumatism and Musculoskeletal Disorders," *Medical Hypothesis* 39, no. 4 (1992): 342–348.

64. R. Della Loggia et al., "Evaluation of the Activity on the Mouse CNS of Several Plant Extracts and a Combination of Them," *Rivista di Neurologia* 51, no. 5 (1981): 297–310.

65. D. D. Jamieson et al., "Comparison of the Central Nervous System Activity of the Aqueous and Lipid Extracts of Kava (*Piper methysticum*)," *Archives Internationales de Pharmacodynamie et de Therapie* 301 (1989): 66–80.

66. S. Witte et al., "Meta-analysis of the Efficacy of the Acetonic Kava-Kava Extract WS1490 in Patients with Non-psychotic Anxiety Disorders," *Phytotherapy Research* 19, no. 3 (2005): 183–188.

67. C. Fiore et al., "A History of the Therapeutic Use of Liquorice in Europe," *Journal of Ethnopharmacology* 99, no. 3 (2005): 317–324.

68. R. V. Farese, Jr., et al., "Licorice-Induced Hypermineralocorticoidism," *New England Journal of Medicine* 325, no. 17 (1991): 1223–1227.

69. M. Duwiejua et al., "Anti-inflammatory activity of *Polygonum bistorta*, *Guaiacum officinale* and *Hamamelis virginiana* in rats," *The Journal of Pharmacy and Pharmacology* 46, no. 4 (1994): 286–290.

70. M. Wiesenauer and R. Lüdtke, "*Mahonia aquifolium* in Patients with Psoriasis Vulgaris: An Intraindividual Study," *Phytomedicine* 3 (1996): 231–235.

71. H. P. Ammon et al., "Mechanism of Antiinflammatory Actions of Curcumine and Boswellic Acids," *Journal of Ethnopharmacology* 38 (1993): 113.

72. S. K. Biswas et al., "Curcumin Induces Glutathione Biosynthesis and Inhibits NF-kappaB Activation and Interleukin-8 Release in Alveolar Epithelial Cells: Mechanism of Free Radical Scavenging Activity," *Antioxidant and Redox Signaling* 7, no. 1–2 (2005): 32–41.

73. R. W. Marz and F. R. Kemper, "Willow Bark Extract—Effects and Effectiveness. Status of Current Knowledge Regarding Pharmacology, Toxicology and Clinical Aspects," *Wiener Medizinsche Wochenschrift* 152, no. 15–16 (2002): 354–359.

74. S. L. Lobo et al., "Use of Theraflex-TMJ Topical Cream for the Treatment of Temporomandibular Joint and Muscle Pain," *The Journal of Cranio-Mandibular Practice* 22, no. 2 (2004): 137–144.

75. N. E. Walsh et al., "Analgesic Effectiveness of D-phenylalanine in Chronic Pain Patients," *Archives of Physical Medicine and Rehabilitation* 67, no. 7 (1986): 436–439.

76. L. W. Blau, "Cherry Diet Control for Gout and Arthritis," *Texas Report on Biology and Medicine* 8 (1950): 309–311.

77. D. Kempuraj et al., "Flavonols Inhibit Proinflammatory Mediator Release, Intracellular Calcium Ion Levels and Protein Kkinase C Theta Phosphorylation in Human Mast Cells," *British Journal of Pharmacology* 145, no. 7 (2005): 934–944.

78. B. Han et al., "Proanthocyanidin: A Natural Crosslinking Reagent for Stabilizing Collagen Matrices," *Journal of Biomedical Materials Research Part A* 65, no. 1 (2003): 118–124.

79. M. Comalada et al., "In Vivo Quercitrin Anti-inflammatory Effect Involves Release of Quercetin, Which Inhibits Inflammation through Down-Regulation of the NF-kappaB Pathway," *European Journal of Immunology* 35, no. 2 (2005): 584–592.

80. A. A. Berbert et al., "Supplementation of Fish Oil and Olive Oil in Patients with Rheumatoid Arthritis," *Nutrition* 21, no. 2 (2005): 131–136.

81. C. L. Curtis et al., "N-3 Fatty Acids Specifically Modulate Catabolic Factors Involved in Articular Cartilage Degradation," *The Journal of Biological Chemistry* 275, no. 2 (2000): 721–724.

82. C. S. Lau et al., "Effects of Fish Oil Supplementation on Non-steroidal Anti-inflammatory Drug Requirement in Patients with Mild Rheumatoid Arthritis: A Double-Blind, Placebo-Controlled Study," *British Journal of Rheumatology* 32 (1993): 982–989.

83. L. P. Hale et al., "Proteinase Activity and Stability of Natural Bromelain Preparations," *International Immunopharmacology* 5, no. 4 (2005): 783–793.

84. J. M. Wallace, "Nutritional and Botanical Modulation of the Inflammatory Cascade—Eicosanoids, Cyclooxygenases, and Lipoxygenases—as an Adjunct in Cancer Therapy," *Integrative Cancer Therapies* 1, no. 1 (2002): 7–37.

85. T. J. De Witte et al., "Hypochlorhydria and Hypergastrinaemia in Rheumatoid Arthritis," *Annals of Rheumatic Diseases* 38, no. 1 (1979): 14–17; K. Henriksson et al., "Gastrin, Gastric Acid Secretion, and Gastric Microflora in Patients with Rheumatoid Arthritis," *Annals of Rheumatic Diseases* 45, no. 6 (1986): 475–483.

Chapter 14. Exercises and Physical Therapies

1. Adaptation of a program designed by Visual Health Information, P.O. Box 44646, Tacoma, WA 98444; tel: 253-536-4922.

2. Sophia Delza, *Tai Chi-Chuan: Body and Mind in Harmony* (Albany, NY: SUNY Press, 1985), 1, 3, 6.

3. Burton Goldberg Group, *Alternative Medicine: The Definitive Guide* (Tiburon, CA: Future Medicine Publishing, 1993), 423–426.

4. A. Thrash and C. Thrash," *Home Remedies: Hydrotherapy, Massage, Charcoal and Other Simple Treatments* (Seale, AL: Thrash Publications, 1981), 102.

5. Gurney's Inn, Resort and Spa Guidebook (Montauk, NY: Holdens Publication, 1997): www.gurneys-inn.com.

6. Ibid.

7. Brian W. Fahey, *The Power of Balance: A Rolfing View of Health* (Portland, OR: Metamorphous Press, 1989), 39.

8. Michael Murray et al., *A Textbook of Natural Medicine: Non-pharmacological Control of Pain IV* (Seattle, WA: Bastyr Publications, 1986), 2.

9. Ron Lawrence and Paul J. Rosch, *Magnet Therapy: The Pain Cure Alternative* (Rocklin, CA: Prima Publishing, 1998), 117.

10. Julie Friedberger, *Office Yoga* (Glasgow, Scotland: Thorsons, 1991), 23.

11. D. L. Berkson, "Osteoarthritis, Chiropractic and Nutrition," Medical Hypothesis 36, no. 4 (1991): 356–367.

Index

A

Acid-forming foods, 91, 226–27, 229
Acupressure, 179–80, 314
Acupuncture, 109, 179–80, 314
Adrenal glands, 56, 206–8, 211
Adrenaline, 23, 56, 206, 207
Adrenal stress index (ASI), 56, 211
Air, indoor, 77
ALA (alpha-linolenic acid), 6, 234–35, 237
Alcohol
  candidiasis and, 130
  gout and, 35
  leaky gut syndrome and, 156–57
Algae, blue-green, 86
Alkaline-forming foods, 226–27, 229
Alkaline salts, 179
Allergens
  definition of, 168
  food, 172–74
  health problems caused by, 168
Allergic reactions
  halting, 179
  immediate vs. delayed, 169

process of, 168–69
symptoms of, 168
Allergies. *See also* Allergens;
  Allergic reactions
  alternative medicine
    therapies for, 167, 178–80
  causes of, 171–72
  cycle of food, 168
  definition of, 168
  food linked to, 172–74
  intestinal mucus and, 92
  leaky gut and, 150
  link between arthritis and, 24, 28, 166, 170–71
  sick building syndrome, 72–73, 178
  success stories, 167, 170, 176–78
  testing for, 57–60, 174–76
Allicin, 132
Alpha-linolenic acid (ALA), 6, 234–35, 237
Alternative medicine. *See also specific therapies*
  benefits of, 9–10
  diagnostic tests in, 43–65
  success stories, 2–6, 10–14
Amino acids, 280–84
ANAs (antinuclear antibodies), 42, 185, 186

Anemia, 40–41, 266
Angelica, 281
Anger, 102
Ankylosing spondylitis (AS)
  bacteria and, 119–20
  detoxification for, 330
  in men vs. women, 35, 36, 120
  pain management for, 327–30
  prevalence of, 38
  sample treatment protocol for, 327–33
  symptoms of, 37–38
Antibiotics, 92–93, 125, 126, 130
Antibodies, 42, 75, 184, 185
Antioxidants, 60, 71, 284, 285
Apples
  Apple Spice Cake with Cranberry Kanten Glaze, 256
  Dr. Zamperion's Zingiber Zing, 246
  Green Mobility Juice, 247
Applied kinesiology, 58–59, 139, 179–80
Arachidonic acid, 36, 161, 229
Arava, 8
Arginine, 75
Aromatherapy, 222–24, 310

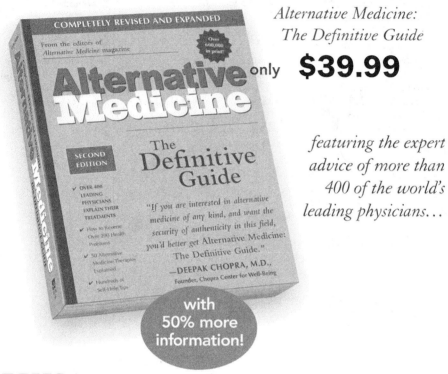
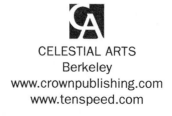